365 Delicious Oat Recipes

(365 Delicious Oat Recipes - Volume 1)

Debra Boone

Copyright: Published in the United States by Debra Boone/ © DEBRA BOONE

Published on December, 07 2020

All rights reserved. No part of this publication may be reproduced, stored in retrieval system, copied in any form or by any means, electronic, mechanical, photocopying, recording or otherwise transmitted without written permission from the publisher. Please do not participate in or encourage piracy of this material in any way. You must not circulate this book in any format. DEBRA BOONE does not control or direct users' actions and is not responsible for the information or content shared, harm and/or actions of the book readers.

In accordance with the U.S. Copyright Act of 1976, the scanning, uploading and electronic sharing of any part of this book without the permission of the publisher constitute unlawful piracy and theft of the author's intellectual property. If you would like to use material from the book (other than just simply for reviewing the book), prior permission must be obtained by contacting the author at author@shellfishrecipes.com

Thank you for your support of the author's rights.

Content

365 AWESOME OAT RECIPES 9

1. Oat Avocado And Green Olive Muffins 9
2. Wheat Bran Bread Loaf 9
3. Ailbhe's Brown Bread 10
4. Airfried Banana Walnuts Oats Muffins 10
5. Almond Butter Date Squares 11
6. Almond Pulp Granola With Dried Cherries 11
7. Almond And Raisin Granola Bars 12
8. Anise Oat Kipferl 12
9. Anzac Bites 13
10. Apple Almond Energy Bars 13
11. Apple Cinnamon Oatmeal Bowls 13
12. Apple Coconut Dream Cake 14
13. Apple Crisp & Quick Crystallized Ginger In A Classic Crisp + Seasonal Fruits 14
14. Apple Oatmeal Mini Muffins 15
15. Apple Streusel Cake 15
16. Apple And Oat Smoothie 16
17. Apple Currant Granola 16
18. Applesauce Coffee Cake 17
19. Apricot Rose Granola 18
20. Apricot And Pistachio Oat Bars 18
21. April Bloomfield's English Porridge 19
22. Autumn Breakfast (or Anytime) Buckle 19
23. Autumn Harvest Slow Cooker Oatmeal ... 20
24. Back To School Raspberry Granola Bars From Karen DeMasco 21
25. Baked Apples Stuffed With Cinnamon Oat Crumble 21
26. Baked Cinnamon Oatmeal Apple 22
27. Baked Pumpkin Oatmeal With Coconut Streusel Topping 23
28. Banana Bread With Chocolate Swirl 23
29. Banana Cake The Fit Version 24
30. Banana Oat Blender Pancakes 24
31. Banana, Blueberry, And Pecan Pancakes .. 25
32. Banana, Date + Walnut Loaf 25
33. Beach Vacation Overnight Oats 26
34. Beet Chocolate Cake 26
35. Berry Breakfast Muslii 27
36. Berry Oatmeal Pie 27
37. Best For Breakfast Apple Chocolate Granola 28
38. Bhutanese Red Rice, Millet, And Oat Breakfast Pudding 28
39. Black Bean And Corn Burgers 29
40. Black Bean And Quinoa Veggie Burgers .. 30
41. Black Pepper Pear Crisp With Salted Oat Streusel 30
42. Blackberry Peach Quinoa Burgers On Sweet Potato Buns 31
43. Blackberry Peach Crumble 32
44. Blood Orange Overnight Oats 32
45. Blood Orange, Cardamom, And Fig Jammy Oat Bars 33
46. Blueberry Muffins 33
47. Blueberry Peach Crumble Ice Cream 33
48. Blueberry Pecan Baked Oatmeal 35
49. Blueberry, Nectarine & Bourbon Crisp 35
50. Bowl A Granola 35
51. Breakfast Cookies 36
52. Breakfast Muesli 36
53. Breakfast Quinoa With Oats And Chia Seeds 37
54. Breakfast Carrot Cake Muffins 37
55. British Flapjacks 37
56. Brown Butter Apple Pie Salad 38
57. Brown Sugar Ice Cream With Oatmeal Raisin Cookie Dough 38
58. Buttermilk Oatmeal Bread 40
59. Butternut Squash Banana Chocolate Chip Muffins 41
60. CARROT NUTMEG PECAN COOKIES 42
61. Caramelized Bananas With Yogurt And Berries 42
62. Caramelized Onion, Ricotta & Steel Cut Oats 43
63. Carr Oatmeal 43
64. Carrot Bean Cakes With Tahini Dressing .44
65. Carrot Cake Balls 44
66. Carrot Cake Cookies 45
67. Carrot Cake Oatmeal With Peanut Butter 45
68. Carrot Cake For A Crowd 46
69. Cashew Butter Bites With Toasted Coconut & Cardamom 46
70. Cavatelli With Asiago Oat Crumbs 47
71. Chai Spiced Porridge With Stewed Apples 47

72. Cheater's Muesli..................................48
73. Cheesecake Cream + Choco Granola 48
74. Cherry Orange Crisp................................48
75. Chewy Crispy Oatmeal Cookies With Chocolate Chips And Dried Cherries................49
76. Chewy Granola Bars 49
77. Chewy Oatmeal Cookies..........................50
78. Chewy Oatmeal Raisin Breakfast Cookies 51
79. Chia Breakfast Bowl 51
80. Chickapea Homemade Meatballs For DOGS..51
81. Choc Chip ANZAC Biscuits......................52
82. Choco Oats Puris (Indian Fried Flat Bread) 53
83. Chocolate Almond Chia Hemp Flax Bars 53
84. Chocolate Cherry Coconut Granola 54
85. Chocolate Chip Cookies 54
86. Chocolate Chip Muffins............................55
87. Chocolate Guinness Stout Oatmeal With Pecans And Greek Yogurt.............................55
88. Chocolate Oatmeal Crepe Cake With Wild Grapes, Berries, And Bananas.....................55
89. Chocolate Raspberry Streusel Muffins 56
90. Chocolate Fruit Pecan Pie 57
91. Chocolate, Oat, And Walnut Slice! 57
92. Chocolatety Almond Super PowerBar 58
93. Chocolatey Banana And Oats 59
94. Chocolaty, Walnut No Bake Brownies......59
95. Cinnamon Cashew Butter Doughnuts 60
96. Classic Homemade Granola 60
97. Coco Ginger Hazelnut Oatmeal................61
98. Coconut Cranberry Muffins 61
99. Coconut Lemon Bombs No Bake Cookies 61
100. Coconut Mango Oatmeal 62
101. Coconut Mocha Oat Cookies 62
102. Coconut Quinoa Porridge With Berry Compote 63
103. Coconut Stovetop Oats With Avocado, Chia, And Almond Butter.............................63
104. Coconut Fig Chunks Of Energy 64
105. Cornflake Crunch Granola 64
106. Cozy Banana Bread Pancakes 65
107. Crab Apple Steel Cut Oatmeal................65
108. Cracklin' Oat Bran Granola....................65
109. Cranberry Ginger Granola.....................66
110. Cranberry White Chocolate Oatmeal Cookies 66
111. Cranberry And White Chocolate Streusel Bars 67
112. Cranberry Cinnamon Baked Oatmeal Topped With Warm Berries And Honey 67
113. Cranberry Oat Pecan Bread 68
114. Crispy Crunchy Oatmeal Cookies 68
115. Crispy Oatmeal Chocolate Chip Cookies..69
116. Crunchies 69
117. Crunchy Berry Breakfast Granola 70
118. Crunchy Pistachio Date Granola 70
119. D.U.M.P. (Don't. Underestimate. My. Peach.) Cake...71
120. Date And Walnut Oatcakes 71
121. Date Squares (revamped) 72
122. Dates And Oats Indian Milk Pudding/Kheer...72
123. Double Chocolate Banana Muffins............73
124. Double Toasted Coconut Oatmeal Shortbreads 74
125. Easiest Ever Banana Bread 74
126. Energy Pretzel Bites (adapted From Pinch Of Yum) 74
127. Everyday Banana Porridge.......................75
128. Everything Breakfast Cookies 75
129. Everything Cookie Ice Cream Sandwich...76
130. Fall Inspired Apple Granola (gluten/dairy/sugar Free) 77
131. Five Minute, No Bake Vegan Granola Bars 77
132. Fruity, Oaty Mini Cake Bites 78
133. Game Changing Pancake Mix 78
134. Gatherer's Pie 79
135. Ginger Rhubarb Crisp (Baby!) 80
136. Ginger, Berry, Nutty Crisp........................80
137. Ginger Apple Crumble Pie (Gluten And Dairy Free)...81
138. Gluten Free Raspberry Oatmeal Bars........82
139. Gluten Free Whole Food Waffles 83
140. Gluten Free Banana, Honey And Almond Loaf 83
141. Gluten Free Buckwheat Scones With Cardamom And Cherries.............................84
142. Gluten Free Chocolate Chip Cookies, With Oat, Buckwheat, Teff, Or Mesquite Flour 84
143. Gluten Free Cornbread Waffles.................85
144. Gluten Free Poppy Seed Rhubarb Bread ..86

145. Gluten Free Strawberry Tart Bars 87
146. Gluten Free Strawberry Rhubarb Almond Crisp 87
147. Gluten Free Sweet Potato Spice Cake With Cream Cheese Frosting 88
148. Gluten Free, Mostly Whole Grain Chocolate Shortbread Cookies 89
149. Gram's Best Oatmeal Cookies 89
150. Grandma's Ranger Cookies 90
151. Granola 90
152. Granola Clusters 90
153. Great Graham Crackers 91
154. Gussied Up Preacher Cookies 92
155. Harry's Favorite Better Than IHOP Multigrain Pancakes 92
156. Healthy Homemade Granola In 30 Minutes 93
157. Healthy Pumpkin Crumble 93
158. Healthy Vegan Cookies 94
159. Hearty Baked Oatmeal 94
160. Heidi Swanson's Baked Oatmeal 95
161. Home Made Organic Maple Granola With Fresh Fruit 95
162. Homemade Cranberry Almond Granola Bars 96
163. Homemade Pizza Crust 96
164. Honey Granola Tart 97
165. Honey Oat Whole Wheat Loaf 98
166. Honey Vanilla Almond Granola 98
167. Honey Oat Crunchies 99
168. Hoppin' John Fritters 99
169. How To Drink Your Way To A Better Night's Sleep 100
170. Iced Oatmeal Pie Bars 100
171. Indian Spiced Porridge 100
172. Irish Oats In Vermont 101
173. Irish Soda Bread With Flax Seeds 101
174. Jasmine Tea Poached Pear Crumble 101
175. LLBT Lemon Lime Souffle Blueberry Tart 102
176. Lemon And Toasted Almond Risotto 103
177. Lemon Curd Tart (V + GF) 104
178. MAPLE OATMEAL NUT GRANOLA BARS: THE PRETTY FEED 104
179. Mama Yoder's Chocolate Chip Cookies . 105
180. Mango Oat Pancakes 105
181. Mango Smoothie Bowl 106

182. Maple Blueberry Granola 106
183. Maple Coconut Spice Granola 106
184. Maple Espresso Baked Oatmeal 107
185. Maple Mulberry Quinoa Oatmeal Bowl . 107
186. Maple Oatmeal Pie 108
187. Maple Pecan Granola 108
188. Maple Quinoa Granola 109
189. Maple Walnut Steelcut Oatmeal With Peach Compote 109
190. Maple Grilled Nectarines & Almond Oat Crumb (gluten Free) 110
191. Maple, Almond, And Cranberry Granola 110
192. Maple, Buckwheat & Nut Brittle 111
193. Marbled Jam Cake 111
194. Marian Burros' Cowboy Cookies 112
195. Masala Chai Tea Oatmeal 112
196. Maya's Chocolate Fudge Sheet Cake 113
197. Mookies (Muffin Top Cookies) 114
198. Morning Person Zucchini Bread 114
199. Muesli Bread With Raisins, Apricot And Almonds 114
200. Multigrain Marmalade Muffins 115
201. Muscovado Baked Beans 116
202. My Coffee Group's Favorite Bircher Muesli 116
203. Nekisia Davis' Olive Oil & Maple Granola 117
204. No Bake Banana Oatmeal Cookies 117
205. No Bake Chocolate, Oatmeal, Peanut Butter Cookies 117
206. No Bake Cookies 118
207. No Bake Peanut Butter Dog Treats 118
208. Nordic Oats With Pumpkin Seed Oil & Booster Topping 118
209. Oat Breakfast Cookies 119
210. Oat Gnocchi With Shaved Asparagus & Brown Butter Vinaigrette 119
211. Oat Porridge Bread 120
212. Oat Streusel Jam Bars 122
213. Oat And Flax Pancakes With Spiced Apple Compote 123
214. Oat And Wheat Sandwich Bread 124
215. Oat And Chocolate Chip Cookies 124
216. Oat Scrambled Eggs 125
217. Oatmeal Cherry Berry Cookies 125
218. Oatmeal Cookies 126
219. Oatmeal Cookies With Sea Salt And Olive

Oil 127
220. Oatmeal Currant Bread 127
221. Oatmeal Ice Cream With Toasted Walnuts 128
222. Oatmeal Pancakes 129
223. Oatmeal Pancakes With Caramelized Bacon And Herbed Crème Fraiche 129
224. Oatmeal Raisin Cookie Porridge 130
225. Oatmeal Raisin Cookies 130
226. Oatmeal Scotchies 130
227. Oatmeal Vanilla Sandwiches 131
228. Oatmeal And Carrots Pancakes Served With Avocado Cream And Poached Peaches 132
229. Oatmeal And Lavender Shortbread With Whipped Goat Cheese And Lemon Coulis 133
230. Oatmeal With Stewed Fruit And Almonds 133
231. Oatmeal With Cinnamon And Apples 134
232. Oaty Brown Sugar Soda Bread 134
233. Olive Oil Braised Broccoli Rabe 135
234. Ooey Gooey Magic Cookies 135
235. Our Best Açaí Bowl 136
236. Overnight Banana Oats 136
237. Overnight Oatmeal Cold Prep 137
238. Overnight Oatmeal Pancakes 137
239. Overnight Oatmeal With Rhubarb Cherry Compote 138
240. Overnight Swiss Style Muesli 138
241. PB&J Granola 138
242. Peach Blueberry Baked Oatmeal 139
243. Peach Cobbler Cake 139
244. Peach Crostata With Spiced Crumble 140
245. Peach Smoothie Popsicles 141
246. Peach Sundaes With Cardamom Gingersnap Topping 142
247. Peach And Plum Muesli Oatmeal 142
248. Peaches And Cream Smoothie Bowl 143
249. Peanut Butter & Jelly Overnight Oats 143
250. Peanut Butter Blondie Brownies 144
251. Peanut Butter Chocolate Balls 144
252. Peanut Butter Chocolate Chunk Cookies 144
253. Peanut Butter Granola 145
254. Peanut Butter Oatmeal Raisin Cookies ... 145
255. Pear Crumble 146
256. Pear Crumble Pie 146
257. Pear Rosemary Galette 147
258. Pearsauce Streusel Bundt Cake 148

259. Perfectly Sweet Seed Bars 149
260. Pomegranate And Plum Yogurt Parfaits 149
261. Porridge In Pink With Raspberries & Greek Yogurt From Maria Speck 149
262. Porridge With Rye Flakes And Abricot Compote 150
263. Poule Au Pot 150
264. Pumpkin Baked Oatmeal With Brandied Cranberries And White Chocolate 151
265. Pumpkin Almond Scones W/ Maple Yogurt Frosting 152
266. Pumpkin Cornbread Muffins 152
267. Pumpkin Maple Oat Rolls 153
268. Pumpkin Pie Oatmeal 154
269. Pumpkin Pie Spice Squares 154
270. Pumpkin Seed Oatmeal Raisin Cookie Bars 155
271. Quick Simple Beef Stew 155
272. Quinoa Porridge 156
273. Quinoa And Oat Breakfast Porridge 156
274. Quinoa, Beet And Chickpea Burgers 157
275. Rainy Morning Oats 158
276. Raisin, Pecan, And Banana Oatmeal With Flax Seeds 158
277. Raspberry Multigrain Muffins 158
278. Raspberry Oat And Yogurt Spelt Muffins 159
279. Raspberry And Honey Cranachan 159
280. Raspberry Rhubarb Crumble With Cracklin' Oat Bran Topping 160
281. Rhubarb Cherry Hibiscus Crumble 160
282. Rhubarb Ginger Downside Up Oatmeal Cake 161
283. Rhubarb, Cherry And Strawberry Crumble 161
284. Rich And Creamy Swiss Style Muesli 162
285. Roasted Squash Salad With Pomegranate And Spiced Oat Clusters 162
286. Rockin RAW Nut Granola The Best RAW Granola….Ever 163
287. Rosemary Cayenne Granola Bars 163
288. Rosemary, Fig, Walnut, And Honey Granola 164
289. Russet Rollscuits With Herbs And Cheese 165
290. SUGAR FREE Barley Oats Quinoa Cashew Orange Cake With Blackberry And Peach Puree

290. 166
291. Salted Caramel Chocolate Protein Bites .. 167
292. Sara's "Granola Bars" 167
293. Savory Breakfast Oat Bowl With Grana Padano 167
294. Savory Oatmeal With Ham, Poached Eggs, And Hollandaise Sauce 168
295. Savory Oats With Roasted Red Pepper Sauce, Baby Broccoli And Poached Eggs 169
296. Savory Ris Oat To With Poached Egg 169
297. Savory Oat, Leek, And Pecorino Scones 170
298. School Morning Muesli 170
299. Silly Good Oatmeal Cookies With Golden Raisins (flourless And Vegan) 171
300. Simple Gifts Granola 171
301. Slow Cooker Granola With Spicy Molasses Glazed Nuts 172
302. Smoked Apple Streusel 172
303. Soda Bread With Walnuts And Rolled Oats 173
304. Soft Oat Cookies 174
305. Spiced Cranberry Orange Maple Breakfast Porridge 174
306. Spicy Shorties 175
307. Steel Cut Oats Mash Up 175
308. Steel Cut Oats With Baked Apple 175
309. Strawberry Goat Cheese Oat Pie With Whipped Goat Cheese 176
310. Strawberry Oatmeal Breakfast Shake 176
311. Strawberry Oatmeal Cookie Cobbler 177
312. Strawberry Rhubarb Crisp 177
313. Strawberry Rhubarb Crumble Parfait 178
314. Strawberry And Almond Crumble (gluten Free) 179
315. Summer Berry & Fig Muffins 179
316. Sundried Tomato And Olive Bread 180
317. Susan's Health Bomb Muffins 180
318. Sweet Potato Banana Pancake & Strawberry Glaze 180
319. Sweet And Savory Whole Oats And Sweet Brown Rice Porridge 181
320. Thai Inspired Turkey Burgers 181
321. The Best Breakfast Pancakes To Touch My Lips 182
322. The Easiest, Creamiest (One Ingredient!) Homemade Oat Milk 183
323. The Healthiest Pumpkin Pie Ever 184
324. The Pantry Cookie 184
325. The Toast With The Most Toasted Oat Sourdough 185
326. The Treasure Loaded Peanut Butter Cookie 186
327. Throwback Oatmeal Muffins 186
328. Toasted Oat & Pecan Oatmeal 187
329. Toasted Oatmeal With Fruit & Spice 187
330. Toasty Brown Butter Steel Cut Oats 188
331. Trail Mix Oatmeal 189
332. Tuna Tartare With Cottage Cheese And Crumble 189
333. Ultimate Superfoods Breakfast Bars 190
334. Underrated Oats Peanut Ginger Eggplant And Sweet Potato With Coconut Oats 190
335. Vanilla Berry Baked Oatmeal 191
336. Vanilla Porridge 191
337. Vanilla Spice Granola 192
338. Vanilla Bean Oatmeal Ice Cream With Oat Cookie Crumbs 192
339. Vegan Almond And Toasted Oat Jam Bars 193
340. Vegan Apple Crisp 193
341. Vegan Banana Chocolate Muffins 194
342. Vegan Beetloaf 194
343. Vegan Chocolate Chunk Cookies With Flaky Sea Salt 195
344. Vegan Cookie Dough Pops 195
345. Vegan Dark Chocolate And Gogi Berry Oatmeal Cookies 196
346. Vegan Dark Chocolate Gingerbread Thumbprint Cookies 196
347. Vegan Strawberry Cream Pie 197
348. Vegan Sweet Potato Casserole 198
349. Vegan Coconut Chocolate Chip Oat Cookies! 199
350. Vegan, Gluten Free And Refined Sugar Free Granola Bars With A Chocolate Dip 199
351. Vegetable Crumble With Chorizo 200
352. Very Almond Raspberry Oatmeal Bars (Gluten Free) 200
353. Walnut, Oat & Apricot Squares 201
354. White Bean & Chicken Sweet Potato Casserole 201
355. Whole Bean Vanilla Almond Granola 202
356. Whole Grain Banana Bread 202
357. Whole Grain Sourdough Rye Bread 203

358. Whole Wheat Oatmeal Banana Bread.....204
359. Zucchini Chocolate Espresso Brownies.205
360. Zucchini Sausage Walnut Bread...............205
361. B[EAT] Burgers..206
362. Best Healthier Chocolate Chip Cookies..206
363. Coconut Cashew Oatmeal Cookies| Gf + Vegan..207
364. Orange Oat Cookies....................................207
365. "Fudgy" No Bake Chocolate Oatmeal Cookies...208

INDEX.. 209
CONCLUSION...213

365 Awesome Oat Recipes

***

1. Oat Avocado And Green Olive Muffins

Serving: Makes 12 | Prep: | Cook: | Ready in:

Ingredients

- 1 cup old-fashioned rolled oats
- 1 cup plain flour
- 1 cup thick buttermilk
- 1/4 cup chopped green olives
- 2 teaspoons freshly cracked black pepper
- 1 egg
- 2 teaspoons salt
- 1 teaspoon baking powder
- 1/2 teaspoon soda bicarb
- 3/4 cup mashed ripe avocados

Direction

- Soak the oats in the buttermilk for an hour.
- Grease and prepare 12 muffin molds and preheat the oven to 200 degrees C.
- Sift the flour together with salt, baking powder and soda bicarb.
- In another bowl, beat the egg into the oat mixture followed by the avocados and the flour till just combined.
- Add the pepper and chopped olives, and bake for 15-20 minutes till an inserted toothpick comes out clean.

2. Wheat Bran Bread Loaf

Serving: Makes 2 loaves | Prep: | Cook: | Ready in:

Ingredients

- 350 gr all-purpose flour
- 200 gr whole wheat flour
- 100 gr wheat bran
- 1 tablespoon fine salt
- 1 tablespoon honey
- 50 gr unsalted butter, softened
- 330 ml lukewarm water
- 35 gr fresh yeast
- 1 tablespoon sugar
- eggwash
- 1 tablespoon quick oats

Direction

- Add the sugar to the lukewarm water. Dissolve the yeast in the water and allow to foam for 15 minutes
- Combine the flours, the bran and the salt in a bowl and make a well in the middle
- Add the honey. Pour the water with the yeast and knead
- Add the softened unsalted butter and knead until the dough has a uniform texture
- Place the dough in a floured bowl and allow to prove for an hour
- Cut the dough into two pieces and knead with a rolling pin to degas
- Roll into two loaves
- Make a few cuts on the surface, brush with egg wash and sprinkle with quick oats
- Place on a greased, lined baking sheet or tin and allow to prove for 15 minutes
- Allow to cool for 10 minutes and place on a rack

3. Ailbhe's Brown Bread

Serving: Makes a two pound loaf | Prep: | Cook: | Ready in:

Ingredients

- 300 grams   Coarse whole-wheat flour
- 150 grams   White, self-raising flour
- 1 teaspoon   Bicarbonate of soda
- 1 teaspoon   Finely ground salt
- 100 grams   Thick, Greek style yoghurt - Fage works quite well.
- 1   Large, free range egg
- 300 milliliters   Full fat, whole milk
- 2 tablespoons   Good quality honey
- 7 grams   Butter (for greasing)
- 1 handful   Jumbo Oats

Direction

- Preheat your oven to 200 C, or 400 F. Grease a large, rectangular loaf pan, preferably 9 x 5 inches or thereabouts, with butter. Set aside.
- With a scales, measure out 300 grams of whole wheat flour into a large mixing bowl. If it's really coarse, give it a go in the blender or food processor to make it softer. Add the 150 grams of self-rising flour to the bowl.
- To the same bowl, add a teaspoon of bicarbonate of soda and a teaspoon of fine salt. Mix these ingredients together - feel free to use your hands! It's fun!
- In a separate jug, measure out 100 grams of the thickest Greek style yoghurt you can get your hands on - I've used Fage before, with good results. Keeping the scales on, crack an egg into the yoghurt mixture. Add all of the milk, next. Stir them together (but don't use your hands for this bit!) You want the total weight of the liquid ingredients to be around 450mls - a little more or less is no bother; if you use a massive egg, you'll use less milk.
- Add the wet ingredients to the dry - bring them together with a rubber spatula or wooden spoon. As you beat the batter (and it will be a batter, not a dough), add the honey, stirring all the while.
- When there are no dry bits of flour left in the bowl, the mixture will be too wet to knead, and too thick to pour, so help it into the greased loaf tin as quick as you can, toss it into the oven, cross your fingers and hope for the best. Resist the urge to open the oven door. If you so desire, a handful of oats sprinkled over the batter before it cooks gives the bread a lovely rustic look.
- When the bread is finished, it should be hard to the touch on the outside, but with a little give when poked. A knife stuck into it will come out clean, and not gummy. Free the loaf from the tin, place it on a cooling rack, and cover with a tea towel. Let it sit for at least two hours before cutting - if you cut it while it's still warm, you'll end up with delicious crumbs and not much else, and all your hard work will've been for naught.
- Serve with butter and jam, or with fish (not at the same time, though, yuck). Or just eat it however you want, the important thing is that you enjoy it!

4. Airfried Banana Walnuts Oats Muffins

Serving: Serves 2 | Prep: | Cook: | Ready in:

Ingredients

- 4 tablespoons   Refined flour
- 1 teaspoon   Chopped Walnuts
- 1/4 cup   Oats
- 1/4 cup   Unsalted butter
- 1/4 cup   Powdered Sugar
- 1/2 teaspoon   Baking powder
- 1 teaspoon   Milk (optional)

Direction

- Mix butter and sugar together and add mashed banana and walnuts. Mix well.
- In separate bowl, mix refined flour, oats and backing powder. Add these dry ingredients in

- the above mixture and cut and fold the mixture 3-4 times.
- Add little milk if the batter seems to be very very thick. But in general this batter will be thick.
- Grease muffin mold and put the muffin batter in each mold. Some walnuts can be put on top of each mold as well. Bake these muffins in preheated air fryer at 160 degrees for 10 min. Once baked, keep muffins in standby time for another 10 min. Take out all the muffin mold and allow to cool down for 10 min. Once cooled, de-mold all the muffins and serve.

5. Almond Butter Date Squares

Serving: Makes 9-12 squares | Prep: | Cook: |Ready in:

Ingredients

- Date Filling
- 2 1/2 cups medjool dates, pitted and roughly chopped
- 1 cup water
- Almond crust
- 1/2 cup unsalted butter or coconut oil at room temperature, plus more for greasing the baking dish
- 1/2 cup almond butter
- 6 tablespoons maple syrup
- 6 tablespoons granulated sugar
- 1 tsp teaspoons kosher salt
- 2 cups rolled oats
- 1 1/2 cups all-purpose flour or oat flour
- 1 1/2 cups almond flour
- 1 1/2 teaspoons baking powder

Direction

- Heat the oven to 350°F.
- Place the dates and water in a small pot. Bring to a boil, then lower to a simmer. Cook, stirring once in a while, for 10-15 minutes, until the dates are broken up and the mixture becomes thick.
- Grease a 10x10-inch or similar size baking dish and line it with overhanging parchment paper. In a big bowl, combine the butter or coconut oil, almond butter, maple syrup, sugar and salt. In a food processor, pulse the oats, flours and baking powder together for 10 seconds or so, until all the oat flakes are broken up into small pieces. Add the other crust ingredients to the food processor and pulse a few times until crumbly. If you don't have a food processor, I recommend using quick cooking oats and to mix the crust with your hands.
- Press down 3/4 of the crust mixture at the bottom of the prepared pan. Spread the date filling evenly over it. Sprinkle the remaining quarter of the crust over the filling to make a crumble. Bake in the oven for about 60 minutes, until the top is golden brown. Let cool for an hour before cutting the squares.
- Store them at room temperature in an airtight container for up to 4 days.

6. Almond Pulp Granola With Dried Cherries

Serving: Makes about 4 cups | Prep: | Cook: |Ready in:

Ingredients

- 1 1/2 cups fresh almond pulp left over from making almond milk
- 1 1/2 cups old-fashioned rolled oats
- 3 tablespoons sesame seeds
- 3 tablespoons melted unrefined coconut oil
- 1/4 cup honey
- 2 teaspoons vanilla extract
- 1/4 teaspoon sea salt
- 2 handfuls dried cherries

Direction

- Preheat oven to 325F.
- Spread almond pulp in a single layer on a baking sheet. Bake for about 10 minutes, to dehydrate the pulp a little.

- Transfer pulp to a large bowl and toss in oats and sesame seeds. In a small bowl, stir together oil, honey, vanilla and salt. Drizzle over oat mixture and toss to coat evenly. Transfer mixture back to the baking sheet and bake 20-25 minutes, gently tossing once halfway through cooking, until granola is golden brown.
- Remove from oven and let cool completely. Add dried cherries and transfer to an airtight container. Stored in a cool dry place, granola will keep up to one week.

7. Almond And Raisin Granola Bars

Serving: Makes 8 bars | Prep: | Cook: |Ready in:

Ingredients

- 200 grams steel-cut oats
- 140 grams almonds
- 110 grams honey
- 60 grams unsalted butter
- 50 grams brown sugar
- 1/2 teaspoon vanilla essence
- 90 grams raisins
- 1/2 teaspoon salt

Direction

- Toast the oats in the oven at 180C for about 10min or until golden. Make sure to stir halfway through.
- Toast the almonds separately at the same temperature until fragrant.
- Put the honey, butter, brown sugar and vanilla essence in a pot over medium heat until the mix starts boiling.
- Add the rest of the ingredients off the heat in the pot and mix.
- Transfer to a mold lined with baking paper and press down hard. Take your time to do this because on it depends the stability of their shape afterwards.

- Let it cool down to room temperature and then take to the fridge for at least 4 hours.
- Take out using the baking paper and cut into bars.
- Wrap in baking paper and keep in the fridge.

8. Anise Oat Kipferl

Serving: Makes 30 cookies | Prep: | Cook: |Ready in:

Ingredients

- 50g oats
- 140g all-purpose flour
- 45g sugar
- 1 pinch of salt
- 4 teaspoons anise seeds, divided
- 100g cold butter
- 1 egg
- 4 teaspoons sugar

Direction

- Toast all the anise seeds in a dry pan on medium heat until fragrant.
- Place the oats and 2 teaspoons of the anise seeds in a food processor and process until coarsely ground.
- Place the ground oat mixture, flour, sugar and salt in a bowl and form a well.
- Add the cubed butter and, using a knife or a pastry cutter, cut the butter into the other ingredients until the mixture resembles sand.
- Add the egg and quickly combine everything to form a smooth dough. Wrap in foil and let rest in the fridge for about 1 hour.
- Preheat the oven to 170 degrees.
- Using tablespoon-sized chunks of dough, form roughly 30 crescent-shaped cookies, placing them on a baking tray lined with parchment paper. Bake for about 12 minutes, until golden.
- Roll the warm cookies in a mix of the remaining sugar and the remaining anise seeds.

9. Anzac Bites

Serving: Makes 40+ walnut-size cookies (or 20 normal-size cookies) | Prep: | Cook: | Ready in:

Ingredients

- 1/2 cup whole wheat pastry flour
- 1/3 cup caster cane sugar
- 2/3 cup cups dried coconut (shredded are fine)
- 3/4 cup rolled oats
- 1/4 cup butter
- 1 tablespoon syrup (or honey)
- 1/2 teaspoon baking soda
- 2 tablespoons boiling water

Direction

- Preheat oven to 350F.
- Mix together flour, sugar, coconut and rolled oats; set aside.
- Melt butter and golden syrup; dissolve baking soda in the boiling water and add to the butter-syrup mix; stir butter mixture into the dry ingredients, mix well until wet and crumbly.
- Pinch the dough into walnut-size balls and place it onto the greased baking sheet; using the thumb to press onto the ball, flatten it a bit.
- Bake for 6~10 minutes, or until golden brown.
- Enjoy.

10. Apple Almond Energy Bars

Serving: Makes 8 | Prep: | Cook: | Ready in:

Ingredients

- 2 cups gluten free rolled oats
- 1 cup plain almonds
- 1 1/2 cups raisins
- 2 apples, cored and diced
- 1 tablespoon dark brown sugar
- 2 1/2 teaspoons cinnamon
- 1/2 teaspoon nutmeg
- 1 pinch salt

Direction

- Pre-heat the oven to 350. Line a sheet tray and spread the oats and almonds out on it in a single layer. Toast them in the oven for 5-10 minutes, until they get really fragrant. Take the tray out but leave the oven on when they're done. Let them cool for a couple of minutes, then set up a food processor. Combine the oats and almonds in the processor bowl with the raisins, diced apples, brown sugar, cinnamon, nutmeg and salt. Pulse it all together thoroughly until it is a sticky, uniform mixture.
- Get out an 8 x 8 baking dish and line it with parchment paper. Make sure there is enough to have flaps hanging over the sides, which makes lifting the bars out of the pan a cinch. Use a spatula to spread the mixture into a perfect, even layer in the pan. Fold the flaps of parchment paper over the mixture and press it out on the parchment paper so that it isn't too sticky. Bake the mixture for 20 minutes, then take it out and let it cool for 10-15 minutes. Slice the mixture into bars by making 3 equal vertical slices, then making a horizontal cut halfway down. Let them cool completely, then store them in an airtight container in the refrigerator. Enjoy!

11. Apple Cinnamon Oatmeal Bowls

Serving: Serves 1 | Prep: | Cook: | Ready in:

Ingredients

- 1/4 teaspoon olive oil
- 1 apple, cored, peeled and cubed
- 1/4 teaspoon brown sugar
- 1 cup old-fashioned oats

- pinch of coarse salt
- 1/4 cup unsweetened almond milk
- 1 tablespoon maple syrup
- 1 teaspoon cinnamon

Direction

- Drizzle the olive oil into a small sauté pan set over medium heat. Add the apple and the brown sugar and sauté until the apple pieces are almost tender, about 5 minutes.
- Meanwhile, prepare the oats according to the package instructions. Once fully cooked, turn off the heat and add the salt and the almond milk to the oats and stir until the almond milk is well incorporated. Pour the oat mixture into a bowl and add the maple syrup, the cinnamon and the still warm apples. Serve immediately.

12. Apple Coconut Dream Cake

Serving: Makes 1 9in cake | Prep: | Cook: | Ready in:

Ingredients

- 1 cup "quick" cooked oats
- 2 large apples (peeled & chopped)
- 2 1/4 cups flour
- 2 cups packed brown sugar
- 2 large eggs
- 1/2 cup butter at room temp
- 2 tablespoons butter at room temp
- 1 cup agave nectar
- 2 cups shredded coconut
- 1 teaspoon cinnamon
- 1/4 teaspoon nutmeg
- 1 teaspoon baking soda
- 1/2 teaspoon salt
- 2 teaspoons vanilla extract

Direction

- Line a 9in spring form pan with parchment paper and butter and pre-heat oven to 350 degrees
- Cream 1 cup butter, 1 cup brown sugar and 1 cup agave nectar for 2 minutes then slowly add vanilla, eggs and then oats and 1/2 of the chopped apples, mix until combined. Sift together flour, baking soda, cinnamon, nutmeg and salt. Add flour mixture to wet ingredients and mix until combined. Scoop batter into spring form pan and bake for 50 minutes or until toothpick comes out clean. Cool cake completely before topping.
- For the topping: cream 2 tablespoons butter, 1 cup brown sugar and 2 tablespoons agave nectar slowly adding cream. Add the coconut and ½ of the chopped apples, mix until combined. Cover the cake to the rim with the topping and bake until golden brown and set about 30 minutes.

13. Apple Crisp & Quick Crystallized Ginger In A Classic Crisp + Seasonal Fruits

Serving: Serves 4 - 6 or more | Prep: 0hours30mins | Cook: 0hours40mins | Ready in:

Ingredients

- Quick-Crystalized Ginger
- 2 tablespoons chopped ginger
- 2 tablespoons sugar (preferably Demerara)
- 1/4 cup water
- Fruit & Topping
- 4 cups apples*, chopped in chunks
- 1 cup peaches or nectarines*, in chunks
- 1 cup blueberries
- 1/4 cup brown sugar
- 1 teaspoon cinnamon
- 6 tablespoons butter
- 1/4 cup white sugar
- 1/4 cup rolled oats

- 1/4 cup quick cooking oats (or 1/2 cup total of either)
- small amount of butter to grease the pan, sprinkle of salt

Direction

- GINGER: Put the ginger, sugar and water in your smallest pan. Bring to a boil, lower to a fast simmer, cook until the ginger is translucent. (It doesn't take long.)
- FRUIT: Put all the fruit in a good-sized bowl with the ginger syrup, brown sugar and cinnamon. Mix it so everything is evenly distributed.
- Transfer the fruit to an 8 X 8" pan, greased with a little butter. Sprinkle with a little salt. Heat the oven to 350 degrees F.
- CRISP: Cut the sugar into the butter. Sprinkle the oats over, then mix them in with forks (chopping motion) or, quickly so the butter does not get too soft from your body heat, with your fingers.
- Break up the topping evenly over the fruit in the pan. Put it on a shelf in the upper third of the heated oven. Let it bake until the fruit is soft and the topping is browned. Check at 40 minutes, but it may take an hour, depending on the oven.
- NOTE: The apples were commercial Granny Smith, with a waxed peel, peeled; Braeburn from a local farm -- no need to peel. Peaches and nectarines, unpeeled. Choice is yours.

14. Apple Oatmeal Mini Muffins

Serving: Makes 48 | Prep: 0hours20mins | Cook: 0hours15mins | Ready in:

Ingredients

- 2 cups oat flour (crushed oats)
- 1/2 cup old fashioned oats
- 2 cups diced and peeled apples (2 large apples or 3-4 smaller apples)
- 2 eggs
- 1 cup buttermilk
- 1/2 cup butter
- 1/2 tablespoon cinnamon
- 1/8 teaspoon salt
- 3/4 cup brown sugar
- 1 teaspoon baking soda
- 2 teaspoons vanilla extract

Direction

- Preheat the oven to 350 F.
- Peel and dice the apples.
- Using a blender, crush 2 cups of old fashioned oats (to get 2 cups of oat flour, you'll need to crush more than 2 cups) or use purchased oat flour.
- In a medium bowl, mix the oat flour, old fashioned oats, cinnamon, baking soda, and salt.
- In another bowl, beat the eggs and vanilla. Add melted butter and sugar. Mix. Add buttermilk. Mix.
- Add the liquid ingredients to the bowl of dry ingredients. Incorporate but don't over-mix.
- Add the chopped apples.
- Using a small spoon, scoop the muffin batter into buttered mini muffin pans. Cook for about 13 to 15 minutes. If you use a larger muffin pan (not mini), you will need to bake the muffins longer.

15. Apple Streusel Cake

Serving: Makes 1 cake | Prep: | Cook: |Ready in:

Ingredients

- Cake
- 1 1/2 cups whole wheat pastry flour
- 2 teaspoons baking powder
- 1/2 teaspoon baking soda
- 2 teaspoons ground cinnamon
- 1/2 teaspoon ground nutmeg
- 2 eggs

- 1/4 cup nut butter
- 1/4 cup apple sauce
- 1/3 cup honey
- 1 teaspoon pure vanilla extract
- 2 cups grated apple
- Streusel Topping
- 1/2 cup rolled oats
- 1/4 cup whole wheat pastry flour
- 1/4 cup coconut sugar
- 1/4 cup coconut oil

Direction

- Heat the oven to 375F and grease or line a springform pan.
- Begin by making the streusel topping. Add the oats, flour, coconut sugar, and coconut oil to a bowl and mix it all together with your hands. Once it's fully mixed, set it to the side and prepare the cake.
- Combine the flour, baking powder, baking soda, cinnamon, and nutmeg in a large bowl.
- In a medium sized bowl, lightly beat the eggs. Add the nut butter, applesauce, honey, and vanilla.
- Remove the seeds from the apple and cut away any bruises. I didn't peel my apples, but if you're using conventional fruit from the supermarket, remove the skin. Grate with a box grater or with the grating attachment of a food processor. Add the shredded apple to the egg mixture.
- Add the egg and apple mixture to the dry ingredients and stir with a wooden spoon until just combined. Pour into the prepared springform and level the batter. Sprinkle the streusel topping over the cake, and bake at 375F for 30 minutes. It will spring back lightly when touched and the sides will be golden and pulling away from the edges of the pan. Serve with coconut whipped cream.

16. Apple And Oat Smoothie

Serving: Serves 1 | Prep: | Cook: | Ready in:

Ingredients

- 1 apple
- 1 banana
- 2 tablespoons oats (if gluten free use gluten free variety)
- 1 tablespoon chia seeds
- 1 teaspoon goji berries
- 1 teaspoon cinnamon
- 1 cup milk (cows, rice, almond, oat milk)

Direction

- Wash and core the apple, cut into chunks and add to the blender with approx. the 3rd of the milk.
- Blend the apple into a puree.
- Add banana, oats, chia seeds, goji berries, cinnamon, and the rest of the milk.
- Blend again until smooth.

17. Apple Currant Granola

Serving: Serves 8-10 | Prep: | Cook: | Ready in:

Ingredients

- 4 cups rolled oats
- 1 cup slivered almonds
- 2 teaspoons cinnamon
- 1/4 teaspoon ground allspice
- 1 teaspoon Kosher salt
- 3/4 cup unsweetened applesauce
- 1/4 cup maple syrup
- 3 tablespoons honey (omit if vegan)
- 2 tablespoons coconut oil
- 1 teaspoon vanilla extract
- 2 packets (1.2 oz each) Trader Joe's Freeze Dried Fuji Apple Slices, broken into pieces
- 1/2 cup dried currants

Direction

- Heat the oven to 300 degrees F. Line a rimmed baking sheet with parchment paper.
- In a medium saucepan over, combine honey, maple syrup, applesauce and coconut oil.
- Bring the mixture to a boil and immediately turn down to medium-low to simmer for about 5 minutes, stirring often until the mixture thickens just a little. Remove from heat and stir in vanilla.
- Mix the oats, almonds, cinnamon, allspice and salt in a large bowl. Pour the applesauce mixture over the oat mixture. Stir to coat thoroughly, and spread evenly on the baking sheet. Bake the granola for about 45 minutes, stirring every ten minutes, until the granola is golden brown and crisp. Keeping an eye on it towards the end of the baking time.
- Remove from oven, and stir in the dried apples and currants. Let the granola cool completely on the baking sheet. It will crisp up as it cools.
- Store the granola in a large, airtight container.
- Serve with milk or on top of yogurt.

18. Applesauce Coffee Cake

Serving: Makes 1 cake | Prep: | Cook: | Ready in:

Ingredients

- Apple Cider Applesauce
- 1 pound juicy apples (Macintosh work very well) peeled. cored and cut into quarters
- 1/4 cup apple cider
- 1 tablespoon Sugar (white, turbinado or brown any will work)
- pinch of salt
- The Crumble Topping and Cake
- THE CRUMBLE TOPPING
- 4 tablespoons unsalted butter softened
- 1/2 cup dark brown sugar packed
- 1/4 cup old fashioned rolled oats
- 3/4 teaspoon cinnamon
- 1/4 teaspoon salt
- 1 cup toasted pecans chopped (If you have a nut allergy the nuts can be omitted)
- THE CAKE
- 2 cups all purpose flour
- 1 teaspoon baking soda
- 1/2 teaspoon nutmeg
- 2 teaspoons cinnamon
- 1/8 teaspoon cloves (OPTIONAL, I omitted I do not like cloves)
- 1/2 teaspoon salt
- 8 tablespoons 1 stick unsalted butter softened
- 1 cup granulated sugar
- 1/2 cup light brown sugar packed
- 4 large eggs at room temperature
- 1 1/2 cups apple cider applesauce
- 2 small juicy apples (Macintosh work very well) peeled and sliced
- 1/2 cup toasted pecans chopped OPTIONAL

Direction

- Apple Cider Applesauce
- Clean, peel, core and quarter the apples. Add to a medium saucepan. Add the cider, sugar and salt and boil until apples are soft. Remove from heat and mash (I used a potato masher) keep some small chunks of apples. Set aside to cool.
- The Crumble Topping and Cake
- Make your crumble topping. In small bowl combine the butter, sugar, oats, flour, cinnamon, salt and pecans mix with fork or by hand to combine. Set aside.
- Pre-heat oven to 350 degrees. Coat your tube pan with cooking spray or vegetable oil. (I recommend using a nonstick pan)Sift flour, salt, baking soda and spices. Cream butter and white and brown sugar in your electric mixer until smooth about 3 minutes. Add the eggs one at a time make sure egg is incorporated before you add another one. With mixer on low add the applesauce and then the flour mixture. Mix just until combined. Add the optional chopped pecans and fold in.
- Pour batter into oiled pan. Place apple slices on top of cake tucking some into the batter,

- sprinkle on the crumble topping. Bake for 60-70 minutes check by inserting cake tester (I used a bamboo skewer) near the middle of the cake and it should come out clean. Remove from oven and let cake cool in pan on wire rack.
- Remove from pan and if you do not serve immediately wrap in plastic wrap and store at room temperature until ready to serve. NOTE: if you make in a Bundt pan like I do it could take some coaxing to get it out of the pan when cooled. It could be easier to remove from a tube pan because it does not have all the grooves that a Bundt pan does.

19. Apricot Rose Granola

Serving: Serves 6 | Prep: | Cook: |Ready in:

Ingredients

- 2 cups rolled oats
- 1/2 cup unsweetened coconut flakes
- 1/3 cup raw pumpkin seeds
- 1/2 cup sliced almonds
- 1 cup unsulphured apricots, chopped into small pieces (I used Organic Turkish Apricots)
- 1 tablespoon flax seed, ground (yields about 1.5 Tb ground flax) + 3 Tbs water
- 1/3 cup coconut oil
- 1/3 cup brown rice syrup (or honey)
- 1 tablespoon dark brown sugar
- pinch of salt
- 1 orange, zested or julienned & diced into tiny pieces (about 1.5 Tb)
- 1 tablespoon rosewater

Direction

- Combine ground flax seed and water in a small bowl. Set aside.
- Heat oven to 225F convention bake or 250F standard bake.
- In a large bowl, add the dry ingredients: oats, coconut, nuts and apricots. Set aside.
- In a saucepan, combine the coconut oil, brown rice syrup, brown sugar, salt and orange zest. Heat on medium-low and mix until the oil and sugars are thoroughly mixed. Remove from heat and whisk in the flaxseed mixture and rosewater.
- Mix the dry ingredients with the wet ingredients and spread on a parchment lined rimmed baking sheet.
- Press ingredients into a rectangle about ½" thickness.
- Bake for 1 hour. Turn off heat and let cool in oven.
- Break into pieces and store in an airtight container.

20. Apricot And Pistachio Oat Bars

Serving: Makes 16, 2 x 2-inch bars | Prep: | Cook: |Ready in:

Ingredients

- 1/2 cup (70 grams) shelled, unsalted pistachios
- 1 cup (55 grams) rolled oats
- 1 cup (140 grams) flour
- 5 tablespoons (65 grams) light brown sugar
- 1/4 teaspoon kosher salt
- 6 tablespoons (85 grams) unsalted butter, chilled and cubed
- 12 apricots (560 grams/1 1/4 pounds)
- the juice and zest of 1/2 a medium lemon
- 1 1/2 tablespoons (22 grams) sugar

Direction

- Heat the oven to 375F/190C. Line an 8 x 8-inch baking pan with parchment paper.
- Add the pistachios to the bowl of a food processor. Blend for 15 seconds, until the pistachios are reduced to a meal. Add the oats, and blend another 15 seconds. Add the flour, brown sugar, salt, and butter; blend for 15 seconds. Add 2 tablespoons water and blend

until the mix barely binds together. Reserve a heaping 1/2 cup of the mix; dump the rest into the prepared baking pan and, using your fingers, tamp it evenly down to form the base of your bars.
- Halve and pit the apricots. Move them to a large mixing bowl, and hand toss with the lemon juice and zest, and the sugar. Arrange the fruit in the baking pan, on top of the crust. Crumble the remaining pistachio-oat mix on top of the apricots. Bake for 45 minutes. Move the pan to the refrigerator for an hour right out of the oven. Cut into squares and serve.

21. April Bloomfield's English Porridge

Serving: Serves 2 to 3 | Prep: 0hours5mins | Cook: 0hours20mins | Ready in:

Ingredients

- 1 1/2 cups whole milk, plus a few generous splashes
- 1 1/2 cups water
- 1 1/2 teaspoons Maldon, or other flaky sea salt (if using finer salt, start with 1/2 teaspoon and add to taste)
- 1/2 cup rolled oats
- 1/2 cup steel-cut oats
- 2 tablespoons sugar (maple, brown, or white) or maple syrup

Direction

- Combine the milk, water, and salt in a medium pot (a 2-quart pot should do it) and set over high heat. As soon as the liquid comes to a gentle simmer, add both kinds of oats and lower the heat to medium.
- Cook the oats at a steady simmer, stirring frequently and lowering the heat as necessary to maintain the simmer.
- After about 20 minutes at the simmer, the rolled oats will have turned a bit mushy, while the steel-cut oats will be just tender and pop when you bite them.
- Taste for seasoning—it should be on the salty side. Add sugar or syrup. Spoon the porridge into warm bowls and let it sit for a minute. Then carefully pour a little cold milk around the edges of each bowl, so it pools all the way round. Sprinkle a five-fingered pinch of sugar or drizzle the syrup in the center of each and let it melt, then serve right away.

22. Autumn Breakfast (or Anytime) Buckle

Serving: Serves 8 to 10 | Prep: | Cook: | Ready in:

Ingredients

- Streusel
- ¾ cup (3 oz) pecans (or walnuts)
- ¼ cup coarsely chopped crystallized ginger
- ½ cup (4 oz) packed brown sugar
- ½ cup (2 1/8 oz) oat flour* (see note at end of recipe)
- ½ teaspoon cinnamon
- ¼ teaspoon salt
- 4 tablespoons cold unsalted butter, cut into ½-inch slices
- 1 tablespoon buttermilk (plus more if needed)
- Autumn Buckle
- 6 ounces cranberries
- 12 to 14 ounces pears and/or apples
- 1 cup (5 oz) all-purpose flour
- ¾ cup (3 ¼ oz) oat flour*
- 2 ½ teaspoons baking powder
- 1 ½ teaspoons ground ginger
- 1 teaspoon ground cinnamon
- ¼ teaspoon salt
- 1/8 teaspoon ground cloves
- 4 tablespoons unsalted butter
- ¾ cup (6 oz) packed brown sugar
- 1 large egg, cold
- 1 tablespoon molasses
- 1 ½ teaspoons vanilla paste or extract

- 2/3 cup buttermilk, room temperature

Direction

- Streusel
- Pulse pecans and ginger in food processor until no large pieces remain. This should take about 8 to 10 long pulses.
- Add the brown sugar, oat flour, cinnamon, and salt. Pulse several times to combine.
- Add the butter, and pulse until everything is incorporated, and no large chunks of butter remain. Drizzle buttermilk over the mixture, then pulse several times. If the mixture doesn't clump together drizzle in another half tablespoon buttermilk and pulse again.
- Set aside while completing the buckle.
- Autumn Buckle
- Preheat oven to 350º F with a rack in the lower middle position. Butter and flour a 2-inch deep, 9-inch square, 10-inch round, or 11- by 7-inch rectangular pan. Set aside.
- Rinse and pick over the cranberries. If using apples: peel and core then cut into ½- to ¾-inch chunks. If using pears: skip the peeling, but core and cut into ½- to ¾-inch chunks. You should have about 4 cups of fruit in total. If you have more, snack on a few apple/pear chunks. Set aside.
- Combine flours, baking powder, spices and salt in a large bowl. Whisk until well mixed, about 15 seconds. Set aside.
- Place butter in a glass bowl or 4-cup glass measure. Microwave for 25 to 35 seconds, until about half melted. Add the brown sugar, egg, molasses, and vanilla to the bowl, then whisk about 30 seconds. Beat in the buttermilk (if the buttermilk is too cold, the mixture may look a bit curdled, but don't worry.)
- Add the wet ingredients to the dry ingredients, and stir just until the batter is smooth. Fold in the fruit.
- Transfer the batter to the prepared pan, spreading it evenly. Sprinkle with the streusel topping in an even layer. Bake for 40 to 55 minutes (depending on your pan and oven). The top will be golden brown, and a toothpick inserted near the center won't have any batter clinging to it (though it may have fruit or streusel on it). If in doubt, bake a couple minutes longer. The fruit helps to protect it from drying out.
- Let cool on a wire rack for at least 20 minutes before serving. It is not a sliceable dessert, so scoop out servings like you would for a crisp or cobbler. Serve warm or at room temperature, with a generous dollop barely sweetened yogurt (or frozen yogurt, or whipped cream).
- Once cool, can be wrapped and stored at room temperature for 1 to 2 days.
- *NOTE: If you don't have oat flour, but you have rolled oats and a coffee grinder or food processor it is easy to DIY. Just grind or pulse the rolled oats until they become powdery. You can toast the oats first as well, which increases the oat flavor in the final dish.

23. Autumn Harvest Slow Cooker Oatmeal

Serving: Serves 4-6 | Prep: | Cook: | Ready in:

Ingredients

- 1 cup steel cut oats
- 4 small cooking pears (or apples if you prefer), chopped
- 1 cup fresh cranberries
- 1/4 cup raisins
- 3 1-inch pieces of cinnamon sticks
- 1/4 teaspoon ground nutmeg
- 1/8 teaspoon ground ginger
- 1/8 teaspoon ground cloves
- 4 cups water

Direction

- Add all ingredients to slow-cooker and mix to distribute spices. The oats tend to sink while the cranberries float, but that's ok.

- Cover and cook on low for 8-10 hours, depending on how thick you like your oatmeal. I usually do closer to the 10 hours.
- Refrigerate leftovers to enjoy later. Since I'm cooking for one, these can last me a week. Oatmeal can gel a bit in the fridge so, when reheating, add a little warm water. This and some mixing should return your oatmeal to the proper consistency.

24. Back To School Raspberry Granola Bars From Karen DeMasco

Serving: Makes 16 bars | Prep: 0hours10mins | Cook: 0hours40mins | Ready in:

Ingredients

- 1 cup (115g) pecan halves, coarsely chopped
- 1 1/2 cups (190g) all-purpose flour
- 1 1/4 cups (115g) old-fashioned rolled oats
- 1/3 cup (65g) sugar
- 1/3 cup (75g) packed dark brown sugar
- 1 teaspoon kosher salt
- 1/2 teaspoon baking soda
- 3/4 cup (170g) unsalted butter, melted
- 1 cup (320g) raspberry jam

Direction

- Heat the oven to 350°F (175°C), with a rack in the center. Butter an 8-inch (20cm) square baking pan. Line the bottom and sides with parchment paper, leaving a 1-inch (2.5cm) overhang on two opposite sides for easier lifting when the bars are done. Butter the parchment. Spread the pecans in a pie plate or on a rimmed baking sheet and toast in the oven until lightly browned and fragrant, about 5 minutes. Let cool.
- Whisk together the flour, oats, sugars, salt, baking soda, and cooled pecans in large bowl. Pour in the melted butter, and using a wooden spoon or rubber spatula, stir until well combined.
- Press two-thirds of the oat mixture (about 3 cups/470g) into an even, firmly packed layer on the bottom of the baking pan. Using an offset or rubber spatula, spread the raspberry jam evenly across the surface of the dough, leaving a 1/4-inch (6mm) border uncovered at the edges (the jam will melt and spread closer to the edges). Evenly sprinkle the remaining oat mixture over the jam.
- Bake until the top is golden brown, about 40 minutes, rotating the pan halfway through baking. Let the granola bars cool completely in the pan on a rack, about 3 hours. (Or go ahead and sneak one while they're still warm—they'll be a little crumbly but so good.) Lift up the overhanging ends of the parchment paper and transfer the granola almost-bars to a cutting board. Cut into 2-inch (5cm) squares. Store in an airtight container at room temperature.

25. Baked Apples Stuffed With Cinnamon Oat Crumble

Serving: Serves 5-6 | Prep: | Cook: | Ready in:

Ingredients

- 5-6 medium sized apples (I use a mix of mackintosh and cortland). Make sure the apples will fit tightly into your baking dish, I use a 9" square which fits 5-6 depending on their size
- 1/2 cup vegan butter or unrefined coconut oil
- 1/2 cup unrefined sugar
- 1/4 cup brown sugar
- 1/4 cup whole wheat pastry flour
- 3/4 cup rolled oats
- 2 teaspoons ground cinnamon
- 1/2 teaspoon ground sea salt
- 1 teaspoon vanilla bean paste (extract will work, too)

- 1 tablespoon freshly squeezed lemon juice
- 1/4 cup fresh cranberries, halved (optional)

Direction

- Preheat oven to 350 degrees.
- In the bowl of a food processor, combine butter, sugars, cinnamon, salt and vanilla. Pulse until coarse crumbs form. Add flour and rolled oats and process for 30 seconds more. You want some whole oat kernels remaining. Turn mixture out into a large mixing bowl and set aside.
- Core apples all the way through, slicing off about 1/4" of the tops. Scoop out flesh with a large spoon. Leave about 1/4" of flesh on the sides and bottom of apples. Set aside.
- If you do not have an apple corer, simply slice off apple tops as instructed above, scoop out flesh, remove and discard seeds.
- Take the flesh that has been scooped out of apples (plus apple tops) and coarsely chop into 1/4" - 1/2" pieces. Toss with 1tsp fresh lemon juice.
- Place apples, cut side up, into a glass or ceramic baking dish. They should be tightly packed and standing up straight.
- Add chopped apple pieces (and cranberries, if using) to the cinnamon-oat mix. Stir to combine. Spoon mixture into hollowed apples, pressing down to pack tightly. Take any remaining filling and sprinkle around apples.
- Bake at 350 degrees for 30-35 minutes or until apples have softened, flesh is wrinkled and topping is lightly browned. Some of the apples may have begun to split apart as well, this is a good thing! You can test for doneness by inserting a sharp knife into one of their sides. If it goes in like butter, you're golden.
- Cool for 20-30 minutes before serving.

26. Baked Cinnamon Oatmeal Apple

Serving: Serves 6 | Prep: | Cook: | Ready in:

Ingredients

- 6 large apples
- 1 cup old-fashioned rolled oats
- 2 tablespoons brown sugar
- 1/2 cup walnuts
- 1/4 cup raisins
- 1 teaspoon baking powder
- 1 1/2 teaspoons cinnamon
- 1/4 teaspoon salt
- 1 eggs
- 1 1/3 cups milk
- 1/2 teaspoon vanilla extract
- 1 tablespoon unsalted butter, melted

Direction

- Preheat the oven to 325°F. Line a 9-by-13-inch baking dish with parchment paper
- Combine the oats, brown sugar, walnuts, raisins, cinnamon, baking powder, and salt in a medium bowl. Mix well.
- Combine the milk, vanilla, and egg in another bowl and blend well. Add the liquid mixture to the oat mixture, along with the melted butter. Mix well with a large spoon. The mixture will be very liquid.
- Using a paring knife, cut off the top part of the apple with the stem and reserve the tops. Push a paring knife through the apple and cut around the core leaving the bottom 1/2 inch of the apples intact. With a small spoon, dig out the remaining core. Make the holes about 1 inch wide.
- Place the apples on the prepared baking pan. Spoon the oatmeal mixture into the apple cavities, filling them to the top. If you have leftover oat mixture you can just bake it in a little dish.
- Bake until the tops of the apples are golden and the oats are set, about 40 minutes. Serve warm or at room temperature. Store leftover

apples covered in the refrigerator for up to three days.

27. Baked Pumpkin Oatmeal With Coconut Streusel Topping

Serving: Serves 4 | Prep: | Cook: | Ready in:

Ingredients

- 1 cup oats (not quick cooking)
- 1 tablespoon ground flaxseeds
- 2-3 tablespoons maple syrup
- 1/2 teaspoon cinnamon
- scant 1/2 teaspoons salt
- 3/4 cup pumpkin puree
- 3/4 cup milk (steep a chai spice teabag in the milk for 5 minutes)
- 1 scant tablespoons butter (melted)/coconut oil (melted)/almond oil
- 1/2 teaspoon vanilla
- 2 tablespoons unsweetened coconut
- 2 tablespoons chopped almonds/nut of your choice
- 2 teaspoons sugar
- 2 tablespoons cacao nibs (optional)
- 2 teaspoons melted butter/oil of your choice
- tiny pinches salt

Direction

- Preheat the oven to 375F and butter/oil four ramekins (I used my old French onion soup gratin bowls).
- Combine the oats, flaxseeds, maple syrup, cinnamon, and salt in a mixing bowl. TOPPING: In another larger bowl, stir pumpkin puree, milk, butter (or other oil/fat), and vanilla together until smooth. In another small bowl, combine coconut, nuts, sugar, cacao nibs, butter/oil, and salt together.
- Add the dry ingredients to the wet and stir until completely combined. Divide evenly between greased ramekins. Divide the topping evenly between the ramekins.
- Put ramekins on a baking sheet and bake for 15-17 minutes. Cool a bit before serving.

28. Banana Bread With Chocolate Swirl

Serving: Serves 11 | Prep: | Cook: | Ready in:

Ingredients

- 1 natural cooking spray or oil for greasing pan
- 3 medium overripe bananas, mashed
- 1/3 cup canola oil
- 1/2 cup coconut sugar
- 2 large eggs
- 2 tablespoons greek yogurt (plain yogurt works also)
- 2 teaspoons pure vanilla extract
- 1 1/4 cups rolled oats, ground (or just over 1 cup of oat flour)
- 3/4 cup brown rice flour
- 1 tablespoon ground psyllium husk
- 1 teaspoon ground cinnamon
- 1/2 teaspoon ground nutmeg
- 1/2 teaspoon salt
- 1/2 teaspoon baking soda
- 1/2 teaspoon baking powder
- 1/2 cup semi-sweet chocolate chips

Direction

- Preheat oven to 375° F (180° C). Either grease a loaf pan directly with cooking spray or oil, or line the pan with parchment paper and then spray the insides. Be sure to have at least half an inch of parchment paper above the loaf pan.
- In a large bowl, mix the mashed bananas, oil, coconut sugar, eggs, yogurt, and vanilla together.
- In another bowl, mix together the ground rolled oats (or oat flour), brown rice flour, psyllium husk, cinnamon, nutmeg, salt, baking soda, and baking powder.

- Mix the dry ingredients with the wet ingredients. I like to add the flour mixture in three batches.
- In a microwave-safe bowl, melt the chocolate chips. Set the microwave for about a minute and then check the chocolate. Be careful with hot bowls! If the chocolate has barely melted, continue microwaving at 15-second increments until the chips are partially melted and very soft. The chocolate doesn't need to be saucy--just melted enough so that you can stir the chips together into a creamy consistency.
- Pour the banana batter into the loaf pan. Add dollops of the chocolate sauce on top of the batter.
- Using a butter knife, swirl the chocolate around so that you create a nice psychedelic swirl pattern.
- Bake the bread for about 50-55 minutes, or until a toothpick comes out clean when you pierce through the banana bread portions. Try not to test the bread by sticking the toothpick in the chocolate portions, as the toothpick will always come out with gooey melted chocolate.
- Let the bread cool for at least 45 to 50 minutes before taking it out of the pan for slicing.
- Store any leftovers in sealable container. Refrigerate any bread that you haven't finished in several days.

29. Banana Cake The Fit Version

Serving: Serves 8 | Prep: | Cook: | Ready in:

Ingredients

- 1 cup Whole Wheat Flour
- 1/4 cup Plain Oats
- 1/2 cup Vegetable Oil
- 2 Eggs
- 3 Ripe Bananas
- 1/4 cup Milk
- 1 teaspoon Baking Powder
- 1 teaspoon Baking Soda
- 1 teaspoon Vanilla Essence
- 1/2 cup Honey (Optional)
- 3 tablespoons Chocolate Chips
- 3 tablespoons Walnuts Chopped

Direction

- For the wet mixture, whisk in the eggs, oil, mashed bananas & vanilla essence together preferably with an electric beater.
- Sieve together wheat flour, baking powder, baking soda and fold this dry mixture into the wet mixture one spoon at a time.
- Add oats & milk to the mixture as you fold in. Mix well. Check for pouring consistency and if necessary add more milk. You can also add honey if you think the bananas weren't as ripe to produce the necessary sweetness.
- Grease the microwave bowl/cake tin with oil. Pour in a layer of half of the mixture in the tin.
- Add half of the chocolate chips and pour in the rest of the cake mixture. Garnish with oats, chocolate chips & chopped walnuts all over the top. More the garnish, the merrier and rich the cake.
- Microwave for 4-6 mins. Post 4 mins keep checking for a good bake of the cake by inserting a pointed toothpick/knife. If you wish to use an oven, then preheat the oven to 325º F/ 160º C beforehand and bake for 30 mins.
- Let the cake cool down to room temperature before you go for diving in ▢. PS: It tastes excellent when served warm for breakfast or as an evening snack with tea.

30. Banana Oat Blender Pancakes

Serving: Serves 2 | Prep: 0hours5mins | Cook: 0hours20mins | Ready in:

Ingredients

- 1 cup non-dairy milk
- 2 cups rolled oats

- 1 medium ripe banana
- 2 teaspoons baking powder
- 1/2 teaspoon baking soda
- 1/2 teaspoon cinnamon
- 1 pinch salt
- Optional: Favorite topping like fresh fruit, jam, chocolate chips, etc

Direction

- Add the rolled oats to your blender and blend until you have a fine flour (1-2 mins)
- Toss in all other ingredients and blend until smooth.
- Heat a pan or skillet.* Pour or scoop out approximately ¼ cup of batter. When the edges start to become solid and bubbles form, flip! Repeat for the remaining batter. Plate and tops with more banana, syrup or your favorite toppings!

31. Banana, Blueberry, And Pecan Pancakes

Serving: Makes 8 little pancakes | Prep: | Cook: | Ready in:

Ingredients

- For the batter:
- 100 grams oats
- A good handful of pecan nuts (about 50g), roughly chopped
- 1 teaspoon baking powder
- A pinch of sea salt
- 1 ripe banana, peeled and mashed
- 150 milliliters coconut milk or almond milk
- A punnet of blueberries (about 200g, or use frozen)
- To serve:
- 2 bananas, peeled and cut into thin slices
- A little coconut oil or butter, a few crumbled pecan nuts, lime wedges, and honey or agave syrup

Direction

- First turn the oven to 120°C/fan 100°C/gas 1/2 to keep everything warm.
- Blitz the oats until you have a scruffy oat flour. Add to a bowl with the pecans and throw in the baking powder and salt.
- Mix the mashed banana with the milk (you can do this by blitzing them together in the food processor, if you like). Beat the banana mixture into the flour and leave the batter to sit for a few minutes.
- Heat a non-stick pan on a medium heat, then add the banana slices and fry on both sides in the dry pan until brown and caramelized. Keep warm in the oven.
- Put the pan back on a medium heat and add a little coconut oil or butter. Drop in a healthy tablespoonful of batter for each pancake. Once the sides are cooked and bubbles have risen to the top, scatter over a handful of blueberries and flip the pancake over. Cook for another couple of minutes on the other side. The pancakes will stay a little moist in the middle because of the banana, so don't worry. Keep them warm in the oven while you cook the rest.
- Serve the pancakes piled with the banana slices. Add some crumbled pecans and a squeeze of lime, and, if you like, a little touch of honey, agave or maple syrup.

32. Banana, Date + Walnut Loaf

Serving: Makes 1 loaf | Prep: | Cook: | Ready in:

Ingredients

- 1/2 cup walnuts, roughly chopped
- 1/2 cup gluten-free oats
- Olive oil
- Maple syrup
- Salt
- 3 overripe bananas
- 2 teaspoons real vanilla extract

- 1/2 cup almond milk
- 6 Medjool dates
- 1 1/2 cups all-purpose, gluten-free flour
- 1/2 cup white rice flour
- 2 teaspoons baking soda
- 2 teaspoons baking powder
- 1 teaspoon xanthan gum

Direction

- Preheat your oven to 425°F and line a baking sheet with parchment paper.
- In a mixing bowl, stir together the walnuts and oats with a tablespoon of olive oil, a tablespoon of maple syrup and a pinch of salt. Place half the mixture onto the prepared sheet pan and reserve the other half. Place the sheet pan in the oven and roast the nut mixture until browned and crunchy, about 10 minutes. Set the roasted mixture aside and turn the oven down to 350°F.
- Combine the bananas, vanilla, almond milk and dates together in a blender along with 1/4 cup maple syrup and 1/4 cup plus 2 tablespoons of olive oil. Blend until completely smooth.
- Meanwhile, whisk together the flours, the baking soda and powder and the xanthan gum together in a large mixing bowl with a healthy pinch of salt. Stir in the banana mixture from the blender. Fold in the reserved toasted walnut mixture and transfer the batter to a nonstick loaf pan or a greased loaf pan. Scatter the reserved untoasted walnut mixture on top of the loaf.
- Bake the banana bread until a wooden skewer tests clean and it's just firm to the touch, 50 minutes. Remove the loaf from the oven and let it cool completely before eating. If you're a flexible vegan, a swipe of cream cheese is really welcome on each bite.

33. Beach Vacation Overnight Oats

Serving: Serves 1 | Prep: 0hours0mins | Cook: 0hours0mins | Ready in:

Ingredients

- 1/2 cup rolled oats
- 1/2 cup orange juice
- 1/2 cup plain yogurt (vanilla is great, too, but a bit too sweet for me)
- 1 tablespoon chia seeds
- 1/3 cup mango chunks, fresh or frozen
- 2 tablespoons almonds or macadamia nuts, chopped

Direction

- The night before, mix together the rolled oats, orange juice, yogurt, and chia seeds (preferably in the container out of which you'll eat it!).
- If your mango is frozen, add it to the top of the oat mixture. If your mango is fresh (lucky you!), hold off and add it in the morning.
- Put the container in the fridge overnight (or for a few hours at a minimum). The oats will soften up and the mixture will thicken.
- In the morning, check the consistency (if it's too thick, add a bit more juice or yogurt), then give it a stir and top with almonds or macadamia nuts.
- Dream of digging your toes into the sand.

34. Beet Chocolate Cake

Serving: Serves 10 | Prep: | Cook: | Ready in:

Ingredients

- 1 tablespoon chia seeds
- 1 + 1/2 cups oat flakes
- 1/4 cup cacao powder
- 1 tablespoon baking powder
- a pinches salt

- 2 raw peeled beets
- 50 grams dark chocolate
- 1/3 cup extra virgin olive oil
- 1/3 cup coconut flower nectar (or other liquid sweetener)
- 100 grams apple sauce (about 1/4 cup + 1 tbsp)

Direction

- Preheat oven at 350° F / 175° C. Mix chia seeds with water and set aside.
- In a high-speed blender or a mill reduce oats into a flour. Add it into a bowl along with cacao, baking powder and salt.
- Grate beets and add them to the bowl and stir.
- In a saucepan melt chocolate with oil, add coconut flower syrup, applesauce, soaked chia seeds and stir until smooth. Add this liquid to the bowl and stir well.
- Pour the batter into the greased cake pan - a 7 inch / 18 cm round cake pan - and bake for about 30 minutes.

35. Berry Breakfast Muslii

Serving: Makes 1 | Prep: | Cook: |Ready in:

Ingredients

- 1/3 cup rolled oats
- 1 cup sweetened almond milk or 2%milk
- 4 almonds
- 1 oz. cranberries
- 1 teaspoon agave nectar or honey
- 1 tablespoon chia seeds
- 1/2 cup fresh mixed berries or any fruit you like!

Direction

- Place the oats into a food safe container with a sealable lid. Pour the milk over the oats. Add the nuts and cranberries. Stir, seal and refrigerate overnight.
- When ready to eat add the remaining ingredients and enjoy!

36. Berry Oatmeal Pie

Serving: Serves 8 | Prep: | Cook: |Ready in:

Ingredients

- Vanilla Walnut Oatmeal
- 1 cup Quick oats
- 1/2 cup Walnuts
- 2 cups Whole Milk
- 1 teaspoon Real Vanilla Extract
- 1 tablespoon Brown Sugar
- 1 9 inch shortbread pie crust
- Berry Glaze
- 2 cups Fresh blueberries, rinsed
- 2 cups Fresh raspberries, rinsed
- 1 cup Sugar
- 2 teaspoons Lemon juice
- 4 tablespoons Corn starch

Direction

- Preheat oven to 350f.
- Raspberries: Add 1/2 cup sugar to a medium fry pan, cook over medium heat for 1 min & stir with spatula, add rinsed raspberries & stir as they cook down. Once a syrup begins to form, add 2 tbsp. cornstarch, 1 tsp lemon juice & stir well. Once thickened, add to bottom of pie crust, evenly spreading over entire crust.
- Oatmeal: In a medium saucepan, combine all ingredients & cook over low heat, occasionally stirring. When oats begin to stick to your spoon, remove from heat & let sit. Once cooled, stir egg in & add to pie, on top of raspberries.
- Blueberries: Add 1/2 cup sugar to a medium fry pan, cook over medium heat for 1 min & stir with spatula, add rinsed blueberries & stir as they cook down. Once a syrup begins to form, add 2 tbsp. cornstarch, 1 tsp lemon juice

& stir well. Once thickened, add top of oatmeal, spreading evenly over entire pie.
- Bake at 350F for 30 minutes. Let cool for 15 minutes, cook, serve & enjoy.

37. Best For Breakfast Apple Chocolate Granola

Serving: Makes 4,5 cups | Prep: | Cook: | Ready in:

Ingredients

- 2 cups oats
- 1/3 cup roughly chopped almonds
- 1/3 cup roughly chopped dates
- 1/2 cup dried cranberries
- 1 tablespoon chia seeds
- 1 tablespoon flax seeds
- 1 1/2 tablespoons sesame seeds
- 2 big apples cut in halves
- 1 tablespoon honey
- 3 tablespoons olive oil, plus a little more
- 1 teaspoon cinnamon
- 1/2 teaspoon ground ginger
- 1/2 teaspoon ground cloves
- 2 tablespoons cacao powder
- 1 teaspoon sea salt

Direction

- Preheat the oven to 180 C. Roast your apples for 40-45 minutes until they soften.
- Oil a baking tray lined with parchment paper. Toss your oats, almonds, chia seeds, flax seeds and sesame seeds in a bowl and transfer them to the baking tray. Toast them for 10 minutes until they get a nutty flavor. Turn the heat down to 150 C.
- In a food processor puree your roasted apples, then add honey, spices, cacao and salt. Pour the mixture over the oats and mix evenly, then add dried fruit.
- Bake for ~1 hour until the granola gets golden color stirring every 10-12 minutes to make sure all sides of granola get toasted.

- Store your granola in airtight containers.
- The beauty of home-made granola is that you totally adjust it to your taste picking the ingredients you love. You can make it with apples, or pumpkin, or maple syrup, add any nuts you love, pick any dried fruit, add your favorite spices and certainly omit excess sugars and fat. It's all about your fantasy: if you love the ingredients you picked then you'll love your granola! Bon Appétit!

38. Bhutanese Red Rice, Millet, And Oat Breakfast Pudding

Serving: Serves 6-8 as a sweet part of a festive breakfast | Prep: | Cook: | Ready in:

Ingredients

- Make red rice and millet the night before:
- 2/3 cup Bhutanese red rice
- 1/3 cup millet
- 2 1/2 cups water
- 1 cinnamon stick, broken in half
- 1 black cardamom pod (or 2-3 green cardamom pods)
- 2 bay leaves
- In the morning:
- 1 1/2 tablespoons unsalted butter
- 2/3 cup unsalted roasted cashews, broken in half with fingers
- 2 teaspoons turbinado sugar
- 1/2 cup Bob's Red mill Gluten free old-fashioned rolled oats (or regular old-fashioned rolled oats if you do not have any GF guests)
- 1/2 cup dried currants
- 2 ripe bananas, mashed (for about 1 cup)
- 2 cups of half-and-half
- 2 large eggs
- 3 tablespoons brown sugar
- Pinch ground ginger
- Pinch ground cloves
- 3/4 teaspoon salt
- 1/2 teaspoon vanilla

Direction

- Make red rice and millet the night before:
- In a small saucepan (or electric rice cooker, as I did) combine Bhutanese red rice, millet, water, cinnamon stick, cardamom and bay leaves; allow grains/spices to soak for at least 20 minutes before cooking. Cover and bring to a boil. Reduce to a simmer, being careful mixture does not boil over. Cook until grains are tender, about 25 minutes. Pick out whole spices and discard. Cool and transfer cooked grains to an airtight container and refrigerate overnight.
- In the morning:
- Preheat the oven to 350 degrees. Spray or butter a 2 quart round ceramic baking dish. Set aside.
- Make cashews: In a small pan, melt butter over medium heat until beginning to brown. Add cashews, shaking pan or stirring occasionally, being careful not to burn them as they cook quickly. You want most of the pieces golden brown on both sides. Remove pan from heat and add turbinado sugar, tossing to combine. Set aside.
- In a large bowl, gently break up the cooked grains with a spoon. Fold in the oats, and currants (breaking up any clusters, with your fingers), to evenly incorporate.
- In a separate bowl (I used my quart Pyrex), using a fork or whisk, combine mashed bananas, half-and-half, eggs, brown sugar, spices, salt and vanilla.
- Pour liquid mixture into grain/currant mixture and stir. Transfer to prepared baking dish. Top with toasted brown butter cashews. Bake for 40-45 minutes until top is golden and puffed up. Serve immediately, with a dollop of crème fraiche or yogurt, if desired. Enjoy and then eat something savory!

39. Black Bean And Corn Burgers

Serving: Serves 4 to 6 | Prep: 0hours20mins | Cook: 0hours50mins | Ready in:

Ingredients

- 1 small yellow onion, chopped
- 1 clove garlic, minced
- 1 tablespoon olive oil
- 3 cups (or 2 cans) cooked black beans, divided
- 1 1/2 teaspoons cumin powder
- 1/2 teaspoon smoked paprika
- 1 teaspoon chili powder
- 1 teaspoon sea salt
- 1 pinch black pepper or red pepper flakes, to taste
- 2/3 cup quick oats or bread crumbs, plus extra as needed
- 3/4 cup fresh (or frozen and thawed) corn

Direction

- Sauté onion and garlic in the olive oil for eight to ten minutes, or until golden, soft, and fragrant.
- Add 2 cups of the beans, the cumin, the paprika, the chili powder, the sea salt, and pepper to taste. Stir in the sauté pan till all is warm.
- Preheat your oven to 350° F.
- Add the oats to the bowl of a food processor and pulse them a few times. Add the onion, garlic, and bean mixture. Process everything together, until it's well combined but still has texture.
- Transfer mixture to a mixing bowl. Add the last cup of black beans and the corn and mix well with your hands. Check for seasoning and season to taste. If the mixture is too mushy to form into patties, add a little more oats or bread crumbs.
- Shape mixture into four large or six smaller patties. Transfer burgers to a baking sheet and bake for 30 to 35 minutes (or until golden), flipping once through. Alternately, you can chill them for twenty minutes before transferring them to a grill and cooking

through. You can also pan fry them in olive oil until golden on each side.

40. Black Bean And Quinoa Veggie Burgers

Serving: Makes 6-8 burgers | Prep: 12hours15mins | Cook: 0hours50mins | Ready in:

Ingredients

- Patties
- 1/2 cup quinoa
- 1 teaspoon olive oil
- 1 small red onion, chopped
- 3 cloves garlic, minced
- 1 pinch Kosher salt
- 2 cans (15.5 ounces each) black beans, rinsed and drained
- 2 tablespoons tomato paste
- 1 large egg
- 2/3 cup cooked corn (fresh or canned)
- 1/4 cup chopped cilantro
- 1 tablespoon minced chipotles in adobo
- 1 1/2 teaspoons ground cumin
- 1 cup rolled oats, ground into crumbs
- Yogurt Sauce
- 1/2 cup fat-free Greek yogurt
- 1 teaspoon minced chipotles in adobo
- 1/2 teaspoon adobo sauce
- 1 teaspoon honey
- 1/2 teaspoon dijon mustard
- 6 multigrain hamburger rolls
- 1 handful Lettuce, avocado slices, and tomatoes, for topping (optional)

Direction

- Place the quinoa in a small saucepan along with 1 cup of water. Bring the water to a boil then reduce heat to medium low and cover the pan. Cook 10 to 15 minutes until the water is absorbed and quinoa is cooked. Remove from heat.
- Heat the oil in a small sauté pan over medium heat and add the onion and garlic. Season them with a pinch of salt and sauté until onions are softened, 5 to 6 minutes. Place the mixture into a large bowl. Add approximately 1 1/2 cans of black beans to the bowl and, using a potato masher or fork, mash all of the ingredients together until a pasty mixture forms. Stir in the remaining beans along with the tomato paste, egg, corn, cilantro, chipotles, cumin, and 1/2 teaspoon salt. Stir in the cooked quinoa and ground oats until evenly distributed.
- Form the mixture into 6 equal patties, compacting them well with your hands as you form them. Place the patties on a baking sheet, cover them with plastic wrap, and refrigerate for at least a few hours or overnight.
- To make the yogurt sauce, stir the yogurt, chipotles, adobo sauce, honey, and mustard together in a small bowl.
- When ready to eat, preheat the oven to 400° F. Spray a baking sheet with nonstick cooking spray and place the patties on the sheet. Cook 10 to 12 minutes, until the patties are golden brown and crispy, then carefully flip them over and cook another 10 minutes. You can also fry the patties in a pan with a small amount of oil. Serve patties on the buns with the yogurt sauce and toppings of your choice.

41. Black Pepper Pear Crisp With Salted Oat Streusel

Serving: Serves 6 to 8 | Prep: 0hours0mins | Cook: 0hours0mins | Ready in:

Ingredients

- Crisp
- Unsalted butter, for greasing
- 4 firm d'anjou pears (about 2 1/2 pounds), chopped into 1" chunks (about 5 1/2 cups)
- 1/2 cup sugar
- 2 1/2 tablespoons cornstarch

- 1 tablespoon apple cider vinegar (or lemon juice)
- 1 teaspoon freshly ground black pepper
- 1/4 teaspoon kosher salt
- Heavy cream, for serving
- Streusel
- 1 1/2 cups rolled oats, divided
- 1/2 cup whole-wheat flour
- 1/2 cup brown sugar
- 1 1/2 teaspoons kosher salt
- 6 ounces (1 1/2 sticks) unsalted butter, very cold, cubed

Direction

- Crisp
- Preheat the oven to 375° F. Grease a 9" cake pan with unsalted butter. Set it on a lined sheet tray.
- Make the fruit filling. Combine the pears, sugar, cornstarch, vinegar, black pepper, and salt in a bowl. Gingerly toss with a spoon (or your hands!) until combined. Pour into the prepared cake pan.
- Streusel
- Add 1 cup oats, plus the flour, sugar, and salt to a food processor. Pulse a couple times just to combine. Sprinkle the butter evenly over the dry ingredients. Continue to pulse until a dough just begins to form—sort of like a shaggy cookie dough. Transfer to a bowl and stir in the remaining 1/2 cup oats by hand.
- Evenly distribute the streusel on top of the fruit. Don't worry if its texture is uneven—big clumps here, little crumbs there—that's just what we want.
- Bake for about 50 minutes until the streusel is deeply browned and the fruit juice is bubbly and slightly thick. Wait at least 20 minutes to serve warm. Or, let sit out for hours and serve at room temperature. Or, if any leftovers last until tomorrow morning, meet your new favorite breakfast. In any case: serve with lots of cream.

42. Blackberry Peach Quinoa Burgers On Sweet Potato Buns

Serving: Serves 4 | Prep: | Cook: | Ready in:

Ingredients

- For the burgers:
- 1 ripe peach
- 1 cup blackberries
- 1/2 cup quinoa
- 1/2 cup buckwheat flour
- 1 tablespoon tamari
- 1 tablespoon tahini
- 1 tablespoon apple cider vinegar
- 1 pinch salt & pepper (to taste)
- For the buns:
- 1 1/2 cups gluten-free oat flour
- 1/2 cup sweet potato puree
- 1 tablespoon coconut oil
- 1/4 teaspoon nutmeg
- 1/2 teaspoon sea salt

Direction

- For the burgers:
- Cook your quinoa in 1 cup water on the stovetop until the water is all absorbed, about 10-15 minutes.
- While that cooks, add your blackberries to a large mixing bowl and mash them pretty well with the back of a fork.
- Then add the rest of your ingredients, along with the quinoa once it's cooked.
- Scoop up about 1/4 of the mix with your hands and form a patty. Repeat with the other 3 burger patties.
- Give the burgers a good sear in a lightly oiled skillet over medium-high heat until each side is nice & dark & crispy-like.
- Then put them on a greased cookie sheet in the 350 oven from whence the buns came, and cook for another 15 minutes.
- For the buns:
- Preheat your oven to 350 F and grease a baking sheet.

- Mix your ingredients in a large bowl until combined. You should end up with a big ball of dough that you can roll out and cut. If it's too sticky, add a little more flour a bit at a time.
- Sprinkle some oat flour on the paper or counter and on a rolling pin. Then roll your dough out to about 1/2 inch of thickness.
- Once you have a nice flat sheet of dough, use a round cookie cutter – or rim of a drinking glass as an impromptu one – to cut nice even round shapes out of the dough. Place these on your greased baking pan.
- Once you've cut out all the biscuits you can, smoosh the dough back together and roll it out again and repeat. When you can't possibly roll out another bun, you'll be good to bake!
- Place your cookie sheet of buns in the oven for 15 minutes or until golden and firm. Remove from the oven and let cool.
- Put one bun on a plate, then your burger, then top with whatever you like. Repeat with the other guys and you'll be ready for this veggie burger feast!

43. Blackberry Peach Crumble

Serving: Serves 4 | Prep: | Cook: | Ready in:

Ingredients

- Fruit Filling
- 4 medium to large ripe peaches, sliced into wedges
- 7 ounces blackberries
- 1 tablespoon lemon juice
- 1 vanilla bean, beans scraped out OR 1 tspn vanilla bean paste
- 4 tablespoons raw sugar (or vegan sub)
- 2.5 tablespoons cornflour
- Crumble
- 3/4 cup natural oats
- 2.5 tablespoons whole wheat flour
- 2.5 tablespoons dried coconut flakes
- 2 tablespoons brown sugar (or vegan sub)
- 1/4 cup (scant) macadamia nuts, coarsely chopped
- 1/2 teaspoon mixed spice
- 2 tablespoons pure maple syrup
- 2 teaspoons vanilla extract
- 4 tablespoons coconut oil, at liquid temperature
- Fresh fruit, to decorate
- Cream, ice cream or custard, to serve

Direction

- Preheat oven to 180C. Grease a 20cm baking dish (I used an enamel pie tin). Place onto a large, flat baking pan.
- Place fruit into a large bowl; add lemon juice and vanilla bean paste and toss gently to combine; add the remainder of the ingredients then fold through until combined. Spoon into prepared baking dish and spread out evenly.
- Add the first 6 crumble ingredients to another large bowl and stir until combined. Whisk maple syrup, vanilla and coconut oil until combined then add to oat mixture and stir through until everything is coated well. Scatter topping evenly over the fruit.
- Bake for 35-40 minutes, or until the crumble is golden brown and the filling is bubbling hot.
- Sit for 10 minutes then serve with ice cream, cream or custard.

44. Blood Orange Overnight Oats

Serving: Serves 1 | Prep: | Cook: | Ready in:

Ingredients

- 4-5 tablespoons rolled oats
- 200 milliliters coconut rice milk or other milk alternative
- 1 blood orange
- 1 handful strawberries, fresh or frozen
- a couple frozen raspberries
- 1 teaspoon strawberry jam

Direction

- Place rolled oats into a jar, add rice milk or other drink alternative, close the jar and shake well to combine. Place in refrigerator overnight.
- In the morning, take oats out of the fridge and place them into a bowl. You can warm up the oats on the stove beforehand, if you like your breakfast warm.
- Peel and thinly slice 1 blood orange and add a few slices to the bowl. Add some berries (fresh or frozen) and top with 1 teaspoon of strawberry jam for sweetness. Serve.

45. Blood Orange, Cardamom, And Fig Jammy Oat Bars

Serving: Makes 24 bars | Prep: | Cook: |Ready in:

Ingredients

- 1 cup AP Flour
- 3/4 cup whole wheat pastry flour
- 1 cup light brown sugar, firmly packed
- 1/4 teaspoon salt
- 1/2 teaspoon baking soda
- 1 1/2 cups whole, rolled, oats
- 1 tablespoon blood orange zest, piled high
- 3/4 cup butter, melted and slightly cooled
- 1-1 1/2 cups fig jam

Direction

- Preheat the oven to 350° F. Line a 9x13 inch half pan with foil or parchment paper being sure to leave a 3 inch overhang on all sides. This will enable easy unfolding when the bars have cooled.
- Mix together the flours, brown sugar, salt, baking soda, oats and zest in a medium bowl. Add the melted butter and incorporate into dry ingredients, forming a wet-sand-like "dough" and eliminating any dry pockets.
- Press 2/3 of the dough firmly into the prepared pan. Starting with 1 c, spread jam evenly over the unbaked crust. Add up to 1/2 cup more of jam depending on how jammy you want your bars. Sprinkle remaining dough/crumble over the jam layer and gently press down.
- Bake until golden brown and jam is bubbly around edges, 20-25 minutes. Cool on completely on rack then cut into bars and enjoy!

46. Blueberry Muffins

Serving: Serves 6 | Prep: | Cook: |Ready in:

Ingredients

- 100 grams spelt flour
- 1 teaspoon baking powder
- 60 grams muscobado sugar
- 100 grams yogurt
- 20 milliliters soy milk
- 30 milliliters evo
- 1 egg
- 100 grams blueberries
- 40 grams oat flakes

Direction

- Mix flour, baking powder and sugar.
- Combine yogurt, soy milk, evo and 1 egg.
- Coat blueberries in flour before adding them to the muffin mix.
- Sprinkle oat flakes over muffins before baking.
- Preheat oven to 180C, bake for 25 minutes.

47. Blueberry Peach Crumble Ice Cream

Serving: Serves 8-10 | Prep: | Cook: |Ready in:

Ingredients

- For the Ice Cream Base & Maple Oat Crumble
- 2 cans of full fat coconut milk
- 1/2 cup pure maple syrup
- 1 pinch xanthan gum (optional)
- 1 vanilla bean (or 1 tbsp vanilla extract)
- 2/3 cup gluten free rolled oats
- 2 tablespoons quinoa flakes
- 2 tablespoons coconut oil
- 3-4 tablespoons pure maple syrup (depending on how sweet you want it)
- 1 pinch sea salt
- Blueberry Peach Swirl & Putting the Ice Cream Together
- 2 peaches, diced
- 1 cup blueberries
- 2-4 tablespoons coconut sugar or sucanat (depending on the sweetness of your fruit)
- 1/2 teaspoon cinnamon
- 2 teaspoons coconut oil
- 1 pinch xanthan gum (optional)

Direction

- For the Ice Cream Base & Maple Oat Crumble
- Make the vanilla bean ice cream base: Add the coconut milk, the 1/2 cup of maple syrup, and xanthan gum to a bowl. Scrape the seeds from the vanilla bean into the bowl, then whisk the mixture until smooth. The vanilla flecks should be evenly distributed. Add the leftover vanilla bean to the mixture, then cover it and chill it at least 4 hours in the fridge.
- Make the Maple Oat Crumble: While the ice cream base is chilling, heat a skillet or pan over medium heat. Add the oats and quinoa flakes to your dry skillet and toast them for a few minutes until light golden brown. Once they are toasted and fragrant, add the coconut oil, maple syrup, and sea salt and stir the mixture so that the maple syrup coats the oats and quinoa. Keep stirring until the mixture starts to stick together and turns a deeper golden brown. Remove the crumble from the heat and spread it onto a parchment lined sheet. Put the sheet in the fridge or freezer to set and cool. Once cooled, break the crumble up into small pieces and set it aside.
- Blueberry Peach Swirl & Putting the Ice Cream Together
- Make the blueberry peach swirl: In a skillet over medium heat, warm the coconut oil. Add the fruit, coconut sugar, and cinnamon and stir to coat. Stir the fruit regularly as it cooks so it doesn't stick to the bottom of the pan. As the fruit begins to soften, mash it to break down the large pieces. Continue to stir and mash the fruit as it cooks. Once the mixture has thickened a bit, stir in the xanthan gum. Remove from the heat and allow to cool completely before mixing into the ice cream base.
- Make the Ice Cream: Remove the chilled ice cream base from the fridge. Fish out the vanilla bean and discard it. (Or, you can save it for homemade vanilla extract or vanilla sugar! Just rinse it and then it's good to go.) The coconut cream will have settled at the top so whisk the mixture until it is smooth. Process the mixture in your ice cream maker according to the directions that came with it. During the last few minutes of churning, sprinkle in about 2/3 of the crumble. When the ice cream is ready (it will be very soft like soft serve), get out the container you will keep it in. I tend to use my smaller ovenex loaf pan as it's easy to scoop from, but any relatively flat vessel will work. Working quickly, spread roughly 1/3 of the ice cream mixture on the bottom of your container, then dollop a few spoonfuls of the fruit swirl on it and drag your spoon around so that the fruit swirls into the ice cream. Continue this process with the rest of the ice cream. When finished, sprinkle the remaining crumble on top. Cover and freeze at least 4 hours to allow it to firm up. At this point you can enjoy it anytime! I find it's easiest to let it soften 10-15 minutes at room temperature before scooping. Makes roughly 1 quart of ice cream with a bit of leftover fruit swirl.

48. Blueberry Pecan Baked Oatmeal

Serving: Serves 6-8 | Prep: | Cook: | Ready in:

Ingredients

- 2 1/2 cups Rolled Old-Fashioned Oats
- 2/3 cup Chopped Pecans
- 1/2 cup Dried Blueberries
- 1 teaspoon Baking Powder
- 1 teaspoon Ground Cinnamon
- 1/4 teaspoon Salt
- 1 2/3 cups Almond Milk
- 1/4 cup Honey
- 2 Large Eggs
- 1 teaspoon Vanilla Extract
- 3 tablespoons Coconut Oil, Melted

Direction

- Preheat oven to 350 degrees. Spray an 8x8-inch baking dish with non-stick cooking spray, set aside.
- In a medium mixing bowl whisk together oats, pecans, dried blueberries, baking powder, cinnamon and salt. In a separate mixing bowl stir together mashed bananas with almond milk, maple syrup, eggs, and vanilla extract and whisk until very well blended. Stir in coconut oil. Pour milk mixture into oat mixture and stir to combine. Pour mixture into prepared baking dish. Bake in preheated oven until set, about 30 minutes. Serve warm.

49. Blueberry, Nectarine & Bourbon Crisp

Serving: Serves about 8-10 servings (depending on size per serving) | Prep: | Cook: | Ready in:

Ingredients

- 1 pint fresh blueberries
- 2-3 ripe, large nectarines (or other stone fruit) sliced into wedges
- 1/4 cup good bourbon
- 1/4 cup brown sugar
- 1 cup cold butter, cut into small cubes
- 1 cup flour
- 1 cup sugar
- 1 cup old-fashioned oats
- 1/2 teaspoon cinnamon

Direction

- Preheat oven to 400 degrees. In a medium-sized bowl, mix the fruit, the bourbon and the brown sugar until the fruit is well-coated. Set aside and allow to macerate for at least ten minutes.
- In another medium-sized bowl, add the butter, flour, sugar, oats and cinnamon. Squeeze all ingredients through your palms until the mixture is well-incorporated and breaks apart into large pieces (see details in the above post).
- Add the fruit and any liquid to the bottom of a cake pan. Add the crumble mixture to the top of the fruit. Do not press the crumble down; instead, generously pile it on top of the fruit until all the fruit is totally covered. Bake for 40 minutes or until the crumble mixture is a nice, golden brown. Carefully remove from the oven and allow to cool slightly before serving.

50. Bowl A Granola

Serving: Serves 6 | Prep: | Cook: | Ready in:

Ingredients

- 4 cups Thick Rolled Oats
- 4 cups Barley Flakes
- 1 cup Chopped Crystallized Ginger
- 1 cup Dried, Unsulphured Apricots
- 1 cup Dried Apple
- 1 cup Chopped Almonds
- 1 cup Walnuts
- 1 cup Dried Bananas

- 1 dash Cinnamon
- 1 cup Pumpkin Seeds
- Brown Rice Syrup

Direction

- Preheat oven to 295 degrees.
- Combine oats and barley. Place on cookie sheet and heat in oven for 20 minutes.
- While oats and barley are lightly toasting, chop all nuts and fruit. Combine into one large mixture and add cinnamon.
- Remove oats and barley from oven after 20 minutes. Drizzle and dollop brown rice syrup on oats and barley. Stir oats and barley around on pan, replace in oven for 15 minutes.
- Repeat step 4 as many times as necessary to get the consistency of granola that you would like.
- Once the granola is chunky enough to your liking, remove from oven and add fruit and nut mixture. Drizzle combination with brown rice syrup one final time, mix, and place back in oven for 5-8 minutes.
- Turn oven off and leave granola in the oven over night. (This step can be reduced to a few hours, but fox maximum crunch I advise to leave overnight.)
- Enjoy!

51. Breakfast Cookies

Serving: Makes 13 large cookies | Prep: | Cook: | Ready in:

Ingredients

- 5 ounces unsalted butter, at room temperature
- 3/4 teaspoon kosher salt
- 5 ounces brown sugar
- 4 ounces raw cane sugar
- 1 large egg, at room temperature
- 1 teaspoon vanilla or almond extract
- 8 ounces organic sprouted wheat flour
- 1 teaspoon baking powder
- 1 teaspoon baking soda
- 2 ounces old-fashioned rolled oats
- 2 ounces walnuts, roughly chopped
- 2 tablespoons golden flax seeds
- 10 ounces dark chocolate, chopped

Direction

- In the bowl of a stand mixer fitted with a paddle attachment, cream together the butter, salt, and sugars until well-incorporated and airy.
- Add in egg and vanilla and beat until the mix resembles a smooth buttercream.
- Add the flour, baking soda, and baking powder and mix on a low speed until just combined.
- Using your hands, fold in oats, walnuts, flax seeds, and chocolate.
- Roll into 3-ounce balls, then chill dough for at least 30 minutes. The longer you chill it, the less it will spread during cooking. I chilled mine for about 8 hours.
- Preheat oven to 350° F. Bake for 15 to 16 minutes, then let them sit on the pan for 10 minutes before transferring to a cooling rack. They won't look done when you pull them out of the oven, but the residual heat from the pan will give them just the right amount of gooey-ness as they rest.

52. Breakfast Muesli

Serving: Serves 2 | Prep: | Cook: | Ready in:

Ingredients

- 1/2 cup old-fashioned rolled oats
- 3/4 cup plain Greek yogurt
- 1/2 cup orange juice
- 1 apple, diced (I like gala or Jonagold)
- 1/4 cup raisins
- 2 tablespoons honey
- generous sprinkling cinnamon & nutmeg
- 1/4 cup slivered almonds

Direction

- Prepare oats (soak in orange juice for 1 hour, or cook in microwave per instructions above).
- In a large bowl, combine diced apple, raisins, yogurt, honey, cinnamon, and nutmeg. Add oats. Mix thoroughly, and adjust ingredients per taste-test.
- Sprinkle mixture with almonds, and enjoy!

53. Breakfast Quinoa With Oats And Chia Seeds

Serving: Serves 1 | Prep: | Cook: | Ready in:

Ingredients

- 1/4 cup cooked quinoa
- 1/4 cup uncooked rolled oats
- 1/2 cup milk (I used 1%)
- 2/3 cup water
- 1 tablespoon chia seeds
- 1/4 teaspoon ground cinnamon
- 1 packet Truvia or 1 tablespoon brown sugar
- 1/4 teaspoon vanilla extrac
- 1 medium banana, sliced
- 1/4 cup chopped pecans

Direction

- In a small saucepan over medium heat, combine the cooked quinoa, rolled oats, milk, water and chia seeds. Cook for 5 to 6 minutes, until oats and chia seeds have absorbed most of the moisture and the mixture is thickened. Add in the cinnamon, Truvia or brown sugar and vanilla extract. Cook for 30 seconds more. Remove from heat and stir in the banana slices. Spoon into a bowl and top with the chopped pecans.

54. Breakfast Carrot Cake Muffins

Serving: Makes about 12 muffins | Prep: | Cook: | Ready in:

Ingredients

- 60 milliliters olive oil or butter
- 70 milliliters maple syrup
- 1 banana
- 150 grams plain yoghurt
- 1 egg
- 1 apple
- 2-3 carrots
- 1 teaspoon baking powder
- 1 teaspoon cinnamon
- 100 grams rolled oats
- 150 grams spelt flour
- 100 grams chopped almonds
- walnuts for topping

Direction

- Blend yoghurt, banana, maple syrup and oil or melted butter with a blender. Whisk in the egg. Also using a blender, blend the oats so you get oat flour. Mix oat flour with spelt flour, salt, cinnamon, baking powder and optionally cardamom and almond flour. Peel carrots and the apple and grate finely.
- Add the flour-mixture to the yoghurt-egg-mixture and fold in carefully. Add grated carrots and apple as well as the chopped almonds. Place the batter in 12 muffins tins. If you like you can add some chopped walnuts on top.
- Bake the muffins in the preheated oven at 175°C (347 °F) for about 20 minutes.

55. British Flapjacks

Serving: Makes 8 flapjacks | Prep: | Cook: | Ready in:

Ingredients

- 1/2 cup (1 stick) unsalted butter, cut into pieces
- 1/2 cup brown sugar
- 1/4 cup golden syrup
- 2 1/3 cups quick-cooking oats

Direction

- Preheat the oven to 350 degrees Fahrenheit. Line an 8x8 inch with parchment paper, or grease heavily with butter.
- In a large pot, heat the butter, brown sugar, and golden syrup over medium heat, stirring constantly, until the butter is melted and the sugar has dissolved.
- Remove from heat and stir in the oats until coated.
- Pour the mixture into the prepared pan and spread out evenly. Bake for 25 minutes, or until golden brown (the edges will be slightly darker). Remove from heat and slice into 8 triangles. Let cool completely before removing from pan.

56. Brown Butter Apple Pie Salad

Serving: Serves 4 | Prep: | Cook: | Ready in:

Ingredients

- 1/4 cup all purpose flour
- 1/4 cup raw pumpkin seeds
- 1/3 cup rolled oats
- 1 heaping tablespoon brown sugar
- 1/2 teaspoon kosher salt
- 3 tablespoons cold unsalted butter, diced
- 4 tablespoons unsalted butter
- 1 small shallot, minced
- juice of half a meyer lemon (about 2 tablespoons)
- few pinches finely chopped fresh marjoram (sub: fresh thyme)
- kosher salt and black pepper, to taste
- 1 head red leaf lettuce, washed and torn into bite sized pieces
- 1 honeycrisp (or other sweet-tart) apple, cored and sliced thin
- 2 ounces fresh chevre

Direction

- Make the Pumpkin Seed Streusel: Preheat oven to 350 degrees. Combine the flour, pumpkin seeds, oats, brown sugar, salt, and 3 tablespoons of butter in a small bowl. Use your fingers to blend the ingredients, until you're left with large streusel-y crumbles. Spread the streusel on a parchment paper-lined baking sheet and bake for 20-30 minutes, or until lightly browned and crisp. Cool slightly.
- Make the Brown Butter Vinaigrette: Melt the remaining 4 tablespoons of butter in a small pan over medium-low heat. Watch the butter carefully- when the foaming has subsided and the butter has started to brown, add the minced shallot and soften for one minute. Remove from heat, and transfer to a small bowl. Whisk in the juice of half a meyer lemon, a sprinkling of fresh marjoram, and season to taste with salt and pepper.
- Assemble the Salad: Toss the lettuce, sliced apple, and chevre with a few tablespoons of the brown butter vinaigrette. Add dressing as needed until leaves are nicely coated. Sprinkle liberally with the pumpkin seed streusel. Enjoy!

57. Brown Sugar Ice Cream With Oatmeal Raisin Cookie Dough

Serving: Makes about 1 1/2 quarts | Prep: | Cook: | Ready in:

Ingredients

- Oatmeal Raisin Cookie Dough
- 1/4 cup chopped walnuts
- 1/2 cup rolled oats or quick-cooking oats
- 5 tablespoons unsalted butter

- 1/2 cup flour
- 1/4 cup plus 2 tablespoons dark brown sugar
- 1/4 teaspoon salt
- 1/2 teaspoon plus 1/8 teaspoon ground cinnamon
- a few pinches grated fresh nutmeg
- 1/2 tablespoon malted milk powder (optional)
- 3 tablespoons skim milk
- 1/2 teaspoon plus 1/8 teaspoon vanilla extract
- 1/4 cup finely chopped raisins
- Brown Sugar Ice Cream
- 2 cups heavy whipping cream
- 1 cup skim milk plus 1 1/2 tablespoons skim milk, divided
- pinch salt
- 1/2 tablespoon cornstarch
- 3/4 cup dark brown sugar
- 1 1/2 tablespoons molasses
- 1 tablespoon light corn syrup (if unavailable, can substitute 2 teaspoons sugar)
- 6 large egg yolks
- 1 teaspoon vanilla extract

Direction

- In a large skillet over medium heat, add walnuts and oats. Toast for 4-5 minutes, stirring frequently. Transfer walnuts and oats to food processor; process until finely ground.
- Add butter to skillet over medium heat. Cook for 5 minutes until butter has turned light brown and has a "nutty smell."
- In a medium mixing bowl, combine walnut and oats mixture, flour, brown sugar, salt, cinnamon, nutmeg, and malted milk powder (optional); mix until well combined. Stir in browned butter, milk, and vanilla. Mix until well-combined. Stir in raisins. Cover, and transfer to refrigerator.
- Place Ice Cream Maker Freezer "Bowl" in freezer at least 8 hours before using.
- Combine heavy cream, 1 cup milk, and salt in a medium saucepan over medium heat. Bring to a simmer.
- In a small bowl, combine 1 1/2 tablespoons milk and cornstarch; stir thoroughly until there are no lumps. Add to the simmering cream mixture and cook for 5 minutes (at a simmer or light boil). (This whole step with the cornstarch is optional).
- Meanwhile, in a medium mixing bowl, beat the brown sugar, molasses, and corn syrup into the egg yolks.
- When the cream mixture is warm, slowly pour about 1/3 to 1/2 of the cream mixture into the sugar & egg yolk mixture, stirring frequently while you are pouring (stirring keeps the eggs from scrambling). Transfer all of the mixture from the bowl back into the medium saucepan. Turn heat to low. Stir frequently with a wooden spoon, for about 5 minutes, until custard thickens slightly (you do not want to the mixture to get too hot, or the eggs will scramble). Transfer the mixture to a medium mixing bowl. Stir in vanilla extract. Cover with plastic wrap. Transfer to refrigerator to cool for at least 4-5 hours (can accelerate process by placing in freezer for 1 hour and then transferring to refrigerator). Can leave in refrigerator 1-2 days, if necessary.
- Before you are ready to make the ice cream, transfer the mixing bowl with the ice cream mixture to the freezer for 30-40 minutes, stirring every 15-20 minutes in order to keep the edges from freezing (you don't actually want the mixture to freeze, just to get colder before putting it in the machine).
- Transfer the mixture to the Ice Cream Maker Freezer "Bowl." Place the bowl in the machine and churn the ice cream. It should take approximately 25 to 30 minutes. It will not necessarily get totally "hard."
- Transfer some of the ice cream to the container(s) you are going to store it in. Working as quickly as you can, add little chunks of the Oatmeal Raisin Cookie Dough into the ice cream, and use your spatula to make sure everything is well distributed. Add another layer of ice cream, another layer of cookie dough chunks, and distribute. Repeat until you have transferred all the ice cream

and used most of the cookie dough chunks. Smooth out the top. Sprinkle with remaining cookie dough chunks (you may have some leftover cookie dough). Place in the freezer (preferably, put the container directly in the ice bin, if you have one, nestled in the ice, so that it will cool as quickly as possible). Freeze for at least 5 hours.

- Before serving, let ice cream rest for 5 minutes at room temperature, where it should just being to start to melt (you don't want to eat ice cream straight from the freezer—it is too hard and to cold—you want it to warm up a little bit so it is slightly softened).

58. Buttermilk Oatmeal Bread

Serving: Serves one good-sized loaf | Prep: | Cook: | Ready in:

Ingredients

- 1 teaspoon of sugar
- 2 ¼ teaspoons active dry yeast, or 1 ½ teaspoons of "rapid-rise" or instant yeast
- 7/8 cup buttermilk (lowfat is fine)
- ½ cup rolled oats (old fashioned or quick)
- 2 tablespoons melted butter
- 3 tablespoons honey
- 1 ½ teaspoon salt
- 3 – 3 ¼ cup bread flour (You may need just a bit more for kneading.)
- 1/4 teaspoon baking soda
- Olive oil for brushing the dough before baking

Direction

- Proof the yeast by putting it in a small measuring cup with 3 tablespoons of water that is warm (no hotter than 115 degrees Fahrenheit), with a pinch of sugar. Set it aside for at least ten minutes.
- (Please see the note below about kneading. You don't have to mix and knead this dough by hand, if you don't care to do so.) Mix together the buttermilk, oats, melted butter, salt, honey, 1 cup of flour and the baking soda. Beat well until combined.
- Beat in another half cup of flour, then add the yeast and water mixture along with another half cup of flour, and beat some more, until combined. The dough should start to feel a bit stretchy.
- Stir in another half cup of flour as best you can and then dump the contents of the bowl onto a lightly floured work surface.
- Set the remaining ¾ cup of flour close to your work area. Knead, adding flour a bit at a time as necessary, using a bench scraper to lift from your work surface any dough that is sticking.
- Knead for about ten or twelve minutes, adding only as much flour as you need to keep the dough from sticking hard to your hands. You don't need to add the entire amount stated in the ingredients list. Remember, this dough has oatmeal in it, which will continue to soak up the liquids in the bread during the rise. (I put a small pile of flour – no more than a few tablespoons – off to the side, and use my bench scraper to pull over a teaspoon or two at a time, as needed.)
- Let the dough rest for a few minutes while you prepare the bowl and your rising area, if necessary. (See note below about the latter.)
- Wash in hot water the same bowl that you used for mixing the dough. Dry it and drizzle in the bottom a teaspoon or two of good, fruity olive oil. You can also use butter to coat the bowl, if you prefer.
- If proofing in your microwave or in your oven, prepare as suggested in Step 17.
- Gently form the dough into a ball, put into the bowl topside down, and then flip it over to coat with the oil.
- Cover the bowl with a piece of parchment and a tea towel. Allow to rise until doubled, for about an hour to an hour and a half.
- Punch down gently, knead a few times, and set aside on the parchment you used to cover the bowl.
- Allow to rise a second time about 45 minutes or until nearly doubled in size. (If you want to

use this bread for sandwiches, you may find it beneficial not to let it rise quite as much. A loaf that's a bit more dense is easier to slice, and holds up better when constructing sandwiches.) See notes below about shaping, and about using a clay pot for loaf bread.
- Brush with olive oil, slash the dough a few times with a sharp knife, and bake at 350 Fahrenheit (for regular ovens) for about 55 minutes, or until the loaf sounds hollow when the bottom is gently tapped.
- Allow to cool on a rack for about an hour before slicing.
- Enjoy!!
- A Note about Rising: If your house is drafty and/or cold (like mine, most of the year) and you don't have all day or overnight to allow your dough to rise, put a small cup of water in your microwave, and turn it on high for two minutes. It should feel ever so slightly warm. (You don't want it too hot, because a quick rise can make the bread coarse.) Remove the cup and put your covered bowl of dough, or your shaped loaf on the parchment in the case of the second rise, in there and shut the door. Instruct all members of your household, in no uncertain terms, that if they need to use the microwave, they may do so only if they remove the dough, gently, and replace it, with the door shut, when done. Or, you can warm up your regular oven to no more than 100 degrees (turning it off immediately so it doesn't get any hotter), leave the door open for a minute or so, then put your dough in there.
- A Note about Clay Pots: This recipe works well either as a free-standing oval on a pizza stone, or in a loaf pan. If using a standard metal pan, lightly oil it before putting the dough into it for the second rise. If you are using a clay pot, please remember that (i) it benefits from soaking in water before using; and (b) you can't put it, while cold, into a hot oven. So fill up the clay pot about ¾ with water and put it into the oven; about twenty minutes before the time you expect to put the bread in the oven, turn it on (325 degrees Fahrenheit for a convection oven, or 350 for a regular oven). When the dough has completed its second rise, remove the hot pan from the oven, discard the hot water – I use it for cleaning the oily bowl– and then place the dough in the clay pot, using the parchment on which the dough rose. You can oil clay pots, but they don't absorb as much water during the soak. The absorbed water creates steam in the oven, which improves the crust.
- A Note about Browning: Check the loaf after about 25 minutes. Convection ovens tend to make the crust a bit dark – especially those with milk and butter in them -- so if the crust looks done after 25 or 30 minutes, cover it very lightly with a piece of foil.
- A Note about Kneading: This dough does not necessarily have to be kneaded by hand, if you have another method that you prefer, and are able to make adjustments accordingly. I happen to like stirring and kneading, because I rely on my hands to tell me when the correct amount of flour has been added. Plus, there's nothing quite like the satisfaction of using your own hands to turn a shaggy, floury mass of not-quite combined ingredients into the most glorious, smooth, shiny and supple ball of dough. I do some of my best thinking while kneading, too.

59. Butternut Squash Banana Chocolate Chip Muffins

Serving: Makes 15 | Prep: | Cook: | Ready in:

Ingredients

- 2   medium very ripe bananas, mashed
- 1/2 cup canned butternut squash puree
- 2   egg whites
- 1/2 cup coconut oil
- 1/2 cup reduced sugar maple syrup
- 1/2 teaspoon ground cinnamon
- 1/4 teaspoon ground ginger
- 1/8 teaspoon ground nutmeg

- 1/2 teaspoon sea salt
- 1 teaspoon baking soda
- 1 cup GF flour or whole wheat if not gluten intolerant
- 2/3 cup GF oat flour
- 3/4 cup GF rolled oats
- 1/2 cup mini chocolate chips

Direction

- Preheat oven 375 degrees
- Prepare a muffin tin with cooking spray
- In a large bowl, add bananas, egg whites, canola oil, maple syrup & butternut squash
- Using a hand mixer, combine wet ingredients
- To the wet add the dry ingredients (except oats & chocolate chips)
- Combine all ingredients thoroughly with the mixer
- Add oats & chocolate chips to the batter & combine by hand
- Fill muffin cavities with batter 3/4 full
- Bake 15 minutes
- Remove from the oven & cool on a baking rack

60. CARROT NUTMEG PECAN COOKIES

Serving: Makes 26 cookies | Prep: | Cook: | Ready in:

Ingredients

- 100 grams plain flour
- 100 grams rolled oats
- 40 grams ground almonds
- 1 teaspoon ground nutmeg
- 1 teaspoon baking powder
- 1/2 teaspoon sea salt
- 2/3 cup chopped pecans
- 1 cup grated carrot
- 1/2 cup honey or real maple syrup
- 1/2 cup butter, melted

Direction

- Preheat oven to 180C fan bake. Line 2 baking trays with baking paper.
- In a large bowl, combine flour, oats, ground almonds, nutmeg, baking powder and salt. Add pecans and carrot and mix well. Gradually add honey/maple syrup and melted butter and mix until a sticky dough is formed.
- Drop tablespoons of mixture onto baking sheets and flatten with your fingers. They won't spread much so 2cm between each cookie is fine.
- Bake for 10-12 minutes or until the cookies are golden on top and bottom.
- Allow to cool and firm on the baking tray for 10 minutes before transferring to a rack. Store in a cool, dry place in an airtight container or cookie jar for up to a week.

61. Caramelized Bananas With Yogurt And Berries

Serving: Serves 1 | Prep: | Cook: | Ready in:

Ingredients

- 1 tablespoon butter or coconut oil
- 1 banana (not very ripe, with slightly green stem)
- 1/8 cup quick oats
- Pinch of sea salt
- 1 tablespoon maple syrup
- Fresh berries (raspberries, blueberries, or blackberries)
- 1 tablespoon roasted walnuts, chopped

Direction

- In a small frying pan heat butter or oil over medium heat. Slice banana in half lengthwise and cut into quarters. With flat side facing down place the banana quarters into the pan. They should make a sizzling noise. Reduce heat to medium low and allow the bananas to brown. Flip onto other side.

- Toss the rolled oats around the bananas and sauté. Sprinkle everything with a pinch of salt.
- Drizzle maple syrup over the bananas and oats and sauté until bananas are browned and caramelized on the bottom as well.
- Place bananas onto plate and top with rolled oats. Garnish with a generous dollop of plain yogurt, fresh berries, and roasted walnuts.

62. Caramelized Onion, Ricotta & Steel Cut Oats

Serving: Serves 2 | Prep: | Cook: | Ready in:

Ingredients

- For the steel cut oats
- 1 cup steel cut oats (not quick cooking)
- 4 cups water
- pinch of salt
- Caramelized Onions, Ricotta & Steel Cut Oats (makes 2 servings)
- 1 teaspoon extra-virgin olive oil
- 1 small onion, thinly sliced
- Salt and freshly ground pepper, to taste
- 1/2 teaspoon molasses
- 1 cup cooked steel cut oats (see step 1)
- 2 tablespoons fresh ricotta

Direction

- To make the oats, bring water to a boil in a deep pot. Add oats and salt, and cook until they begin to thicken. Reduce to a simmer, and continue cooking, uncovered, until grains are slightly tender and water has mostly absorbed, about 15 to 20 minutes. Turn off heat, cover pot and let sit for 5 minutes before serving.
- Heat olive oil in a skillet over medium-high heat. Add onions and season with salt and pepper. Sauté until they begin to soften and become golden, about 5 minutes. Stir in molasses, and a touch more olive oil if necessary. Cover skillet and reduce heat to medium-low. Cook, covered, until onions are very tender, about 10 more minutes.
- Divide the cooked oatmeal among two bowls. Top with equal amounts of caramelized onions and fresh ricotta. Stir together with your spoon before digging in.

63. Carr Oatmeal

Serving: Serves 1 or 2 | Prep: | Cook: | Ready in:

Ingredients

- 1/3 cup rolled oats (aka "old fashioned" or "5 minute")
- 1 teaspoon ground flaxseed meal
- 2 teaspoons oat bran
- 1/3 cup finely shredded carrot
- 1 1/2 cups cool water
- 2 dried black mission figs, chopped fine (discard stem)
- 2 pitted dried dates, chopped fine
- 1/4 teaspoon cinnamon
- Dash nutmeg
- Dash cardamom
- Pinch sea salt
- 2 tablespoons green pumpkin seeds
- Splash cream, milk or soy milk

Direction

- To toast the pumpkin seeds, heat a skillet dry for a few minutes, then add them and shake the pan every minute until they toast and start to pop. Remove from heat. You could substitute pepitas (already roasted and salted pumpkin seeds), just omit the salt from the recipe.
- Combine oats, oat bran, flax meal, shredded carrot, chopped dried fruit, spices and water in small saucepan.
- Cook over medium-low heat, stirring with a wooden spatula (to keep bottom from sticking). The flax and bran will start to bind the mixture as it heats, so keep re-

incorporating and stirring to keep everything smooth. (You can go get some coffee and come back, this is not a high-maintenance oatmeal. If at any point during cooking the mixture starts to bubble and boil rapidly, turn down your heat, stir really well, and keep cooking, add a little extra water if it's clumpy). After about 12 minutes, the mixture will be velvety, with no visual distinction between liquid and solid ingredients and the bubbles should rise and pop slowly. Remove from heat, give it a few more vigorous stirs, and turn into a serving bowl.

- Sprinkle a little salt and the roasted pumpkin seeds over the oatmeal. Drizzle a few teaspoons of medium-colored honey over top (don't overpower the carrots with sweetness, but this helps enhance their flavor). Splash some milk around the outside edge of the oatmeal. The oatmeal is sort of thickened like a pudding, so I like to drag spoonful through the honey and milk to really make it feel gourmet as I eat.

64. Carrot Bean Cakes With Tahini Dressing

Serving: Serves 4-6 | Prep: | Cook: | Ready in:

Ingredients

- For the carrot bean cakes
- 3 large carrots
- 4 tablespoons canola oil
- 1 14-ounce can chickpeas, drained and rinsed
- 1 medium onion
- 1/2 cup rolled oats
- 1 teaspoon cumin
- 1/2 teaspoon cayenne, or to taste
- salt and freshly ground pepper
- 1 egg
- 1/4 cup panko bread crumbs
- Tahini dressing
- 1/4 cup plain low-fat yogurt
- 2 tablespoons tahini
- 1 tablespoon freshly squeezed lemon juice
- 1 clove garlic, minced
- salt and freshly ground pepper

Direction

- Preheat oven to 425 degrees. Cut carrots into spears about 3 inches long and 1/2 inches wide. Toss with 1 tbsp. canola oil and salt and pepper and roast on a baking sheet for 30-40 min, until golden brown and tender.
- Combine roasted carrots, oats, beans, onion (quartered), egg, cumin, cayenne, salt and pepper in a food processor and pulse until chunky (leaving some small pieces visible), and then transfer to bowl. Add panko bread crumbs to the bean mixture so that it is firm enough to form patties.
- Using wet hands, shape mixture into small patties, cover, and refrigerate for at least 30 min.
- Add canola oil to skillet and turn heat to medium. When oil is hot, add bean patties and cook until golden brown on each side, about 3-5 min.
- For the tahini dressing, combine yogurt, tahini, lemon juice, garlic, salt, and pepper in a small bowl and mix well. Spread dressing on each bean cake after frying.

65. Carrot Cake Balls

Serving: Makes 8 | Prep: 0hours45mins | Cook: 0hours5mins | Ready in:

Ingredients

- 1 1/2 ounces (40g) desiccated/dried unsweetened shredded coconut, for coating
- 1 ounce (25g) quinoa flakes or jumbo rolled oats
- 1 small carrot, about 1 3/4 ounces (50g), sliced

- 3 1/2 ounces (100g) soft dried apricots, roughly chopped
- 1 tablespoon almond or cashew butter
- 1 teaspoon mixed/apple pie spice
- 1 tablespoon vanilla protein powder (optional)
- 1 tablespoon hulled hemp seeds

Direction

- First toast the desiccated/dried unsweetened shredded coconut. Place the coconut in a large, dry frying pan/skillet over a medium-low heat and cook for a couple of minutes, tossing the pan regularly, until light golden — take care as the coconut burns easily. Tip the toasted coconut onto a large plate and set aside while you make the balls.
- Put the quinoa flakes (or oats) and carrot in a food processor and process until very finely chopped. Add the apricots, nut butter, mixed/apple pie spice, and protein powder (if using), and process again to a thick smooth-ish paste, occasionally scraping down the mixture from the sides when needed. Stir in the hemp seeds.
- With damp hands, shape the carrot mixture into 8 large, walnut-sized balls, then roll each one in the toasted coconut until coated all over (any leftover coconut can be used in another recipe). Chill in the fridge for 30 minutes to firm up. Store in the fridge in an airtight container for up to 2 weeks.

66. Carrot Cake Cookies

Serving: Makes 24 | Prep: | Cook: | Ready in:

Ingredients

- 2 bananas, mashed (1 cup)
- 2 carrots, grated (1 cup)
- 1/4 cup butter or coconut oil, melted
- 1/4 cup sugar or other sweetener
- 2 teaspoons vanilla extract
- 1 cup oats
- 1/2 cup almond flour
- 1/2 cup brown rice flour
- 2 teaspoons baking powder
- 1/2 teaspoon salt
- 1 tablespoon cinnamon
- 1 teaspoon ground ginger
- 1 cup toasted nuts, dried fruit chocolate chips, or a combination (optional)

Direction

- Preheat oven to 350F. Toast nuts if using.
- Mix together banana, carrot, butter sugar and vanilla.
- Add oats, flours (can sub 1 cup wheat flour if desired), baking powder, salt, and spices. Add nuts/fruit/chocolate if using.
- Form tablespoons into balls and flatten. Bake 12 minutes. Cool on wire rack.

67. Carrot Cake Oatmeal With Peanut Butter

Serving: Serves 1 | Prep: | Cook: | Ready in:

Ingredients

- 1/3 cup old-fashioned oats
- 1 large carrot, grated
- 1/2 teaspoon cinnamon, preferably the oil-rich and spicy-sweet Saigon variety
- 3 egg whites
- 1 cup water (or milk of your choice)
- 1 tablespoon peanut, almond, or cashew butter
- sweetener, to taste (I love brown sugar)
- 1 teaspoon vanilla extract

Direction

- Add the carrot and oats to a small sauce pot with the water, and bring to a boil. Stir for about a minute, then reduce the heat to low. Cover the pot and let it simmer for another 2

minutes. Remove the lid and increase the heat until the carrots are cooked down and the oatmeal has thickened.
- Reduce the heat to low and add the egg whites, stirring to thoroughly incorporate. Cover the pot and let the whites cook through.
- Remove the lid and stir; the oatmeal should be thick. Turn off the heat and add the cinnamon, vanilla, and sweetener of your choice. Pour the oatmeal into a warm bowl and top with the nut butter.

68. Carrot Cake For A Crowd

Serving: Serves 10-12 | Prep: | Cook: | Ready in:

Ingredients

- Carrot Cake
- 1 3/4 cups flour
- 1/2 cup old-fashion rolled oats
- 1 1/2 teaspoons salt
- 1 1/2 teaspoons fennel seed
- 1 teaspoon cinnamon
- 1/2 teaspoon ginger
- 1/4 teaspoon nutmeg
- 1 1/4 cups vegetable oil
- 1/4 cup olive oil
- 2 cups sugar
- 4 eggs, at room temperture
- 3 cups freshly grated carrot
- 1/2 cup golden raisins
- 1/2 cup pecans, chopped
- 1 teaspoon orange zest
- Cream Cheese Frosting
- 2 cups confectioners sugar
- 1 8-ounce block of cream cheese
- 1 stick butter
- 1 teaspoon vanilla extract or vanilla bean paste

Direction

- Preheat oven to 350°F.
- In a medium-size bowl, whisk together the flour, oats, baking soda, salt, fennel seed, cinnamon, ginger and nutmeg. Set aside.
- In the bowl of a stand mixer fitted with the paddle attachment, mix both oils with the sugar. Once combined, add in the eggs one at a time. Next, add the flour mixture in batches on low speed. Once fully combined, turn off the mixer and remove the bowl from the stand. Using a rubber spatula, fold in the carrots, raisins, pecans and orange zest.
- Pour the batter into a prepared 13x9-inch baking pan and bake 45-50 minutes. Remove cake from oven and let cool.
- Place the cream cheese and butter into the mixer bowl and beat with a paddle attachment until smooth. With the mixer on low speed, add the remaining two cups of confectioners' sugar a spoonful at a time until completely incorporated. Once all the sugar has been added, add the vanilla and salt. Spoon the cake over top of the cake and then spread evenly with a spatula.

69. Cashew Butter Bites With Toasted Coconut & Cardamom

Serving: Makes 24 | Prep: | Cook: | Ready in:

Ingredients

- 1 cup cashew butter
- 1 1/4 cups gluten-free oats
- 1/2 cup maple syrup
- 2 cups sweetened coconut flakes
- 1/4 teaspoon salt
- pinch cardamom

Direction

- First, toast 1 cup coconut. Lay flat on a piece of parchment paper, and toast for 8-10 minutes in a 300 F oven, until just golden and toasty. Watch carefully- coconut burns quickly. Set aside to cool.

- For the bites: stir together cashew butter and maple syrup in a medium microwave safe bowl. Microwave for 20 seconds, remove and stir. Microwave for another 20 seconds, remove and stir.
- Whisk wet mixture together with 1 1/4 cup GF oats, remaining 1 cup coconut, salt, and pinch cardamom. Scoop out of the bowl with a spoon, and using your hands, quickly roll into balls and place on parchment paper. Place in refrigerator to chill for at least an hour.
- Remove from the refrigerator and roll balls in toasted coconut. Enjoy a bite now, then pop the rest back in the fridge. Makes 24 bites.

70. Cavatelli With Asiago Oat Crumbs

Serving: Serves 6-8 | Prep: | Cook: | Ready in:

Ingredients

- 8 ounces old fashioned rolled oats
- 8 ounces Asiago cheese, finely grated
- 6 ounces butter, softened
- 16 ounces cavatelli (farfalle, spaghetti, pappardelle and fettuccine also work well)
- Freshly ground pepper
- Red pepper flakes (optional)

Direction

- In a food processor, grind the oats until powdery.
- In a large bowl, mix the oat powder, Asiago and butter. Mix well and knead with your hands for a couple of minutes until it comes together into uniform dough. Press the dough into a disk (or cube, or any other shape of your liking) and refrigerate for about 2 hours, until very firm.
- Preheat the oven to 350F. Line a large baking sheet with parchment paper. Remove the dough from the fridge, and using a cheese grater, grate the dough over the baking sheet. (Make sure the gratings are uniformly distributed).
- Bake for about 25-30 minutes. Remove the sheet from the oven, and leave the gratings on it to crisp.
- In the meantime, cook your pasta to al dente. Drain the pasta and arrange it on individual plates. Pour the crumb mixture over the top, and season to taste with pepper and red pepper flakes (this is optional -- I like them, but my husband does not). Toss well and serve very hot.

71. Chai Spiced Porridge With Stewed Apples

Serving: Serves 2 | Prep: | Cook: | Ready in:

Ingredients

- for the stewed apples:
- 1 pound apples
- 1 tablespoon water
- 1 tablespoon light brown sugar
- 1/2 teaspoon cinnamon
- for the chai-spiced porridge
- 1 cup porridge oats
- 2 1/2 cups milk
- 2 tablespoons light brown sugar
- 3/4 teaspoon cinnamon
- Pinch ground ginger
- Pinch ground cloves
- Pinch ground nutmeg

Direction

- First, to make the stewed apples, peel and core the apples, then cut them into bite-sized pieces. Place in a small saucepan and add the water, brown sugar and cinnamon, stirring to combine. Bring to a boil, then reduce the heat to medium. Cook for about 10 minutes, stirring occasionally, until the apples are soft and the juices are syrupy. Remove from the heat and set aside.

- To make the porridge, in a saucepan, combine the oats, milk, brown sugar and spices. Stir well to combine. Bring to the boil and cook briskly for 3 minutes, stirring all the time (or cook according to your porridge oats packet instructions). Remove from the heat.
- To serve, divide the porridge between 2 bowls and spoon the stewed apples on top. Any leftover stewed apples can be kept in the fridge in an airtight container for up to 1 week.

72. Cheater's Muesli

Serving: Makes however much you want it to make | Prep: | Cook: |Ready in:

Ingredients

- Old-fashioned oats
- Walnuts, lightly crushed with your hands
- Cinnamon
- Good flaky salt

Direction

- Combine all ingredients but the salt in a dry skillet, adapting the nut-oat ratio depending on your preference. Start with just a shake of cinnamon. Toast over low heat, stirring or shaking, until the oats turn a light golden color and you can smell the nuts toasting. Add a good pinch of salt.
- Sprinkle this over a bowl of yogurt, and stir in some fresh fruit or jam. If you can get your hands on savory yogurt or labneh, try it drizzled with best-quality olive oil. (And maybe even some roasted carrots?)

73. Cheesecake Cream + Choco Granola

Serving: Serves 12 | Prep: | Cook: |Ready in:

Ingredients

- for the cream
- 1 1/2 cups raw cashews
- 0.8 pounds medjoul dates
- 1/4 cup maple syrup
- 1/2 cup coconut oil, melted
- 1 pinch salt
- 1/4 cup almond milk
- for the granola
- 1 cup rolled oats
- 1 cup raw buckwheat
- 1/2 cup raw almonds, chopped
- 1 tablespoon chia seeds
- 1 pinch salt
- 1/4 cup cacao powder
- 1/4 cup coconut oil, melted
- 1/4 cup maple syrup

Direction

- For the cream
- Soak cashews overnight, than wash, drain and put them in a high-speed blender with all other ingredients.
- Blend until smooth and reserve in fridge.
- For the granola
- Preheat the oven at 350°F / 175°C.
- In a bowl mix oat flakes, buckwheat, almonds, chia seeds, salt and cacao powder.
- In a little bowl mix coconut oil and maple syrup and pour them over the dry ingredients. Stir until well combined.
- Spread the mixture on a baking dish covered with parchment paper and bake for about 25 minutes or until it starts to be crunchy, but pay attention because cacao burns pretty suddenly!
- Let it cool and reserve in a jar.
- Serve a quenelle of cream and sprinkle with - a lot of - granola!

74. Cherry Orange Crisp

Serving: Serves 6 | Prep: | Cook: |Ready in:

Ingredients

- For the filling:
- 4 cakes cherries, pitted and quartered
- 1 shot sugar
- 1 teaspoon orange zest
- 1 1/2 teaspoons vanilla bean paste (extract will work too)
- For the crumb topping:
- 1/3 cup flour
- 1/3 cup brown sugar
- 1/3 cup old fashioned oats
- 3 tablespoons softened butter
- 1/4 teaspoon cinnamon
- 1/4 teaspoon cardamom
- 1 pinch salt

Direction

- Mix the cherries, sugar, zest, and vanilla in a bowl, and spread evenly in a heavy baking dish. Set aside while you make the topping.
- Combine the flour, oats, sugar, and spices.
- Add the butter, and mix with your fingers until it becomes a crumb texture.
- Bake at 400 for 45 minutes, or until the topping is golden brown and crispy, and the cherries are bubbling up at the sides. Tip: put a baking sheet on the rack below, so any spills don't burn onto the bottom of the oven.

75. Chewy Crispy Oatmeal Cookies With Chocolate Chips And Dried Cherries

Serving: Makes 24 cookies | Prep: | Cook: | Ready in:

Ingredients

- 1 cup light brown sugar
- 3/4 cup unsalted butter, softened
- 1 egg
- 1 teaspoon vanilla extract
- 3/4 cup flour
- 1/2 teaspoon salt
- 1/2 teaspoon baking soda
- 1/2 teaspoon cinnamon
- 3 cups rolled or old fashioned oats
- 1 cup dried cherries
- 1 cup bittersweet chocolate chips

Direction

- Preheat oven to 350 degrees. Beat butter and sugar until creamy in a large bowl.
- Add egg and vanilla and beat to combine.
- Whisk together flour, salt, baking soda, and cinnamon in a medium bowl.
- Add dry ingredients to the wet and beat to combine.
- Stir in oats, cherries, and chocolate chips. This will take some doing, but the batter should combine to a sticky, chunky mass of oaty cookie dough.
- Line two baking sheets with parchment paper. Dollop the dough in heaping tablespoons in evenly spaced mounds on the sheets.
- Wet your fingers and compress the dough into little domes. They don't need to be perfect. The dough won't expand too much as they cook, so don't worry if the cookies seem close together.
- Bake 12 - 15 minutes.

76. Chewy Granola Bars

Serving: Makes 20 smallish bars | Prep: | Cook: | Ready in:

Ingredients

- 2 cups rolled oats
- 1 cup whole wheat pastry flour
- 1/4 cup ground flax seed
- 1/4 cup chia seeds
- 2 teaspoons ground cinnamon
- 1/2 cup dried cranberries, chopped
- 1/4 cup mini chocolate chips or cacao nibs
- 1/4 cup sunflower seeds
- 1/4 cup pumpkin seeds
- 1/2 teaspoon salt

- 1/2 cup dates, pits removed (about eight)
- 1/2 cup honey
- 1/4 cup applesauce
- 1/4 cup coconut oil, melted
- 2 teaspoons pure vanilla extract

Direction

- Heat the oven to 350F and line a 9x13 baking sheet with parchment paper.
- Mix the oats, flour, flax, chia, cinnamon, cranberries, cacao nibs, sunflower seeds, pepitas, and salt in a large bowl.
- In a high-speed blender or food processor, blend the dates, honey, applesauce, coconut oil, and vanilla until it becomes a paste.
- Add the paste to the dry ingredients and mix with a wooden spoon or your hands. It takes a while with a spoon, so I usually just get in there and squish everything together with my hands.
- Press the mixture into the lined baking sheet and bake for 22-25 minutes, or until the edges are slightly browned. If you over bake it, it'll be dry.
- Let the sheet cool on a rack for ten minutes before lifting the granola bars out. You can cut them now, but if you let them cool completely first you'll get a nice clean cut and nicer looking bars. Store them in the fridge or freezer if you don't plan on eating them within a few days.
- Notes: You don't have to melt the coconut oil before blending, but it makes it a lot easier to mix in. You can change up the add-ins (sunflower seeds, cranberries) as you see fit. Use whatever you have on hand. Want to use 1 cup of chocolate chips and leave out the rest? Go for it.

77. Chewy Oatmeal Cookies

Serving: Makes 18 large cookies | Prep: 0hours20mins | Cook: 0hours15mins | Ready in:

Ingredients

- 2 sticks (227 g) unsalted butter, at room temperature
- 1 cup (213 g) light brown sugar
- 1/3 cup (66 g) granulated sugar
- 2 large (113 g) eggs
- 1 teaspoon (5 g) vanilla extract
- 1 3/4 cups (210 g) all purpose flour
- 1 teaspoon (6 g) baking soda
- 1/2 teaspoon (2 g) baking powder
- 1 teaspoon (4 g) fine sea salt
- 1 teaspoon (2 g) ground cinnamon
- 2 cups (199 g) old fashioned oats

Direction

- Preheat the oven to 350° F with racks in the upper and lower thirds. Line two baking sheets with parchment paper.
- In the bowl of a stand mixer fitted with the paddle attachment, cream the butter and sugars on medium-low speed until light and fluffy, 4-5 minutes
- Add the eggs one at a time, mixing on medium speed until each one is fully incorporated. Add the vanilla and mix to combine. Scrape the bowl well.
- In a medium bowl, whisk together the flour, baking soda, baking powder, salt, and cinnamon. Add to the butter mixture and mix on low speed until incorporated, 1 to 2 minutes. Add the oats and mix on low speed to combine, 30 seconds to 1 minute. Scrape the bowl well.
- Use a 1/4 cup (#16 scoop) to portion the cookie dough onto the prepared baking sheets. Stagger the cookies, leaving 1 1/2 inches between them to allow for spreading.
- Bake the cookies, rotating the sheets from front to back and top to bottom at the halfway mark, until evenly golden brown, 14-16 minutes. Transfer the cookies to wire racks to cool.

78. Chewy Oatmeal Raisin Breakfast Cookies

Serving: Serves 12 | Prep: | Cook: |Ready in:

Ingredients

- 1 cup oat flour
- 1/4 cup raisins
- 1/3 cup chopped almonds
- 1/2 cup oats
- 1/2 cup coconut oil, melted and cooled
- 1/2 cup maple syrup
- 1/4 cup nut butter
- 1 egg
- 1 teaspoon vanilla extract
- 3/4 teaspoon baking soda
- 1/2 teaspoon cinnamon
- 1/4 teaspoon nutmeg
- 1/4 teaspoon ginger

Direction

- Combine the dry ingredients - flour, oats, almonds, raisins, spices, and baking soda - in a large bowl and stir.
- In a small bowl, whisk together the wet ingredients - coconut oil, nut butter, maple syrup, and egg - and pour into the dry. Stir until just incorporated. Refrigerate for 45-60 minutes.
- Preheat the oven to 350F and line a baking sheet with parchment paper. Scoop large spoonfuls of dough onto the sheet, about 2 inches distance between each portion.
- Bake for 15-17 minutes or until golden brown around the edges. Remove from oven and let cool on the baking sheet - this allows them to firm up a bit.
- Serve immediately and store leftovers in a covered container with a small opening for air - this prevents them becoming mushy.
- Enjoy!

79. Chia Breakfast Bowl

Serving: Serves 2 | Prep: | Cook: |Ready in:

Ingredients

- 2 bananas
- 4 tablespoons chia seeds
- 2 packets instant oats (original)
- 1.5 cups coconut milk (or whatever kind of milk you prefer)
- 2 scoops of protein powder (I prefer chocolate)
- 1 splash vanilla extract
- 1 handful almonds (or whatever kind of nuts you prefer)
- 1 handful raspberries (or whatever kind of berries you prefer)
- 2 tablespoons coconut flakes

Direction

- Mash bananas in a medium sized bowl with a fork.
- Add in chia seeds. Stir to combine.
- Add in instant oats. Stir to combine.
- Pour in milk. Stir to combine.
- Add in protein powder. Stir to combine.
- Add in vanilla extract.
- Add in nuts, if desired. Cover bowl and put in fridge overnight. A few minutes before eating, add in berries and coconut flakes.

80. Chickapea Homemade Meatballs For DOGS

Serving: Makes roughly 120 mini meatballs | Prep: | Cook: |Ready in:

Ingredients

- 28.2 ounces (800 grams) of boneless, skinless chicken thighs (approx 6 thighs), cut into small pieces
- 6.3 ounces (180 grams) of chicken liver

- 1 granny smith apple (140 grams), cored and cut into small pieces
- 1 small carrot (140 grams), peeled and cut into small pieces
- 1 cup (140 grams) of frozen peas
- 1 cup of rolled oats
- 1/4 cup (40 grams) of flaxseed
- 2 tablespoons of sesame oil
- 2 tablespoons safflower oil (or flaxseed oil)
- 1/2 teaspoon of salt

Direction

- Preheat the broiler on high.
- In a food-processor, pulse and grind the chicken thighs and chicken liver until smoothly ground/pureed (if you have a small food-processor, you may do this in 2 batches). Make sure there are no large chunks left when you do this, and transfer the ground meat into a stand-mixer bowl. Then add the granny smith apple and carrot in the food-processor (no need to wash), pulse until finely minced, and transfer to the stand-mixer bowl as well. Grind the flaxseeds with 1/2 cup of rolled oats in a spice-grinder. Rinse the frozen peas through a sieve to make sure they are separated WITHOUT any ice-cubes attached, dry thoroughly on a kitchen towel. Add everything along with the remaining 1/2 cup of rolled oats, sesame oil, safflower oil and salt to the stand-mixer bowl.
- With a stand-mixer, beat the mixture with a paddle-attachment on high speed for about 5 min, until thick and sticky. What this does is it binds the excess water in the mixture with protein, and gives you springy meatballs that won't release water during baking. You can do this by hand with a wooden spoon, but expect really sore muscles. If you want to skip this step, be warned that you might get watery meatballs in the oven.
- Line baking sheets with parchment paper, and make mini meatballs the size of a large melon-baller, with 1? (3 cm) space in between. Place the baking sheet on the middle-upper rack in the oven, about 3 1/2? (9 cm) below the broiler. Bake for 15 min, but remember to shake the baking sheet every 5 min in between to roll the meatballs around for even browning. Prepare another sheet of meatballs while the first batch is baking, then after 15 min, move the first batch to the lower rack in the oven for another 5 min to finish cooking, and place the second batch on the middle-upper rack to brown. Repeat the same process with every batch.
- After each batch has been baked on the middle-upper rack for 15 min, then the lower rack for another 5 min, you can remove it from the oven and let then cool on a cooling-rack. Store them in an air-tight container in the fridge for up to 5 days, or freeze them for up to 2 months. Reheat in the microwave to bring them back to room-temperature (but not hot!) before giving them to some seriously wagging tails.

81. Choc Chip ANZAC Biscuits

Serving: Makes 25 - 28 | Prep: | Cook: |Ready in:

Ingredients

- 1 cup organic flour
- 1 cup organic rolled oats
- 1/2 cup Organic Times Rapadura Sugar
- 1 cup organic desiccated coconut
- 140 grams Organic Times Salted Butter
- 1 tablespoon water
- 1/2 teaspoon bi-carb soda
- 1/4 - 1/2 cups Organic Times Choc Drops

Direction

- Preheat the oven to 180 C / 350 F, non-fan forced.
- Line 2 baking trays with baking paper.
- In a saucepan on low heat, place the golden syrup, water and butter.
- In a heatproof bowl place the flour, sugar, oats and coconut.

- Once the butter has melted and is bubbling with the syrup, add your bi-carb and stir through thoroughly.
- Tip saucepan contents into the dry ingredients and mix thoroughly.
- Once mixed, add your choc drops and mix again.
- Shape mixture into walnut-sized balls and pop well-spaced onto the baking tray. Use a fork to flatten slightly.
- Bake for 12-15 minutes, or until golden brown.
- Take out of the oven and cool completely before eating. These biscuits get harder as they cool and will keep in an air tight container for 4 days.

82. Choco Oats Puris (Indian Fried Flat Bread)

Serving: Serves 5 | Prep: | Cook: | Ready in:

Ingredients

- 1 1/2 cups Maida (All Purpose Flour)
- 1 cup Oats
- 1/4 cup Sugar
- 1/2 cup Grated Chocolate
- Oil for frying

Direction

- Take flour, add 2 teaspoon oil, grated chocolate, and knead dough.
- Take another bowl and mix sugar and oats into it.
- Make small balls and deep it into the oats so that oats and sugar sticks to the ball. Roll small puris of about 2 inch diameter from it. Spread it separately on the paper or muslin cloth. Prepare all the puris.
- Take oil in frying pan and deep fry all the puris. Start frying in batches after all the puris are rolled so that it gives some time for drying. Fry it on medium flame. The puris then will turn out to be crispy.
- Don't put too many puris in frying pan otherwise it will not become crispy. Drain it and put it on the paper napkin separately to remove excess oil. Let it cool completely. You can store this puris for about 8-10 days.

83. Chocolate Almond Chia Hemp Flax Bars

Serving: Makes 18 | Prep: | Cook: | Ready in:

Ingredients

- 1 cup GF rolled oats
- 1 cup raw almonds
- 15-18 medjool dates
- 2 tablespoons golden flax meal
- 1 tablespoon hemp seed hearts
- 2 tablespoons chia seeds
- 1/2 cup unsweetened shredded coconut flakes
- 1/2 teaspoon sea salt
- 1/4 cup coconut oil
- 1/2 teaspoon almond extract
- 2 tablespoons mini chocolate chips

Direction

- In a food processor layer dates, almond & oats then blend them roughly, pulsing the blender a few times
- Then add coconut oil, salt, almond extract, flax, hemp, chia & coconut
- Blend until a sticky mixture forms
- If a sticky mixture doesn't form, add more dates until it does
- Remove mixture from blender into a mixing bowl
- Add chocolate chips & mix by hand by hand
- Prepare an 8"x8" square baking dish with parchment paper leaving it hang over the sides of the baking dish
- Add batter to baking dish, pressing firmly into the pan to flatten out into the shape of the pan
- Refrigerate overnight

- In the morning, remove from the baking dish by lifting the sides of the parchment paper
- Cut into bars with a pizza cutter
- Keep in the fridge in a storage container up to a week, keep in a storage bag in the freezer up to a month

84. Chocolate Cherry Coconut Granola

Serving: Makes about 16 cups | Prep: | Cook: |Ready in:

Ingredients

- 3 cups old-fashioned large flake rolled oats
- 1 cup wheat germ
- 1/2 cup oat bran
- 1/2 cup wheat bran
- 2 1/2 cups all bran flakes
- 2 cups bran buds
- 1 1/2 cups Kashi 7 Whole Grain Cereal
- 1 cup slivered almonds
- 1 cup flaked coconut
- 1 cup cocoa powder
- 1 1/2 cups dried cherries
- 1 cup brown sugar
- 3/4 cup butter
- 1/2 cup water
- 1 teaspoon pure vanilla extract

Direction

- Preheat oven to 350°F.
- In a large mixing bowl, combine the oats through to the cocoa powder. Stir or use hands to mix thoroughly.
- In a pot over medium heat, melt the butter until it lightly browns, then add the brown sugar, water and vanilla. Simmer until the brown sugar has melted.
- Pour the liquid over the dry ingredients. Put everything in a large roasting pan that has been sprayed with Pam.
- Bake for 20-25 minutes for a softer textured granola, 30 minutes to make it crunchy. Stir every 10 minutes to ensure all of the granola browns evenly.
- Remove from heat and stir in dried cherries.

85. Chocolate Chip Cookies

Serving: Makes 3 dozen | Prep: | Cook: |Ready in:

Ingredients

- 1 cup flour
- 1/2 teaspoon baking soda
- 1/4 teaspoon baking powder
- 1/2 cup butter, softened
- 1/2 cup granulated sugar
- 1/2 cup brown sugar
- 1 egg
- 1 teaspoon real vanilla extract
- 3/4 cup old-fashioned oats
- 1 1/4 cups semi-sweet chocolate chips

Direction

- Preheat the oven to 350 degrees. Cover two baking sheets with foil and spray with cooking spray.
- With a stand or hand mixer, cream butter and sugars on medium high speed for 3 minutes. Add the egg and vanilla and beat for 1 minute more, until light and fluffy. Sugar and butter creamed after 3 minutes of beating on medium-high speed. After adding egg and vanilla, the batter is light and creamy.
- Add the flour, baking soda, baking powder and pinch of salt, each slowly and on low speed. Add the oats and combine, and then the chocolate chips and combine - all on low speed.
- Using a half-tablespoon, drop 12 cookies, evenly spaced, onto one cookie sheet. Bake cookies for 10 minutes, turning halfway through. While they cook, drop 12 more cookies on second sheet.
- When first round of cookies are done, pull them out and let them cool 2-3 minutes before

moving to a cooling rack. Pop the second sheet in and repeat with remaining 12 cookies and cooling.

86. Chocolate Chip Muffins

Serving: Makes 12 regular sized muffins | Prep: | Cook: | Ready in:

Ingredients

- 1 cup oat flour
- 1 cup multigrain flakes (like oatmeal flakes but multigrain)
- 3/4 cup melted, but cooled, butter
- 3/4 cup darkest brown sugar
- 1 teaspoon baking powder
- 1/4 teaspoon baking soda
- 1/2 teaspoon salt
- 3/4 cup applesauce
- 3/4 cup chocolate chips
- 1 egg

Direction

- Preheat oven to 350 degrees.
- Place silicone or paper muffin liners in muffin pan.
- Combine oat flour, sugar, butter, egg, baking powder, baking soda, salt and applesauce in a mixing bowl.
- Mix well
- Fold in the multigrain flakes and chocolate chips.
- Divide batter evenly amongst the muffin cup liners and bake for 23 minutes.

87. Chocolate Guinness Stout Oatmeal With Pecans And Greek Yogurt

Serving: Serves 1 | Prep: | Cook: | Ready in:

Ingredients

- 1 cup Guinness Stout
- 1/2 cup milk of choice, or water
- 1/2 cup old-fashioned oats
- 1 dash salt
- 1 handful crushed pecans, plus more for topping
- 1 tablespoon cocoa powder
- 1/4 teaspoon vanilla extract
- 1 tablespoon maple syrup
- 2-3 Greek yogurt

Direction

- In a small saucepan, heat the Guinness over low heat so that it comes to a gentle simmer. Keep it steady, giving it the occasional stir. Let it boil until you are left without half the original amount, more or less. (The more you boil, the more concentrated the flavor.)
- Add in the milk/water, oats, and salt. Bring to another boil over medium heat, folding the oats into the stout mixture.
- When the oats start to thicken, about 3 minutes, stir in the cocoa powder, vanilla, and maple syrup. Make sure that there are no clumps of cocoa remaining. Add in the nuts, so they begin to soften with the heat, and release their aroma.
- When the oatmeal has reached the desired consistency (usually about 5-7 minutes), transfer to a bowl or dish.
- Top with Greek yogurt, and more pecans. Enjoy.

88. Chocolate Oatmeal Crepe Cake With Wild Grapes, Berries, And Bananas

Serving: Makes about 15 crepes | Prep: | Cook: | Ready in:

Ingredients

- 1 3/4 cups oats
- 1 pinch salt
- 1/4 cup unsweetened cocoa powder
- 4 egg whites
- 2-3 tablespoons maple syrup or honey, plus more to top
- 1/4 teaspoon vanilla extract
- 1 1/2 cups milk of choice
- 1 sliced banana
- 1 handful berries, nuts, fruit, toppings of choice, etc.

Direction

- In a blender, grind the oats so that they are powdery, like the consistency of coarse flour. (I did this in two batches.) Add in the salt and cocoa powder and blend so that everything is sifted together.
- Crack the egg whites into the blender, or over a bowl if you're not confident in your cracking skills. Transfer to the blender, along with the vanilla, maple syrup, and 1 cup of milk. Blend, occasionally scraping down the sides.
- When everything is a nice, even color, transfer the blender to the refrigerator and let chill for about 30 minutes up until an hour. Take out once chilled, and stir in the other 1/2 cup of milk. The batter should be the consistency of heavy cream or syrup. If it's too thick or gloppy, add a tablespoon more of milk, and stir.
- Spray a sauté pan with cooking spray, and begin to heat the empty pan on low. When it starts to sizzle a bit, drop a little less than 1/4 cup of the batter into the hot pan, and swirl around so that a nice circle forms. Remember that there are supposed to be thin!
- After about 1 minute, the edges should start to set and curl. Gently move the crepe around the pan and gently lift up one edge. Roll the crepe over to the other side, and cook for about half as long. There will likely be air bubbles so that you know it's done.
- Repeat until all of the batter is gone.
- Stack the crepes, one on top of the other, occasionally throwing in some fruit and drizzling on some sweetness to keep it moist. Continue stacking until all of the crepes are gone.
- Serve with berries, nuts, chocolate, maple syrup, cinnamon, powdered sugar, etc. Enjoy!

89. Chocolate Raspberry Streusel Muffins

Serving: Makes 8 large muffins | Prep: | Cook: | Ready in:

Ingredients

- Struesel
- 1/2 cup (60 g) all purpose flour
- 1/3 cup (33 g) old fashioned oats
- 1/4 cup (53 g) dark brown sugar
- pinch salt
- 5 tablespoons (70 g) cold unsalted butter, but into 1/2 inch cubes
- Muffins
- 2 cups (340 g) raspberries
- 2 1/4 cups (269 g) all purpose flour, divided
- 1/4 cup (22 g) good qaulity cocoa powder (such as Valrhona)
- 1 tablespoon (12 g) baking powder
- 1/2 teaspoon (3 g) baking soda
- 1/2 teaspoon (2 g) fine sea salt
- 1/2 cup (113 g) unsalted butter, melted and cooled slightly
- 1 cup (198 g) granulated sugar
- 2 large (113 g) eggs, at room temperature
- 1 1/2 teaspoons vanilla extract
- 1 cup (226 g) buttermilk, at room temperature

Direction

- Make the streusel: in a small bowl, stir the flour, oats, brown sugar, and salt to combine. Add the butter and mix with your fingers until the mixture forms large crumbs. Set aside.
- Preheat the oven to 350°F. Place 8 freestanding paper baking cups on a baking sheet (see headnote).

- In a medium bowl, toss the raspberries with 1/4 cup (30 g) of the flour. Set aside.
- In a small bowl, whisk the remaining flour, cocoa powder, baking powder, baking soda, and salt to combine.
- In a medium bowl, whisk the melted butter and sugar to combine. Add the eggs one at a time and mix well to incorporate. Beat in the vanilla extract.
- Add the flour mixture and mix well to combine (I usually switch to a silicone spatula at this point).
- Add the buttermilk and mix until fully incorporated. Fold in the raspberry mixture.
- Divide the batter between the baking cups - filling about 2/3 of the cup. Sprinkle the surface of each generously with the prepared streusel.
- Bake until a toothpick inserted into the center comes out clean (or with a few moist crumbs), 17-20 minutes.
- Transfer to a wire rack to cool.

90. Chocolate Fruit Pecan Pie

Serving: Makes 8 | Prep: | Cook: | Ready in:

Ingredients

- 1 cup oat flour
- 1 cup apple sauce
- 1 teaspoon baking powder
- 1 teaspoon baking soda
- 1 mango
- 2 banana
- 4 tablespoons cacao
- 6-8 dates
- 1½ cups pecan and hazelnut mix
- 4 tablespoons Agave syrup

Direction

- Pre heat the oven at 375 °F
- Put the nut mix in a kitchen machine and blend finely
- Put into a bowl
- Add 4 tbsp. of Agave syrup and mix through the nut mix
- Put mixture in a spring form and press the crust finely
- Put all of the fruit in a blender and blend into a smooth mixture
- Divide in half
- Add the oat flour, baking powder, baking soda and cacao and stir through thoroughly.
- Put this mixture on top of the pecan hazelnut crust
- Add the remaining fruit mixture on top of the pecan hazelnut crust
- Bake the pecan pie about 40 to 45 minutes
- Bake the pecan pie about 40 to 45 minutes

91. Chocolate, Oat, And Walnut Slice!

Serving: Makes 25 large pieces | Prep: | Cook: | Ready in:

Ingredients

- Base and topping
- 2 cups Brown Sugar
- 250 grams Butter, melted
- 2 Eggs
- 2.5 cups Self Raising Flour
- 3 cups Rolled Oats
- Chocolate walnut filling
- 300 grams Milk Chocolate
- 400 grams Condensed milk (can)
- 30 grams Butter
- 1 cup Walnuts, chopped
- 2 teaspoons Vanilla Essence

Direction

- Base and topping
- Lightly grease a large, deep slice tin. About 23cm X 32cm. Line with greaseproof paper.
- Combine butter, sugar, eggs and essence in a bowl. Add sifted flour and rolled oats. Mix

well. Press two thirds of this mixture evenly over the base of tin. Save the remainder for the topping.
- Chocolate walnut filling
- Combine chocolate, condensed milk, and butter in a saucepan over a low heat. Stir until chocolate has melted. Add nuts and vanilla. Mix well. Spread onto the base.
- Crumble remaining base, evenly over the filling. Bake in a moderate oven for about 30 minutes, or until just golden. Remove from the oven and cool on a rack. When cool, refrigerate until cold, then cut into yummy slices!!

92. Chocolatety Almond Super PowerBar

Serving: Makes 10 bars | Prep: | Cook: | Ready in:

Ingredients

- 1 tablespoon coconut oil (and more to coat the pan)
- 2 cups rolled oats (not instant, gluten-free if needed)
- 1/2 cup raw sliced almonds
- 1/2 cup walnut halves, finely chopped (pulsed in food processor works well)
- 1/4 cup raw wheat germ (see note; for gluten-free, substitute oats pulsed fine in the food processor)
- 4 tablespoons raw unsweetened shredded coconut
- 2 tablespoons flax seed meal
- 1/4 cup honey (or sub maple syrup or rice syrup for vegan)
- 1 teaspoon ground cinammon
- 1 teaspoon vanilla extract
- 1/4 (heaping) teaspoons coarse salt
- 1/2 cup dried sweetened sour cherries
- 1/2 (packed) cups pItted dates (about 14 small dates)
- 1 1/4 cups semi-sweet or bittersweet chocolate chips
- 1 1/4 cups creamy natural almond butter

Direction

- Heat the oven to 350° with a rack in the middle. Coat an 8-by-8-inch baking pan with coconut oil or Pam and set aside.
- In a large bowl, combine oats, almonds, walnuts, wheat germ, coconut, and flax seed meal. (Note, if using wheat germ that is already toasted, add it to the mix after the toasting step) Transfer to a rimmed baking sheet and spread in an even layer. Bake, stirring halfway through, until almonds are light golden brown, about 12 minutes. Transfer to a wire rack. Reduce the oven temperature to 300°F. Transfer the toasted mixture back to the large bowl when cool enough to handle.
- Add cherries and dates to the food processor bowl and process until the fruit forms a dough-like ball; transfer to a medium size microwave-safe bowl. Add almond butter, honey, salt, cinnamon and coconut oil and microwave until everything is warm and soft, about 1-2 minutes. Add the vanilla extract and mix well.
- Fold the wet ingredients into the dry until well-incorporated (the mixture will be a bit clumpy). Fold in the chocolate chips.
- Transfer mixture to your oiled pan and spend a good couple of minutes pressing the mixture down with a spatula until it is firmly and evenly compacted together.
- Pop the pan back into the oven until fragrant and chocolate has melted, about 10 minutes. Place the pan on a wire rack and repeat the pressing and smoothing process again (this ensures the bar will stick together).
- Allow the pan to cool to the touch (about 20 minutes), but still slightly warm and melty. Use a knife to pull the bars away from the sides slightly, then place a cutting board over the top and invert to release the bars. If the

chocolate solidifies it will stick to the pan and be a bit more difficult to coax out.
- Place the bars (on the cutting board) in the fridge until cold (about 20 min). Use a nice sharp chef's knife to cut the block in half, then each half into 5 even bars. Wrap in plastic wrap and store in the fridge or freezer (let come to room temp before eating).

93. Chocolatey Banana And Oats

Serving: Serves 1 | Prep: | Cook: |Ready in:

Ingredients

- 1/2 cup vanilla flavored almond milk
- several dashes cinnamon
- 1 tablespoon almond or peanut butter
- 1/4 cup old fashioned oats
- 1 teaspoon chia seeds
- 1 tablespoon raw cacao
- 1/2 banana, sliced
- nuts of your choice - I like walnuts and almonds

Direction

- Heat the milk on high with several dashes of cinnamon in a small saucepan several minutes until steaming. Once steaming, turn the heat off and stir in the nut butter.
- In your breakfast bowl, pour in the oats, chia seeds, and cacao. Top with the milk mixture and stir. Add banana and nuts and serve.

94. Chocolaty, Walnut No Bake Brownies

Serving: Makes 12 | Prep: | Cook: |Ready in:

Ingredients

- Brownie Filling
- 2 cups oat four*
- 2 cups walnuts
- 1/2 cup organic maple syrup
- 2 tablespoons black chia seeds
- 4 tablespoons carob powder
- 2 tablespoons cacao powder
- 4 tablespoons melted coconut oil
- 2 teaspoons vanilla extract
- 2 pinches salt
- Brownie Frosting
- 4 tablespoons melted coconut oil
- 4 tablespoons organic maple syrup
- 4 tablespoons cacao powder
- 1/4 cup walnuts
- 1/4 cup walnuts for garnish

Direction

- Brownie Filling
- *If you can't find oat flour, use normal or gluten-free oats, put them in a food processor and break them down until they become a fine powder*
- Place all ingredients into a food processor.
- Process until all ingredients are well combined and form a big doughy ball. It's good to process just to nice and combined, you still want a bit of texture in the mixture.
- Press down with your fingers, spoon or spatula to create a smooth surface.
- Place brownie filling into the fridge to set while you're making the frosting.
- Brownie Frosting
- Place all ingredients, accept walnuts, in a bowl and mix together.
- Fill a plastic zip-lock bag with 1/4 walnuts. Using a rolling pin or any round item break down the walnuts into smaller pieces. You could also do this in a food processor or with a mortar and pestle.
- Take first brownie layer out of the fridge, and if went touched, is nice and firm, pour over half the frosting.
- Spread the frosting so it covers the entire brownie layer. Add the crushed walnut pieces onto of the frosting layer and place back in the fridge to harden.

- Repeat the brownie filling then brownie frosting steps so you create a filling, frosting, filling, and frosting layered effect
- Before you put the last layer of frosting into the fridge to set crumble over some walnuts as a topping
- Slice and enjoy!! - would be super yummy with ice-cream or even a layer of smooth peanut-butter spread right on top

95. Cinnamon Cashew Butter Doughnuts

Serving: Makes 6 | Prep: | Cook: | Ready in:

Ingredients

- Cinnamon Cashew Butter Doughnuts
- 1⅓ cups oats
- 12 medjool dates
- 3 tablespoons pure maple syrup
- 1 cup cashew butter
- 1 teaspoon vanilla extract
- 1 teaspoon cinnamon
- Cinnamon Cashew Butter Glaze
- 4 tablespoons cashew butter
- 2 tablespoons maple syrup
- ½ teaspoons cinnamon
- 2 tablespoons cacao powder
- 2 tablespoons liquid coconut oil

Direction

- Cinnamon Cashew Butter Doughnuts
- Blend the oats in a food processor until they are roughly ground (not dust-like).
- Add the dates and process until combined with the oats.
- Place cashew butter, vanilla, cinnamon and maple syrup in the food processor and pulse until the ingredients stick together in a dough-like substance.
- Firmly press the dough into the doughnut pan.
- Stick the tray in the freezer so that the doughnut can firm-up, which takes roughly fifteen minutes.
- Remove the doughnuts from the pan. They pop out pretty easily if you place a knife down the side.
- Cinnamon Cashew Butter Glaze
- Place cashew butter, vanilla, maple syrup, cacao and cinnamon in a bowl and stir to combine.
- Add in the coconut oil and stir to combine.
- Generously drizzle the glaze on top of each doughnut and place on a parchment paper-lined tray.
- Place tray in the freezer for at least 2 hours to harden before eating (if you can wait that long).

96. Classic Homemade Granola

Serving: Serves 10 | Prep: | Cook: | Ready in:

Ingredients

- 3 cups Gluten Free Rolled Oats
- 1 1/2 cups walnuts
- 1/2 cup pecans
- 1/2 cup flaked coconut
- 1/2 teaspoon kosher salt
- 2 teaspoons ground cinnamon
- 1/2 cup canola oil
- 1/2 cup maple syrup
- 1/2 cup dried tart cherries
- 1/2 cup golden raisins

Direction

- Preheat oven to 350 degrees F. Line a baking sheet with parchment.
- In a large bowl, stir together oats, walnuts, pecans, coconut, salt, and cinnamon until combined. Add the oil, and maple syrup and stir until the oats and nuts are fully coated. Spread into an even layer on the prepared baking sheet.

- Bake for about 25 minutes, stirring after 15. Add the dried fruit. Stir it in and bake for 5 additional minutes. The granola should be fragrant, golden brown and toasted. Cool completely on pan. May be stored in an airtight container (I used zipper bags) for up to 2 weeks at room temperature.

97. Coco Ginger Hazelnut Oatmeal

Serving: Serves 4 | Prep: | Cook: |Ready in:

Ingredients

- 1/4 cup hazelnuts
- 1 cup rolled oats
- 2 cups water
- 1 teaspoon grated fresh ginger root
- 2 tablespoons chia seeds
- 1-2 tablespoons maple syrup
- 1/4 cup almond milk or light coconut milk

Direction

- Toast and chop hazelnuts. In a baking sheet, lay hazelnuts in toaster oven and toast for 2-3 minutes, until skins begin to blister and hazelnuts become a light golden brown. Or toast in oven at 350 for 10-15 minutes. Remove from heat and let cool. Wrap in a clean, dry kitchen towel and rub hazelnuts until all skins fall off. Roughly chop skinned hazelnuts.
- In a medium saucepan, bring water and oats to a boil.
- Reduce heat to medium, add ginger, chia seeds, coconut, hazelnuts, and maple syrup. Cook for about 5 minutes until thick and creamy. Add almond milk and stir for about a minute, until heated through.
- Serve, and top with a bit more chopped hazelnuts and coconut for garnish. Enjoy!

98. Coconut Cranberry Muffins

Serving: Makes 15 | Prep: | Cook: |Ready in:

Ingredients

- 8 egg whites
- 1/2 cup plain, nonfat Greek yogurt
- 1/2 cup honey
- 1/2 cup coconut oil
- 1 cup coconut flour
- 1/2 cup Gluten Free oat flour
- 1/2 teaspoon sea salt
- 1/2 cup reduced sugar craisins
- 2 teaspoons baking soda
- 2 teaspoons hemp seed hearts for sprinkling

Direction

- Preheat oven 350 degrees
- In a large bowl or stand mixer, add egg whites & whisk quickly until fluffy
- To the eggs, add Greek yogurt, honey, coconut oil & sea salt and stir to combine
- Add baking soda, oat flour and coconut flour
- Gently fold into batter to combine, do not over mix
- Add craisins & combine gently
- Add muffin liners to a muffin tin or spray with cooking spray
- Add batter to muffin cavities
- Top with sprinkles of hemp seeds
- Bake 25 minutes then remove muffin tin from oven
- Allow muffins to cool in the tin 20 minutes prior to removing & enjoying

99. Coconut Lemon Bombs No Bake Cookies

Serving: Makes 12-14 | Prep: 0hours0mins | Cook: 0hours0mins |Ready in:

Ingredients

- 1 cup cashews
- 1/3 cup buckwheat grouts
- 1/3 cup old fashioned rolled oats
- 1/4 cup unsweetened shredded coconut
- juice of one lemon
- 7-8 medjool dates, pitted and chopped
- 1/4 - 1/2 cups shredded coconut, for rolling

Direction

- Place cashews, buckwheat groats and/or oats in food processor and blend until a medium to fine grind (doesn't have to be perfect). The buckwheat may stay a bit chunky so if you're looking for a smooth center use all oats.
- Add rest of ingredients and blend until combined and you have a doughy consistency. If you find your dough is a bit too dry try adding fresh squeezed lemon juice, 1 tablespoon at a time.
- Chill dough for about 20-30 minutes.
- Roll into 1 inch balls then roll in coconut flakes.
- Store in air tight container in refrigerator for up to two weeks.

100. Coconut Mango Oatmeal

Serving: Serves 1 | Prep: | Cook: | Ready in:

Ingredients

- 1/2 cup rolled oats, gluten-free preferred
- 1/2 cup full-fat coconut milk
- 1/2 cup water
- 1 pinch salt
- 1/2 teaspoon honey, or agave if vegan
- 1/2 cup diced fresh mango
- 1 tablespoon coconut butter
- 1 tablespoon unsweetened shredded coconut, lightly toasted
- 1 tablespoon chopped, unsalted cashews, lightly toasted

Direction

- Add the oats, coconut milk, and water to a saucepan. Bring to a boil, then reduce heat to a simmer and cook for 8-10 minutes, stirring often. Cook until oats have softened and desired consistency is reached.
- Remove oats from the heat, sprinkle in the pinch of salt. Stir in the 1/2 teaspoon of honey and tablespoon of coconut butter.
- Pour into a bowl and top with mango, coconut flakes, and cashews. Enjoy!

101. Coconut Mocha Oat Cookies

Serving: Makes 3-4 dozen | Prep: | Cook: | Ready in:

Ingredients

- 3/4 cup coconut oil, softened
- 1-3/4 cups light brown sugar
- 2 eggs
- 2 cups whole wheat pastry flour
- 2 tablespoons oat bran
- 3 tablespoons stong brewed coffee or espresso, cooled
- 2 cups semisweet or other nondairy chocolate chips
- 1/4 cup coconut milk
- 1 cup hazelnuts or macadamia nuts, toasted and chopped (optional)
- 2 teaspoons baking soda
- 1 teaspoon cinnamon
- 4 cups oats

Direction

- Preheat oven to 375 and grease cookie sheets or line with parchment paper.
- Cream softened coconut oil, sugar and coconut milk together, then add eggs and beat well.
- In a large bowl, sift together flour, baking soda, and oat bran. Mix in the wet ingredients, then stir in coffee, chocolate chips, oats and nuts.

- Scoop out 2 tablespoon-sized portions of cookies, spacing them out on the cookie sheets and slightly pressing them flat. Bake 14-18 min or until lightly golden. Let cool and serve!

102. Coconut Quinoa Porridge With Berry Compote

Serving: Makes 4 servings | Prep: | Cook: | Ready in:

Ingredients

- Porridge
- 1 cup oats
- 1/2 cup quinoa
- 6 cups coconut water
- 1 pinch salt
- Compote
- 3 cups mixed berries, such as strawberries, raspberries, blueberries and blackberries
- 1 teaspoon sweetener, such as coconut sugar
- 1 teaspoon vanilla

Direction

- Porridge
- Measure the oats and quinoa and place into a medium sized saucepan.
- Add the coconut water.
- Bring the porridge to a simmer over a low heat.
- Allow to simmer for 10-15 minutes, stirring frequently. It's ready when the porridge is smooth and you can see the quinoa grains starting to open up.
- Compote
- If using strawberries, cut them in half so they're about the same size as the other berries.
- Combine the berries, sweetener, and vanilla in a medium sized saucepan.
- Heat the berries slowly over a low flame.
- Allow to simmer for 10-15 minutes, stirring frequently. It's ready when the compote has created a sauce, but you can still see some whole berries.
- Top the porridge with compote, then drizzle with maple syrup or your favorite sweetener. Leftover porridge and compote can be stored in the fridge for a few days. To reheat the porridge, just add a little bit of extra water and reheat on the stove.

103. Coconut Stovetop Oats With Avocado, Chia, And Almond Butter

Serving: Makes 1 bowl | Prep: 0hours0mins | Cook: 0hours0mins | Ready in:

Ingredients

- 1/2 cup oats
- 3/4 cup coconut milk
- 1 tablespoon chia seeds
- 1/2 avocado, sliced
- 1/2 tablespoon almond butter
- Sprinkle of coconut flakes
- Dash of cinnamon

Direction

- Combine 1/2 cup oats cooked with 3/4 cup coconut milk over stovetop. Bring to a boil, then stir until oats are softened.
- Add in 1 tablespoon chia seeds and 1 tablespoon almond butter once oats are cooked.
- Transfer ingredients into a bowl, and top beautifully with the sliced avocado, sprinkle of coconut flakes, and a dash of cinnamon (and a little drizzle of almond butter).

104. Coconut Fig Chunks Of Energy

Serving: Makes 40 pieces | Prep: | Cook: | Ready in:

Ingredients

- 30 dried figs, stems removed
- 5 dried dates, pitted
- 1/2 cup walnuts, roughly shopped
- 2 tablespoons unsweetened shredded coconut, plus additional for rolling
- 3 tablespoons whole grain oats
- 3 tablespoons smooth almond butter
- 2 teaspoons dairy-free dark chocolate chips
- 1 teaspoon ground flax seeds
- 1 1/2 teaspoons vanilla extract
- dash of salt

Direction

- Line a 9×9 baking pan or loaf pan with parchment paper, allowing enough for overhang on the two larger sides. Set aside.
- Using a kitchen mixer, such as a Cuisinart fitted with a blade attachment, add the figs, dates, walnuts, 2 tablespoons coconut, oats, almond butter, chocolate chips, flax feeds, vanilla extract and salt. Mix on high for 1-2 minutes until well blended. The mixture should resemble coarse sand.
- Place the mixture into the prepared pan. Using a small glass or jar, press the mixture firmly and evenly making it as flat and uniform as possible.
- Refrigerate for 1 hour to set.
- To finish the power bites, place about 1/2 cup of shredded coconut on a small plate and set aside.
- Gently lift the parchment paper out of the pan and place on a cutting board. Using a slicer knife, cut into small, 1-inch squares. Roll the bites in shredded coconut evenly to coat.
- Store the power bites in an airtight container in the refrigerator. They should keep fresh for up to two weeks.

105. Cornflake Crunch Granola

Serving: Makes 8 cups | Prep: 0hours15mins | Cook: 0hours35mins | Ready in:

Ingredients

- Cornflake Crunch
- 3 cups cornflakes
- 5 tablespoons unsalted butter – melted
- 1 1/2 tablespoons dark brown sugar – packed
- Granola
- 3 cups old fashioned oats
- 1 1/2 cups slivered almonds
- 3/4 cup unsweetened coconut chips
- 1/4 cup dark brown sugar – packed
- 2 teaspoons cinnamon
- 1/4 cup vegetable oil
- 1/4 cup maple syrup
- 2 teaspoons vanilla extract
- 3/4 teaspoon salt

Direction

- Preheat your oven to 300°F. First, make the cornflake crunch: grab a baking sheet and line it with foil. Add the cornflakes and crush them up with your hands. Melt the butter in a small bowl, then stir in the brown sugar. Pour the mixture onto the cornflakes and toss to coat.
- In a large bowl, combine the oats, almonds, coconut, brown sugar, and cinnamon. In a separate bowl, combine the oil, maple syrup, vanilla, and salt. Pour the wet mixture onto the dry ingredients, then stir to combine. Pour onto a separate foil lined baking sheet and pop both trays into the oven. Bake the cornflake crunch until golden, about 15 min. Bake the granola for 35-40 min, stirring a few times along the way.
- Let both cool off, mix them together, then store in a big container or Ziploc.

106. Cozy Banana Bread Pancakes

Serving: Makes 9-11 | Prep: | Cook: |Ready in:

Ingredients

- 1 cup Gluten Free Oats
- 1/2 cup Hazelnuts, toasted
- 1 teaspoon baking powder
- 1   Ripe Banana
- 1 tablespoon Ground Flax
- 1 cup Unsweetened Almond Milk
- 1 pint Sea Salt
- 1 pinch Vanilla or Cinnamon

Direction

- In a food processor grind the oats into a finely ground flour. Once they are ground, set them aside and grind the hazelnuts into a flour. Add the oat flour back into the food processor along with the salt, banana, flax, milk, hazelnuts, and the optional flavour (cinnamon, vanilla, etc.). Puree the mixture until fully incorporated.
- Set a pan onto medium heat to warm up. Once the pan is warm, add a tsp. of coconut oil, or oil of choice, to coat the bottom. Spoon pancakes into pan (about 2 Tbsp. of batter per pancake) and cook until bubbles form on the top, flip and cook the other side until brown. Because these pancakes are made with oats, they will take a bit longer to cook then ones made with flour, so sit down, brew something warm, pull out a crossword, and relax. It is the weekend after all.

107. Crab Apple Steel Cut Oatmeal

Serving: Serves 4-6 | Prep: | Cook: |Ready in:

Ingredients

- 1 cup steel-cut oats
- 4 cups water
- Pinch salt
- 1   banana, mashed or thinly sliced
- 4-5   crab apples, cored and medium dice
- 1 teaspoon cinnamon
- 1/4 teaspoon ground clove
- 1/4 teaspoon nutmeg
- 1/4 teaspoon allspice
- 1/2 cup raisins and/or goji berries
- 1/2 cup chopped pecans or whole pumpkin seeds
- grass fed milk or almond milk, to serve

Direction

- Bring water, oats and salt to a boil in a covered medium-sized saucepan. Once to a boil, uncover and cook at boiling for about 2 minutes and then turn heat to low.
- Add the crab apples and banana. Cook for 15 minutes, then add spices and raisins. Cook another 10 minutes, or until oats are cooked and most of the water is absorbed. Turn off the heat and stir in nuts.
- Serve with milk or almond milk and enjoy warm.

108. Cracklin' Oat Bran Granola

Serving: Makes 4 to 6 servings | Prep: | Cook: |Ready in:

Ingredients

- 175 grams Cracklin' Oat Bran cereal
- 40 grams unsweetened coconut flakes
- 55 grams sliced almonds
- 2 tablespoons olive oil
- 2 tablespoons coconut oil
- 1 pinch salt
- 1 1/2 teaspoons honey or agave nectar
- 60 grams crystallized ginger, chopped

Direction

- Preheat the oven to 300° F and line a baking sheet with parchment paper. Using a knife or your hands, break the Cracklin' Oat Bran squares into uneven pieces, leaving some whole or halved and breaking others into lentil-sized pieces or smaller.
- Mix the cereal with the coconut and almonds.
- In a small saucepan over low heat, heat the olive oil and coconut oil with the salt and honey until melted.
- Pour the liquid over the cereal and nuts and stir to coat. Spread evenly on the prepared baking sheet.
- Bake for 20 minutes, until the cereal has darkened and feels dry to the touch. Mix in the chopped crystallized ginger.
- Allow to cool, then eat with milk or cereal (or by the handful). Store in an airtight container for up to 1 week.

109. Cranberry Ginger Granola

Serving: Makes 4.5 cups | Prep: | Cook: | Ready in:

Ingredients

- 2 cups old fashioned oats
- 1/2 cup unroasted pumpkin seeds
- 1/2 cup sliced almonds
- 1/2 cup shredded coconut
- 1/2 cup dried cranberries
- 1/2 cup crystallized ginger
- 1/2 cup coconut oil
- 1/2 cup agave syrup
- 10 cardamom pods (or 1 tsp ground)
- 1/2 teaspoon cinnamon
- 1/8 teaspoon allspice
- 1/8 teaspoon salt

Direction

- Warm the oil, syrup, and spices in a small pan. If using cardamom pods, crush them first to open them up.
- Combine the oats, pumpkin seeds, almonds, and coconut in a large bowl.
- Stir in the oil/syrup mixture, straining it if you used cardamom pods. Mix together until it's combined. You don't want to soak the oats, so add the wet ingredients in two or three parts to coat well each time.
- Bake at 300 until golden brown, stirring occasionally. This will take roughly an hour, but remember that it will continue to bake a bit longer once you pull it out of the oven so you don't want to let it get too dark.
- Let cool, then add in the cranberries and chopped ginger.
- Store in an airtight container.
- Enjoy!

110. Cranberry White Chocolate Oatmeal Cookies

Serving: Makes 4 dozen cookies | Prep: | Cook: | Ready in:

Ingredients

- dry mixture
- 3 cups old-fashioned rolled oats
- 1 cup all-purpose flour
- 1 teaspoon baking soda
- 1 teaspoon baking powder
- 1/2 teaspoon ground cinnamon
- 1/2 teaspoon salt
- wet mixture
- 1 cup room temperature unsalted butter
- 1 cup granulated sugar
- 1 cup light-brown sugar
- 2 large eggs
- 1 teaspoon vanilla extract
- 1 cup dried cranberries
- 11 ounces white chocolate chips

Direction

- Preheat oven to 350 degrees F.

- Whisk together oats, flour, baking soda, baking powder, cinnamon, and salt in a large bowl; set aside.
- Put butter, granulated and light-brown sugars in the bowl of an electric mixer fitted with the paddle attachment. Mix on medium speed until pale and fluffy, about 5 minutes.
- Mix in eggs, one at a time and vanilla.
- Reduce speed to low. Add oat mixture; mix until just combined.
- Stir in cranberries and white chocolate chips.
- Using a table spoon or ice cream scoop, drop dough onto baking sheets lined with parchment paper, spacing 2 inches apart.
- Bake until golden and just set, about 14 minutes. Let cool on sheets about 3 minutes.
- Transfer cookies to racks using a spatula; let cool completely.
- Cookies can be stored in airtight containers at room temperature and shared with old friends.

111. Cranberry And White Chocolate Streusel Bars

Serving: Makes 24 bars | Prep: | Cook: | Ready in:

Ingredients

- Cranberry and White Chocolate Streusel Bars
- 1 cup butter, softened and cut into bits
- 2 cups flour
- 2/3 cup oats
- 1/2 cup sugar
- 2 egg yolks
- 1 set of Cranberry filling from 8 oz fresh cranberries (recipe below)
- 1/3 cup chopped walnuts
- 1/3 cup white chocolate chips
- Cranberry Filling
- 8 ounces (2 ½ cups) fresh cranberries
- 2/3 cup sugar
- 3 tablespoons water

Direction

- Preheat oven to 350F. Butter a 7×11 inch pan.
- Prepare the cranberry filling first. - In a medium sized saucepan, place all the ingredients. Then, over medium-high heat, cook the ingredients until boiling. Continue to boil the filling until it becomes thick and syrup, about 5 minutes. Remove from heat and let cool while you make the shortbread.
- In a food processor, mix flour, oats and sugar 10 seconds.
- Add 1 cup butter; mix until mixture forms a ball.
- Set aside ½ cup of mixture.
- Mix in yolks.
- Press yolk mixture into pay. Spread with cranberry filling. Sprinkle walnuts and chocolate chips, then press into dough. Form pea-sizes crumbs with reserved dough mixture, sprinkle over top.
- Bake at 350F until topping is pale gold, about 45 minutes. Cool on rack and cut into 24 bars.

112. Cranberry Cinnamon Baked Oatmeal Topped With Warm Berries And Honey

Serving: Serves 1 | Prep: | Cook: | Ready in:

Ingredients

- 3/4 cup Quaker oats
- 1 cup almond milk
- 2/3 cup Dehydrated cranberries
- 1 tablespoon Cinnamon
- 2 tablespoons Brown sugar
- 1 teaspoon vanilla extract
- 1/2 cup Fresh Berries medley
- 1-2 tablespoons Honey

Direction

- Preheat Oven to 375

- Combine Oats, cinnamon, brown sugar, cranberries in a bowl and mix
- Add almond milk and vanilla and mix well
- Put in an oven safe bowl (Lightly greased to prevent sticking) and bake for 30-40 minutes
- Pull out of oven and flip on serving plate (Let bowl cool to touch in order to prevent burn injury)
- Warm fresh berries medley in a sauce pan until a little juicy
- Top oatmeal with juicy fresh berries medley and drizzle with honey
- Serve warm. Feel free to add some eggnog or warm milk if you want but I wanted just a simple bounty of healthiness this morning!

113. Cranberry Oat Pecan Bread

Serving: Makes 1 loaf | Prep: | Cook: | Ready in:

Ingredients

- 1 cup all-purpose flour
- 3/4 cup whole-wheat flour
- 1 teaspoon baking soda
- 1 teaspoon baking powder
- 1/2 teaspoon salt
- 1/2 teaspoon cinnamon
- 1 egg
- 1 cup milk (low-fat is OK)
- 1 cup old-fashioned oats
- 1/2 cup pure maple syrup
- 1/4 cup light brown sugar (packed)
- 6 tablespoons butter, melted
- 1 cup fresh or frozen cranberries, chopped (if frozen, do not thaw them)
- 1 cup pecans, toasted and chopped
- Demarara sugar, for sprinkling on top of the bread

Direction

- Preheat the oven to 350. Grease a loaf pan. Nut toasting tip: while the oven is heating, put the pecans on a flat baking dish or piece of foil to toast for about 10 minutes (they will be done when you begin to smell them, but be careful not to let them burn).
- In a medium bowl, combine the flours, baking soda and powder, salt and cinnamon.
- In a large bowl, beat the egg until white and yolk are combined. Stir in the milk, oats, maple syrup, brown sugar and melted butter, mixing just to blend completely. Stir in the cranberries and pecans.
- Scrape the batter into the greased loaf pan. Sprinkle the top with demerara sugar if you wish. Bake the bread for 1 hour, or until a tester inserted in the middle comes out clean.
- Cool to room temperature before slicing.

114. Crispy Crunchy Oatmeal Cookies

Serving: Makes about 3 dozen small cookies | Prep: 0hours0mins | Cook: 0hours0mins | Ready in:

Ingredients

- 1 cup all-purpose flour
- 3/4 teaspoon baking powder
- 1/2 teaspoon baking soda
- 1 teaspoon kosher salt
- 1/4 teaspoon cinnamon
- 14 tablespoons unsalted butter, at room temperature
- 1 cup sugar
- 1/4 cup packed light brown sugar
- 1 large egg
- 1 teaspoon vanilla extract
- 2 1/2 cups old fashioned rolled oats

Direction

- Heat the oven to 350° F and arrange a rack in the middle of the oven. Line two baking sheets with parchment paper.

- In a medium bowl, whisk together the flour, baking powder, baking soda, salt, and cinnamon. Set aside.
- In the bowl of a standing mixer, or using handheld beaters, cream the butter and the two sugars until light and fluffy, 3 to 5 minutes. Scrape down the sides of the bowl, add the egg and beat until incorporated, about 30 seconds. Scrape down the bowl and do the same with the vanilla.
- On low speed, add the flour mixture and beat until just combined. Remove the bowl from the mixer and fold in the oats by hand, mixing just until there are no remaining flour pockets.
- Form balls out of tablespoon-sized pieces of dough and place them 2 inches apart on the parchment-lined cookie sheets. Bake one sheet at a time for about 15 minutes, rotating once for even cooking. Let the cookies cool completely on the baking sheets for maximum crispness. The cookies will keep in an airtight container for a week.

115. Crispy Oatmeal Chocolate Chip Cookies

Serving: Makes about 5 dozen small cookies | Prep: 0hours20mins | Cook: 0hours10mins | Ready in:

Ingredients

- 1 1/4 cups all-purpose flour
- 1 teaspoon kosher salt
- 1 teaspoon baking soda
- 1 teaspoon ground cinnamon
- 1/4 teaspoon freshly ground nutmeg
- 1/8 teaspoon allspice
- 2   sticks unsalted butter, softened
- 1 cup packed light brown sugar
- 1/2 cup granulated sugar
- 1   large egg
- 1 teaspoon vanilla extract
- 3 cups rolled oats
- 2 cups semisweet chocolate chips or chunks

Direction

- Heat the oven to 375 degrees F. In a medium bowl, whisk together the flour, salt, baking soda and spices. Set aside.
- In the bowl of a standing mixer, cream the butter and two sugars until light and fluffy, about 3 minutes. Add the egg and vanilla and beat until combined, scraping down the sides of the bowl once. Add the flour and spices in three additions, beating until just combined and scraping down the sides of the bowl after each addition. Do not overbeat!
- Stir in the oats and the chocolate chips, distributing evenly. Drop the dough in heaping tablespoons on parchment-lined baking sheets, keeping the cookies at least 2 inches apart. Flatten gently with the back of a spoon and bake for about 10 minutes, rotating the baking sheets halfway through. The cookies are done when they turn lightly golden around the edges, and the tops look almost dry. Cool on the baking sheets for a minute, then transfer to wire racks to cool completely. The cookies are best still slightly warm, but you can successfully store them in an airtight container for up to a few days.

116. Crunchies

Serving: Makes 8-12 pieces | Prep: | Cook: | Ready in:

Ingredients

- 1 cup shredded coconut
- 1 cup oats
- 1/2 cup brown sugar
- 1 cup cake flour
- 2 tablespoons golden syrup
- 2 teaspoons soda bicarb
- 5 ounces butter

Direction

- Mix dry ingredients-coconut, oats, sugar, flour, salt.
- Boil butter and syrup
- Add soda bicarb.
- Add dry ingredients.
- Mix well.
- Press on to a flat baking tray.
- Bake for 15 mins in a preheated oven at 180C until golden brown.

117. Crunchy Berry Breakfast Granola

Serving: Makes 3 cups | Prep: | Cook: | Ready in:

Ingredients

- 1.5 cups Rolled Oats
- 1/3 cup Dried Berries
- 2 tablespoons Chia Seeds
- 1 teaspoon Orange Zest
- 1 teaspoon Vanilla extract
- 1/2 teaspoon Cinnamon Powder
- 35 grams Slivered Almonds
- 20 grams Unsalted Butter
- 45 milliliters Agave Nectar
- Pinch Salt

Direction

- Line a baking tray with parchment/ baking paper and keep aside. Preheat the oven to 150C for at least 10 minutes.
- Meanwhile mix oats, slivered almonds, dried berries and chia seeds in a bowl and keep aside.
- In another bowl mix melted butter, vanilla extract, orange zest, cinnamon powder, salt and agave nectar and whisk it well to ensure all the ingredients are well incorporated.
- Now pour the wet ingredients into the dry ingredients and with the spoon mix it so that no clumps are formed. I like using my hands and making sure all the elements are well coated and no lumps are formed.

- Now transfer the mixture on to the baking tray and spread out evenly. Put it in the oven and bake at 150C for 18 -20 minutes.
- After 10 minutes take the baking tray out and using a spoon stir the entire mixture so that nothing is overdone or burnt. Put it back in the oven.
- Once done take out the baking sheet from the oven. The mixture won't be crunchy now. Allow it to cool.
- As the mixture cools, it becomes crunchy. Transfer it to an airtight container and you can store it up to 2 weeks in the fridge.

118. Crunchy Pistachio Date Granola

Serving: Makes 6 cups | Prep: | Cook: | Ready in:

Ingredients

- 2 1/2 cups rolled oats
- 1 cup roasted shelled pistachios
- 1/2 cup sunflower seeds
- 2 tablespoons flax seeds
- 1 cup sweetened flaked coconut
- 1/2 teaspoon kosher salt
- 1/3 cup orange blossom or citrus-y honey
- 1/3 cup extra virgin olive oil or canola oil
- 1/2 cup brown sugar
- 1 cup finely chopped pitted dates

Direction

- Preheat the oven to 300 degrees. Line 2 large baking sheets with parchment paper and set aside.
- In a large bowl combine the oats, pistachios, sunflower seeds, flax seeds, coconut and salt. Mix well and set aside.
- In a small saucepan, combine the honey, oil, and brown sugar and heat over medium high heat, stirring occasionally until mixture comes to a rolling boil and the sugar is dissolved. Pour the honey mixture over the oats and stir

until thoroughly combined. Add the dates and mix well.

- Divide the granola between the two sheet pans and spread it out into a single layer. Bake for 10 minutes, stir the granola and arrange in a single layer again.
- Bake for a second 10 minutes and stir. Spread the granola into a single layer and bake for an additional 5-10 minutes until golden brown.
- Add the dates to the granola and toss to combine. Let cool to room temperature until dry and crisp. Store in an airtight container.

119. D.U.M.P. (Don't. Underestimate. My. Peach.) Cake

Serving: Serves 12 | Prep: | Cook: | Ready in:

Ingredients

- 8-10 fully ripe (almost past their prime) peaches
- 1 cup peach nectar
- 1/2-1 cups water
- 1 cup sugar
- 2 cups flour
- 1 teaspoon baking soda
- 1 teaspoon salt
- 1 teaspoon each of cardamon, clove & fresh grated nutmeg
- 1 tablespoon cinnamon
- 1 cup buttermilk
- 1 1/2 sticks of butter, melted
- 1 cup oats
- 1/4 cup brown sugar
- 2 tablespoons melted butter
- 3 tablespoons maple syrup (the best quality you have)
- 1/4 cup pecan pieces
- 1/2 cup heavy cream
- 3 tablespoons maple syrup
- 1 teaspoon cardamon

Direction

- Slice peaches into thick pieces. I usually quarter and then cut each quarter into 3 or 4 slices, depending on your size.
- Butter or spray a 9 x 13 pan. Line the bottom of the pan with overlapping peaches--you don't have to get fancy--it won't be seen as this is a cobbler like consistency and it will get scooped out of the pan! You just want more than enough peaches so there is peach in every bite! Mix nectar and water together, and make sure there is enough liquid covering the peaches.
- If it is winter and you weren't able to can or freeze Mrs.Wheelbarrow's peaches....then you may substitute 2 cans of peach slices with juices and skip the peach nectar/water.
- Mix sugar, flour, baking soda, salt, spices and butter milk together, add 3/4 of the melted butter. Mixture will be very thick. Spoon on top of peaches, smoothing around. Pour remaining melted butter on top of cake mix.
- Make crumble by combining oats, brown sugar, maple syrup with 2 t. of melted butter. Sprinkle on top of cake mix. Sprinkle pecans on top.
- Bake at 350 for 30-35 minutes or until golden brown and bubbly.
- To serve maple-cardamom whipped cream. Put metal mixing bowl and metal wire whisk attachment in freezer for 15 minutes. Add COLD whipping cream, cardamom and maple syrup to bowl, whip until stiff.

120. Date And Walnut Oatcakes

Serving: Makes 12 | Prep: | Cook: | Ready in:

Ingredients

- 2 cups rolled oats
- 1 1/3 all-purpose, spelt, or whole wheat pastry flour (use gluten-free certified oat flour to make the recipe gluten-free)

- 1/2 teaspoon baking powder
- 1/2 teaspoon salt
- 1 teaspoon ground cinnamon
- 1 teaspoon ground ginger
- 1/2 cup chopped walnuts
- 2/3 cup pitted and chopped medjool dates
- 1/2 cup almond milk
- 1/4 cup grapeseed oil (or canola oil, or safflower oil, or melted coconut oil)
- 1/2 cup applesauce
- 1/2 cup maple syrup

Direction

- Preheat your oven to 350° F. Lightly oil 8 muffin cups. Place the oats, oat flour, baking powder, salt, cinnamon, ginger, walnuts, and dates into a large mixing bowl and whisk them all together.
- Whisk together the almond milk, oil, applesauce, and syrup in a separate, medium-sized bowl. Pour these wet ingredients into the dry ingredients and mix evenly. Scoop the mixture by the 1/3 cup into your prepared muffin cups. Bake for 12- to 18 minutes, or until the cakes are lightly golden. Serve.

121. Date Squares (revamped)

Serving: Makes 8x8" pan | Prep: | Cook: | Ready in:

Ingredients

- 1/2 cup coconut oil
- 1/2 cup brown sugar (I think you could cut the sugar down and it would work fine)
- 1 cup flour (all-purpose or whole wheat)
- 1/2 cup wheat germ
- 1/2 cup oat bran
- 1/4 cup rolled oats
- 1/4 cup steel cut oats
- 1 teaspoon salt
- 1 egg, large
- 1 cup toasted hazelnuts, chopped
- 10 ounces dates, medjool if possible (I weighed before I pitted them)
- 1/2 cup water

Direction

- Combine coconut oil, sugar, flour, wheat germ, oats, oat bran and salt in large bowl of a mixer and mix until a crumbly dough forms. Add hazelnuts and stir to combine. Set aside approximately 1 cup of mixture.
- To remaining dough add the egg and beat until dough holds together somewhat. It will look like cookie dough. Press into an 8 x 8" pan lined with parchment and set aside.
- Pit and coarsely chop dates. Cook with water over medium heat until a chunky, very thick jam forms. Spread over top of dough in pan.
- Sprinkle remaining dough over dates and bake in a 350F over for about 30 min. A skewer will come out clean when done. Cool and cut into bars.

122. Dates And Oats Indian Milk Pudding/Kheer

Serving: Serves 3 | Prep: | Cook: | Ready in:

Ingredients

- 1/2 cup Rolled oats
- 1/4 cup Jaggery (unrefined cane sugar)/sugar
- 2 cups Milk
- 10 Dates
- 1/2 teaspoon Cardamom powder
- 10 Almonds for blending
- 10 Almonds for garnishing
- 1 teaspoon Ghee/Clarified butter

Direction

- Soak whole almonds in hot water for about 15 to 20 minutes or give one boil to the water and let the almonds steep in it for about 15

minutes. After 15 minutes, peel the almonds. Chop about half of them (around 10).
- Deseed dates and keep about 4 to 5 for garnishing. Place the rest of the peeled almonds (about 10) and 5 to 6 pitted dates in a blender jar and make a fine paste with a little milk.
- In a saucepan, roast the oats on medium high heat, stirring continuously till you get a nutty aroma; about 2 to 3 minutes. Tip in the milk and the ground almonds-date paste (rinse the jar with additional milk) into the pan and bring to a boil on medium high heat.
- When the jaggery has completely melted into the pudding/kheer, add the cardamom powder, stir and remove from heat. In a small saucepan, heat ghee and roast the chopped almonds till light golden brown. Stir into the cooked pudding/kheer.
- Serve delectable dates and oats kheer piping hot, warm or cold with additional nuts and chopped dates sprinkled on top. Kheer thickens as it cools, so feel free to add more milk when needed.
- Instead of oats, you can use rice or broken wheat/bulgur instead. Rice will need more time to cook. Feel free to add any variety of nuts in this pudding.
- If you do not have jaggery, use brown sugar or plain sugar. For a vegan option, use coconut milk instead.

123. Double Chocolate Banana Muffins

Serving: Makes 12 | Prep: | Cook: |Ready in:

Ingredients

- 1 cup Raw Almonds
- heaping 1/2 cups Gluten Free Rolled Oats
- 2 eggs
- 2 Really Ripe Bananas
- 4-5 tablespoons Real Maple Syrup (more or less depending on how sweet you want your muffins)
- 3 tablespoons Milk (I use 2% but you could use non dairy)
- 2 tablespoons Dark Cocoa Powder
- 1 teaspoon Pure Vanilla Extract
- 1 teaspoon Baking Powder
- 1/2 teaspoon Cinnamon
- 1/2 cup Mini Chocolate Chips plus more for tops

Direction

- Preheat oven to 350 Degrees.
- Add the almonds to the bowl of a food processor and grind until you get a coarse meal.
- Next add the oats and pulse a few times to incorporate. The almonds and the oats will be your "flour".
- Then add the rest of the ingredients except the chocolate chips. Process until combined and smooth.
- Add mini chocolate chips and pulse only 3 times to mix in, you don't want to break them up too much.
- Prepare a muffin tin with liners or grease well. I like the coconut oil spray from Trader Joe's if I don't have liners.
- Using a 1/4 cup measuring cup fill the lined or greased muffin tins. Then top with extra mini chips if desired.
- Bake for 25 minutes and test to see if toothpick comes out clean. If not put back in for 2 minute increments until the toothpick comes out clean.
- Allow to cool completely before storing. I store these in an airtight container on the counter or pop then into the freezer in a zip lock!
- Enjoy!

124. Double Toasted Coconut Oatmeal Shortbreads

Serving: Makes about 44 cookies | Prep: | Cook: |Ready in:

Ingredients

- 1 3/4 cups rolled oats
- 1 1/4 cups all-purpose flour
- 1 cup unsweetened shredded coconut
- 16 tablespoons (2 sticks) butter, softened
- 1/2 cup turbinado sugar
- 1 teaspoon salt

Direction

- Preheat the oven to 325° F convection (or 350° F for a regular oven).
- Spread the oats out on a baking tray and toast in the oven for about 10 minutes. Let the oats cool completely and then process in a food processor, until powdery.
- Spread the coconut out on a baking tray and toast in the oven until golden and crunchy, for about 8 minutes, stirring once or twice. Allow to cool completely.
- Beat the butter with sugar until creamy. Stir in the oats, flour, coconut and salt. Mix on low speed until the dough comes together. Scrape the dough out onto a work surface and pat it into two logs, about 1 1/4 inches in diameter. Wrap the logs up in plastic wrap and refrigerate until very firm, at least two hours.
- Preheat the oven to 325°F convection (or 350°F regular bake). Slice the dough into 1/4-inch thick slices and arrange on a baking sheet lined with parchment paper. Prick the top of the shortbreads with a fork. Bake for about 20 minutes, or until golden. Slide the parchment onto a wire rack and let the shortbreads cool.
- The shortbreads can be kept in an airtight container for about a week.

125. Easiest Ever Banana Bread

Serving: Serves 10 | Prep: | Cook: |Ready in:

Ingredients

- 3 small bananas
- 1/2 cup grapeseed or canola oil
- 3 eggs
- 1/2 cup milk
- 1 cup brown sugar
- 1 cup whole wheat or plain flour
- 1 cup oat bran
- 1 tablespoon baking powder
- 1 tablespoon cinammon
- 1 teaspoon vanilla extract

Direction

- Heat the oven to 350 degrees F, and butter a 5-by-9-inch loaf pan. In a separate bowl mix the dry ingredients. Breaking down the pieces of brown sugar, add the flour and oat bran, the baking powder and the cinnamon.
- In a mixing bowl mash the bananas and add all the liquids (beaten eggs, oil, milk and vanilla) and mix by hand with a fork, you want this mush to have a bit of consistency.
- In a separate bowl mix the dry ingredients. Breaking down the pieces of brown sugar, add the flour and oat bran, the baking powder and the cinnamon.
- Combine the liquids (banana mush) with the flour by hand and transfer to the cake pan. The final consistency should be sticky, but you can add a bit more milk if you find it too hard. Bake for 35-40 minutes et voila!

126. Energy Pretzel Bites (adapted From Pinch Of Yum)

Serving: Serves 25 bites | Prep: | Cook: |Ready in:

Ingredients

- 1 1/2 cups rolled oats
- 1 1/2 cups pretzels
- 1/4 cup chia seeds
- 1/2 cup coconut oil (melted)
- 1/4 cup maple syrup
- 1/2 cup toasted coconut (for topping)
- 1/2 cup nuttela (melted)
- 1/2 cup peanut butter (melted)

Direction

- Place the pretzels in a Ziploc bag and crush with a rolling pin until broken into small bits.
- Place the oats in the processor and pulse until smooth. Then add in the pretzel and pulse together. The mixture should be crushed, ground like texture.
- In a small bowl, mix all ingredients together until combine.
- Dip the bites into melted Nutella chocolate and sprinkle toasted coconut over.
- Chill in the freezer for 20 minutes before serving.
- Bites can be kept in a sealed plastic container in the refrigerator

127. Everyday Banana Porridge

Serving: Serves 1 | Prep: | Cook: | Ready in:

Ingredients

- 3 handfuls oats
- 2 tablespoons buckwheat porridge
- 1 tablespoon cacao powder
- 1 tablespoon dried coconut
- 1 banana
- 1 handful chopped nuts of your choice (I used walnuts)
- cinnamon
- 1 tablespoon peanut butter (optional)

Direction

- In a pan or a small pot, pour boiling water over the oats (water has to cover the oats completely, I usually pour more water after the oats have cooked for a while).
- After the oats have soaked the water a bit (about 5 mins), add the buckwheat porridge, ground coconut, chopped banana, walnuts and cinnamon. Pour more water if it is too thick. Stir and let it cook for about 3 mins.
- After achieving creamy consistency, pour into a bowl and add a tablespoon of peanut butter. Enjoy!

128. Everything Breakfast Cookies

Serving: Makes 32 | Prep: | Cook: | Ready in:

Ingredients

- 5 cups rolled oats (not quick cooking)
- 1/2 cup ground flax
- 1/2 cup brown rice flour
- 1 teaspoon baking soda
- 1 teaspoon cinnamon
- 1 pinch sea salt
- 1/2 cup coconut, shredded and unsweetened
- 1/2 cup nuts, toasted and chopped (I like pecans)
- 1/2 cup chopped dried fruit (I like cranberries or raisins)
- 1/2 cup turbinado sugar or light brown sugar
- 4 eggs
- 1/2 cup canola oil or melted butter or coconut oil
- 1/2 cup milk (as needed)

Direction

- Preheat oven to 350º. Line four baking sheets with parchment paper and set aside.
- Place the oats in the bowl of a large food processor fitted with a steel blade and pulse until oats are roughly chopped.

- In a large bowl, add chopped oats, ground flax, brown rice flour, baking soda, salt, and cinnamon. Stir until well combined and set aside.
- In a medium sized bowl, add canola oil. Beat eggs in one at a time, beating until well combined with the oil. Beat the sugar into the eggs and oil until well combined.
- Stir dried fruit, nuts, and coconut into the wet ingredients until well combined.
- Add wet ingredients to dry until just combined. The dough should be wet enough to hold together -- add milk a couple of tablespoons at a time until the dough is the right consistency.
- Scoop 1/4c of dough using an ice cream scoop or spoon and place on cookie sheet. Pat them to flatten a bit. You can place them fairly close to one another on the baking sheets because they neither spread nor puff up much.
- Bake the cookies for 25 to 30 minutes until golden brown all over and crispy looking. Allow to cool on a rack. I freeze these and microwave them as I need them.

129. Everything Cookie Ice Cream Sandwich

Serving: Makes 6 giant sandwiches | Prep: | Cook: | Ready in:

Ingredients

- 1 cup all-purpose flour
- 2 teaspoons baking soda
- 1/2 teaspoon salt
- 2 teaspoons finely ground coffee
- 1/3 cup crushed original hickory sticks
- 1 cup crushed corn flakes
- 1/3 cup crushed pretzels
- 1/4 cup crushed pecans
- 1/3 cup rolled or instant oats
- 1 cup mini marshmallows
- 2 tablespoons sesame seeds
- 2/3 cup dark chocolate chips
- 1/2 cup butter
- 2 tablespoons duck fat (or more butter)
- 1/2 cup dark brown sugar
- 1/2 cup granulated sugar
- 2 teaspoons vanilla extract
- 1   large egg
- 6 cups of your favorite ice cream

Direction

- In a bowl, whisk together the flour, baking soda, salt and ground coffee.
- To crush the hickory sticks, corn flakes, pretzels and pecans, I placed them in the bowl of a food processor and pulsed a few times. If you don't have a food processor you can also place the ingredients in a ziplock bag wrapped in a towel and crush them with a rolling pin. Transfer to a separate bowl and add oats, marshmallows, sesame seeds and chocolate chips. Toss to mix.
- If your butter is still cold, cut it in cubes of 1-2 cm and heat it in the microwave 10 seconds at a time until softened but not melted. Place the butter, duck fat and both types of sugar in the bowl of a stand mixer or in a big bowl with a hand mixer. Beat on medium-high speed for 3 minutes or until light and fluffy. Add the vanilla extract and the egg and mix for 30 seconds or until the mixture is smooth and uniform.
- Add the flour mixture to the bowl and beat on low speed until there is no more dry ingredients. Top with the rest of the ingredients (hickory sticks, corn flakes, pretzels, pecans, oats, marshmallows, sesame seeds, chocolate chips) and continue mixing, still on low speed, to blend them in evenly.
- Cover the bowl with plastic wrap and place the dough in the fridge for an hour, so that it can firm up and will be easier to roll into cookies.
- 15 minutes before you take the dough out, heat the oven to 350°F. Cover two baking sheets with a Silpat or parchment paper. Place 2 tbsp. of dough per cookie in your hands and

- roll them into a ball. Place a maximum of 6 cookies per sheet. They will spread quite a lot.
- Bake for 12-15 minutes, until the edges are golden brown and the middle is set. Let them completely cool.
- Scoop 1 cup of ice cream on a cookie and top with a second one, now enjoy!

130. Fall Inspired Apple Granola (gluten/dairy/sugar Free)

Serving: Serves 10 | Prep: | Cook: |Ready in:

Ingredients

- 2 cups gluten free oats
- 2 tablespoons coconut oil (kept separate)
- 1 tablespoon cinnamon
- 1 cup walnuts
- 1 apple
- 1 cup cranberries
- 3 tablespoons brown rice syrup
- 2 tablespoons honey
- 1/4 cup apple juice

Direction

- Preheat your oven to 325.
- Chop your apple into 5-6 pieces.
- Put them in a blender with juice, honey, cinnamon, 1 tbsp. brown rice syrup, and 1 tbsp. coconut oil.
- Blend until smooth.
- Combine this mixture in a bowl with your oats.
- Stir well.
- Coat a baking pan with the rest of your coconut oil.
- Put your oats in the pan and bake for 25 minutes
- Remove from oven and add cranberries, walnuts and apricots.
- Turn the oven down to 250.
- Drizzle the rest of your syrup on your granola and mix well.
- Let warm at 250 for one hour.
- Serve and enjoy!

131. Five Minute, No Bake Vegan Granola Bars

Serving: Serves 10 to 12 | Prep: 4hours5mins | Cook: 0hours0mins |Ready in:

Ingredients

- 2 1/2 cups rolled or quick oats
- 1 cup raw pumpkin seeds (pepitas)
- 1/2 cup raisins
- 2/3 cup peanut or almond butter
- 1/2 cup agave nectar or brown rice syrup (increase based on how well things stick together)
- 1/8 teaspoon sea salt (adjust based on which nut butter you use)

Direction

- Mix oats, pumpkin seeds, and raisins in a large bowl.
- Whisk together nut butter, sweetener, and sea salt. Pour into oat mixture, and mix well, till everything is sticky and combined. If it's too dry, add a bit more agave.
- Press mixture into a shallow baking dish that you've lined with foil or saran wrap. Cover with more foil/saran, press well into the baking dish, and refrigerate for 4 hours. Cut into bar shapes, wrap, and keep refrigerated till ready to use. They will last two weeks in the fridge.

132. Fruity, Oaty Mini Cake Bites

Serving: Makes 12-16 | Prep: | Cook: | Ready in:

Ingredients

- 120 grams butter
- 120 grams sugar
- 2 eggs
- 120 grams flour
- 1 teaspoon vanilla extract
- 120 grams rolled oats
- 50-75 grams frozen summer berries
- 1 handful of flaked almonds

Direction

- Pre-heat the oven to 180 degrees Celsius. Generously grease the cups in a cupcake/ muffin tray (depending on how generous you are when portioning the batter later, you might need multiple trays).
- Cream the butter and sugar until light and fluffy.
- Add the eggs one at a time, with a tablespoon of the flour to avoid curdling, mixing thoroughly after the addition of each egg.
- Add the rest of the flour and fold in gently. Add the vanilla extract and fold in gently.
- Add the oats and fold gently. Add the frozen summer berries and, again, fold it all gently until the oats and berries are evenly distributed.
- Using a large serving spoon (or an ice cream scoop!) put the batter into the cupcake/ muffin tray's cups. You want the batter to come about half way up the cup. Sprinkle on a few flaked almonds on the top of each cake (patting them down a little).
- Put the cupcake/ muffin tray (or trays if you had enough batter to fill more than one) into the oven for 20-25 minutes until the tops of the cakes are golden.
- When done, take the trays out of the oven and leave to cool for about 10 minutes. Then use a knife or a spatula to go round the edges of each cake and remove each cake from its cup (they normally pop out pretty easily for me). Leave to cool completely for a few minutes or, if you're like me, consume while still warm and soft.

133. Game Changing Pancake Mix

Serving: Makes 10 cups of dry mix (enough to make about sixty 4-inch pancakes) | Prep: | Cook: | Ready in:

Ingredients

- For assembling pancake mix:
- 2 1/2 cups (255 grams) old-fashioned oats
- 1 cup (117 grams) rye flour
- 2 cups (270 grams) whole-wheat flour
- 2 1/2 cups (300 grams) unbleached all-purpose flour
- 1/4 cup light brown sugar, tightly packed
- 1 tablespoon baking soda
- 1 tablespoon baking powder
- 1 tablespoon plus 1 teaspoon kosher salt
- 1 cup extra-virgin olive oil
- For making pancakes:
- 1 cup pancake mix
- 1 cup buttermilk
- 1 large egg
- Butter, for frying pancakes
- (Makes six 4-inch pancakes; scale as desired)

Direction

- To assemble pancake mix: In a food processor, blitz the oats until they are finely ground.
- Combine the oats and all other dry ingredients in a large mixing bowl. Using the paddle attachment on your mixer, mix together the dry ingredients on low speed, then slowly drizzle the olive oil into the bowl while the mixer is running. Stop the mixer and pinch a small portion of the mix between your fingers. It should barely clump and stay together. If it doesn't clump, drizzle in just enough

additional olive oil until it reaches the right consistency. Store the mix in an airtight jar or container for a few weeks at room temperature, or over a month in the refrigerator or freezer.

- To make pancakes, put 1 cup of the mix in a large bowl and whisk a few times to aerate. Whisk in 1 cup of buttermilk and 1 egg. Let the batter stand for 5 to 10 minutes to thicken up.
- Heat a griddle or nonstick pan over medium heat and grease it with plenty of butter. Ladle the batter onto the griddle using a 1/4-cup measure. When bubbles come to the surface and the edges start to brown, flip the pancakes and cook on the other side until golden brown and crispy around the edges. (If desired, place a cookie sheet in the oven and heat oven to 220° F; as your pancakes are done, transfer them to the cookie sheet to keep them warm while preparing the rest.) Serve with warm maple syrup and softened salted butter.

134. Gatherer's Pie

Serving: Serves 6 | Prep: | Cook: | Ready in:

Ingredients

- for the oats:
- 1 cup oat groats
- 5 cups salted water
- 1 cup yellow onions, minced
- 1 cup button mushrooms, cut into matchstick pieces
- 1 1/2 teaspoons garlic, minced
- 1 tablespoon flat leaf parsley, minced
- 2 tablespoons unsalted butter
- kosher salt and fresh ground pepper
- for the collards:
- 2 pounds collard greens, center stems removed, leaves rinsed and chopped
- 1 pound whole milk cottage cheese, drained
- 1/4 cup onion minced
- 1 tablespoon garlic, minced
- 1 tablespoon unsalted butter
- 3/4 cup heavy cream
- 1/4 cup whole milk yogurt
- 2 egg yolks
- freshly ground nutmeg

Direction

- In a 3 quart sauce pan bring the water to a boil. Add the salt and the oats. Bring it back to a boil and then reduce the heat so the water stays at a low boil to a brisk simmer and cook the grains for 30 minutes or until just tender. Drain the oats.
- While the grains are cooking place a 10 inch sauté pan over high heat. When hot, near smoking, add the butter, swirl it around the pan. It should just start to brown. Add the onions and mushrooms immediately and stir. Add the garlic. Stir. Let the moisture cook out of the mushrooms. Remove from the heat and once it has cooled add the parsley.
- Bring a large pot of salted water to a boil, once again the water should taste salty. Add the greens and stir to make sure all of them are submerged. Cook until just tender, about 3-5 minutes depending on how old the greens are and how big the leaves were. Drain in a colander and immediately rinse with cold running water turning the greens to make sure all of them have cooled. Once they are cool enough to handle collect them into a ball and squeeze as much moisture out of them as you can. Place the ball on a cutting board and chop them again.
- Place a medium sauté pan over medium heat and add the butter. When it starts to melt add the onions and cook them until they just begin to soften. Add the garlic and stir. Cook about a minute more.
- Combine the greens, onion/garlic mixture and cottage cheese in a bowl. Season them with salt and pepper and mix until well combined. Taste and adjust the seasoning.
- Butter an eight by eight three inch deep casserole. Combine the oats with the mushroom mixture and spread it into the

bottom of the casserole. If it looks dry for some reason add a tablespoon or two of water. Next spread the collard greens across the top packing them down a little. At this point you could place it in the fridge for a few hours, or up to a day covered, if you wanted or preheat the oven to 350 degrees and continue.

- In a mixing bowl lightly beat the egg yolks. Bring the cream to a boil in a sauce pan. Add yogurt and bring back to a boil. Immediately temper the eggs by adding a little bit of the cream/yogurt mixture and whisking them. Then add the egg mixture back to the sauce pan with the rest of the cream and yogurt. Place over low heat and stir continuously until it starts to thicken. It should look like thin pancake batter. Remove from the heat and stir in a pinch nutmeg. Pour over the top of the casserole making sure it is spread evenly. Bake in a preheated 350 degree oven for 45 minutes to 1 hour or until bubbly, golden brown and delicious.

135. Ginger Rhubarb Crisp (Baby!)

Serving: Serves 8 | Prep: | Cook: |Ready in:

Ingredients

- Rhubarb Filling
- 6 cups chopped fresh rhubarb (or frozen could work too)
- 1/2 cup maple syrup
- 1/4 cup flour (of your choice, but I used all-purpose)
- 1/2 teaspoon cinnamon
- 1/2 teaspoon dry ginger
- Oatmeal Crisp
- 1 cup large flake oats
- 1/2 cup brown sugar
- 1/2 cup flour (of your choice, but I used all-purpose)
- 1/2 cup melted butter

- 2 tablespoons black sesame seeds

Direction

- For the filling: In large bowl, toss rhubarb, with maple syrup. Add flour, cinnamon, and ginger. Transfer to lightly greased 8-inch square baking pan (I used corning ware passed down from my mum-in-law).
- For topping: Toss together oats, sugar, flour and sesame seeds. Drizzle in butter. Mix well. Sprinkle over rhubarb mixture.
- Bake in preheated 375F oven until golden brown, about 30 minutes. Delicious with vanilla ice cream or plain yogurt!

136. Ginger, Berry, Nutty Crisp

Serving: Makes 16 squares | Prep: | Cook: |Ready in:

Ingredients

- 80 grams Speculoo biscuits (a spicy biscuit)
- 20 grams walnuts
- 190 grams plain/AP flour
- 50 grams oats
- 20 grams ground almonds/almond meal/almond flour
- 1 teaspoon ground ginger
- 150 grams cold, unsalted butter, cubed
- 50 grams 50 g chopped walnuts – reserve for the topping
- For the filling
- 300 grams 50 g chopped walnuts – reserve for the topping
- 1 large egg
- 100 grams light brown sugar
- 1 tablespoon ground almonds/almond meal
- For the Glaze
- 1/2 cup golden icing/super fine sugar
- 2 tablespoons crème fraîche
- 2 teaspoons Yuzu Citrus Seasoning

Direction

- Pre-heat oven to 180 C/350 F, line a 9 inch square tin with greaseproof paper so that the base and sides are covered – use a few dabs of butter to get the paper to stick to the pan.
- While the oven is heating up, place the 20 g of walnuts on a tray and toast for 5 – 8 minutes. Cool, then place in a food processor and pulse until finely chopped. Don't take it too far otherwise you will have a nut paste rather than a nut flour. Set aside.
- Place the Speculoo biscuits in a food processor and blitz to fine crumbs. Add the flour, oats, ground almonds, the ground walnuts and ginger and pulse a couple of times to combine. Add the cold butter and pulse until the mixture looks like coarse, damp sand.
- Set aside 1 cup of this mixture for the topping and tip the rest into the prepared tin. Pat it level – don't press down too hard or it will be tough – then bake for 15 minutes.
- While the base is baking, get the filling ready; sort through the fruit and discard any moldy ones.
- Using an electric mixer and a medium sized bowl, whisk the egg and sugar until coffee colored and creamy – about 2 minutes. Then add the almond meal and salt and whisk again. Fold in the berries.
- After the base has been in the oven for 15 minutes, remove it and top with the filling – covering the hot base as evenly as you can with the fruit. Sprinkle over the chopped walnuts and the reserved topping. Bake for 30-35 minutes until golden brown.
- Cool in the tin for 10 minutes, then using the lining paper as handles, lift out and place on a wire rack to cool completely before glazing.
- Combine glaze ingredients together until smooth and drizzle over the top. Slice into 16 squares (4 x 4)
- Stores brilliantly, covered in the fridge for 4-5 days.

137. Ginger Apple Crumble Pie (Gluten And Dairy Free)

Serving: Makes one 9-inch round pie | Prep: | Cook: | Ready in:

Ingredients

- For the pie dough:
- 1/2 cup sorghum flour
- 1/4 cup brown rice flour
- 1/4 cup gluten-free oat flour
- 1/4 cup arrowroot powder
- 1 teaspoon psyllium husk powder (or xanthan gum)
- 1 teaspoon natural cane sugar
- 1/2 teaspoon fine sea salt
- 1/2 cup unrefined coconut oil, cold
- 3-6 tablespoons ice water
- 1 egg, for brushing (or 1 teaspoon plant-based milk if you are vegan)
- For the filling and crumble
- FILLING
- 5 to 6 Honeycrisp apples
- 1 teaspoon freshly grated ginger
- 1 tablespoon fresh lemon juice
- 1/2 cup coconut sugar (or light brown sugar)
- 1/2 teaspoon ground cinnamon
- 1 tablespoon arrowroot powder
- pinch of salt
- CRUMBLE
- 1/2 cup gluten-free oat flour
- 1/4 cup gluten-free rolled oats
- 1/4 cup almond flour
- 1/4 cup chopped walnuts
- pinch of salt
- 1/4 cup unrefined coconut oil, melted

Direction

- For the pie dough:
- In a large bowl, whisk the dry ingredients together; set aside. Cut the coconut oil the dry ingredients using a pastry cutter until it resembles coarse crumbs. Drizzling in the ice water a tablespoon at a time. Use a wooden spoon to stir gently, adding more water until

dough comes together (squeeze it together -- if it crumbles, you need to add more water). Gather dough together with your hands and shape into a flat disk. Loosely wrap the dough with plastic wrap and refrigerate for 30 minutes.

- Grease a 9-inch pie pan with coconut oil and set aside. Remove dough from fridge, and line a work surface with a large piece of parchment paper. Flour parchment, and place dough on top, then let rest for 5 to 10 minutes. Using a rolling in, roll out dough to an 11-inch round, gently turning and sprinkling with flour to prevent sticking. Place pie pan on top of dough, gently slide one hand underneath the parchment paper. Holding the top of the pie pan with your other hand, swiftly and carefully flip the paper and invert the dough into the pan; gently peel back the parchment. Press the dough into pan and trim edges. If there are any tears, press the dough back together or patch them with trimmed dough. Shape the crust and transfer the pie pan to the refrigerator while you prepare filling and crumble.
- For the filling and crumble
- Peel and core apples. Slice each apple in quarters and then into half-moons with about 1/4-inch thickness. Mix the apples and fresh ginger with the lemon juice and set aside. In a small mixing bowl, mix the sugar, cinnamon, arrowroot, and salt. Sprinkle the sugar mixture over the apples a little at a time and toss until combined. Set aside.
- To make the crumble, mix the oat flour, rolled oats, almond flour, chopped walnuts, and salt; add the coconut oil and mix until mixture resembles wet sand. Set aside.
- Heat oven to 400° F and remove chilled pie shell from fridge. Fill pie shell with the apple mixture, arranging them evenly across pie; evenly distribute crumble topping with your fingers. Using a pastry brush, lightly brush top of pie crust with the egg wash (or milk). Place pie in the center of your oven and bake for 15 minutes. Reduce heat to 375° F and bake for 40 to 45 minutes, until crust and topping are golden brown and apples are tender when pierced with a knife.
- Remove from oven and place on a cooling rack. Let the pie cool completely before serving.

138. Gluten Free Raspberry Oatmeal Bars

Serving: Makes 16 bars | Prep: | Cook: |Ready in:

Ingredients

- 1/2 cup Nutiva Shortening
- 3/4 cup coconut sugar
- 2 eggs
- 1 teaspoon vanilla
- 1 cup gluten free baking mix
- 1/4 cup almond flour
- 1/2 teaspoon baking soda
- 1/4 teaspoon salt
- 1 3/4 cups gluten free old fashioned oats
- 1 cup raspberry preserves

Direction

- Preheat oven to 350 degrees and prepare a 9X9 in pan with cooking spray.
- In a large bowl cream together shortening and coconut sugar until light and fluffy, about 3 minutes. Add in eggs and vanilla and beat just until combined.
- In a small bowl whisk together baking mix, almond flour, baking soda and salt.
- Add the dry ingredients to the wet ingredients and beat until combined.
- Using a spatula, fold in 1 1/2 cups of the oats, setting aside the remaining 1/4 cup.
- Spread 2/3 of the batter into the prepared pan and top with the raspberry jam, spreading evenly.
- Combine remaining 1/4 cup of oats with the rest of the batter. Use your fingers to drop blobs of the dough on top of the raspberry

spread. Note: spread will show through in spots.
- Bake for 25 minutes and cool on a wire rack before cutting.

139. Gluten Free Whole Food Waffles

Serving: Makes 3 waffles. double for more. | Prep: | Cook: | Ready in:

Ingredients

- 6 tablespoons almond meal or almond flour
- 1/4 cup corn flour
- 1/2 cup oat flour
- 1 1/2 teaspoons baking powder
- pinch sea salt
- 1 egg, separate yolk and white
- 3/4 cup milk of choice (I use homemade unsweetened almond milk)
- 1/2 teaspoon vanilla extract
- 2 tablespoons maple syrup
- 1/4 cup coconut oil, melted

Direction

- In a large bowl, whisk together the almond meal, corn flour, oat flour, baking powder, and sea salt.
- In a small bowl, whisk the egg yolk, milk, vanilla, and maple syrup.
- Pour this wet mixture into the dry mixture and whisk to combine. The mixture will be quite runny.
- Pour in the coconut oil and whisk again. Batter will still be runny. Let it sit while you beat the egg white.
- Beat the egg white until it forms firm peaks - this takes about 60-90 seconds. Fold the egg white into the batter. There will still be small lumps of egg white in the batter. This is fine.
- Make sure your waffle iron is hot and grease it with a little coconut oil. Using a ladle, spoon batter onto waffle iron. On my waffle iron I use a medium high setting, cook it for about 5 minutes, and I get three large waffles from this recipe. Make sure waffle is browned and crispy - as shown in my photos - before you remove it from the waffle iron.

140. Gluten Free Banana, Honey And Almond Loaf

Serving: Serves 10-12 | Prep: 0hours15mins | Cook: 0hours45mins | Ready in:

Ingredients

- 100 grams unsalted butter, softened
- 1 cup honey
- 3 eggs
- 1 1/2 cups mashed ripened banana (approx. 3 small bananas)
- 1 3/4 cups self-raising gluten-free flour mix, sifted
- 3/4 cup almond meal, sifted
- 1 teaspoon baking powder
- 1/2 cup milk
- 1/3 cup rolled oats (optional)

Direction

- Pre-heat oven to 180 C. Grease and line a deep straight-sided loaf pan (11.5cm x 20cm base measurement).
- In a large bowl of an electric mixer, beat butter and honey until pale and creamy.
- Beat in eggs, one at a time, until well combined. Gently beat in the mashed banana until just combined.
- Stir in combined sifted flour, almond meal and baking powder, alternating twice with the milk. Mix until just combined. At this stage fold in any additional mix-ins, if using, such as raspberries or chocolate chips.
- Pour the mixture in to the prepared pan and smooth over the top. Sprinkle over the oats, if using.

- Bake for 45 minutes or until a skewer inserted in to the center comes out clean. Remove. Cool for 15 minutes in pan. Turn out onto a wire rack to cool completely.
- You can serve slices of the loaf on their own or toasted with a light spread of butter. Store in an air tight container for up to 3 days.

141. Gluten Free Buckwheat Scones With Cardamom And Cherries

Serving: Makes 10-12 scones | Prep: | Cook: | Ready in:

Ingredients

- 1/2 cup rolled oats (not instant or quick)
- 2 cups buckwheat flour
- scant 1/2 cups natural brown cane sugar
- 1 1/2 teaspoons gluten-free baking powder
- 1 teaspoon ground Guatemalan cardamom
- 1/2 teaspoon baking soda
- 1/4 teaspoon salt
- 5-6 tablespoons unsalted butter, softened and cut into small cubes
- 1 egg
- 1/2 cup buttermilk
- 1 teaspoon pure vanilla extract
- 1/2 cup dried cherries, chopped

Direction

- Preheat oven to 400 F. Line a large baking sheet with a silpat (or parchment or cooking spray) and set aside.
- In a blender, pulverize 1/4 cup of the oats into a rough flour. Put them and the remaining 1/4 cup of unblended oats into a large mixing bowl. Add the flour, sugar, baking powder, cardamom, baking soda and salt, and whisk until well combined. Using two knives or your fingers, blend the butter into the flour mixture until well incorporated.
- In a smaller mixing bowl, lightly beat the egg, and then whisk in the vanilla and buttermilk. Add this to the flour mixture, stirring to combine. Fold in the cherries.
- Using a large spoon (soup spoon or the like), scoop out balls of dough and place in rows on the silpat-lined pan. Flatten slightly. Each should be about the size of your palm. Place pan in the oven and bake 17-18 minutes until scones are firm on top but not hard or crunchy. Cool slightly and serve.

142. Gluten Free Chocolate Chip Cookies, With Oat, Buckwheat, Teff, Or Mesquite Flour

Serving: Makes about fourteen 3-inch cookies | Prep: | Cook: | Ready in:

Ingredients

- 3/4 cup raw pecan or walnut halves
- 8 tablespoons (113 grams) unsalted butter
- 1/2 vanilla bean, split lengthwise and scraped
- 1/2 cup (110 grams) packed light brown sugar (I prefer organic)
- 1/4 cup (50 grams) granulated cane sugar (I prefer organic)
- 3/4 cup plus 3 tablespoons (100 grams) gluten-free oat flour
- 1/4 cup plus 2 tablespoons (45 grams) tapioca flour
- 1/2 teaspoon fine sea salt
- 1/2 teaspoon baking soda
- 1 large egg
- 6 ounces (170 grams) bittersweet chocolate (60 to 75% cacao mass), coarsely chopped (1 1/4 cups)
- Flaky salt such as Maldon for the tops

Direction

- Position racks in the upper and lower thirds of the oven and preheat to 375° F (190° C). Line 2 rimless cookie sheets with parchment paper.
- Spread the nuts on a small, rimmed baking sheet and toast until fragrant and slightly darkened in color, 8 to 10 minutes. Remove and let cool completely, then break into rough quarters.
- Meanwhile, melt the butter and vanilla bean and scrapings together in a small, heavy-bottomed saucepan over medium heat. Continue to cook, swirling occasionally, until the butter turns golden and smells nutty, 3 to 5 minutes.
- Place the sugars in a large bowl and when the butter has browned, scrape it and any browned bits into the sugar immediately to stop the cooking. Let cool, stirring occasionally, 10 minutes. Remove the vanilla pod and discard (or save for making vanilla extract).
- Meanwhile, sift together the oat and tapioca flours, baking soda and salt into a medium-sized bowl. Set aside.
- When the sugar mixture has cooled to warm, beat in the egg until well combined. Use a sturdy wooden spoon to stir the flour mixture into the sugar mixture, stirring until well combined, then continue to stir vigorously for a few more seconds; the mixture will firm up slightly. Stir in the cooled nuts and chopped chocolate until evenly distributed. If the dough is soft, let it sit at room temperature or in the refrigerator to firm up a bit, 15 to 30 minutes (or chill for up to 1 week).
- Scoop the dough into 1 1/2-inch (4-centimeter) diameter balls (about 3 tablespoons; a size 24 or 30 spring-loaded ice cream scoop makes this a snap) and place them on the prepared cookie sheets, spacing them 2 to 3 inches (5 to 7 1/2 centimeters) apart, topping each with a few flecks of flaky salt.
- Bake the cookies until the edges are golden and set and the tops are pale golden but still soft and underbaked, 8 to 12 minutes, rotating the pans back to front and top to bottom after 8 minutes for even baking.
- Remove the cookies from the oven, let cool on the pans for a minute, then pull them, parchment and all, onto cooling racks to stop the cooking. They will be very soft and fragile at first, but will firm up when cool. Let cool to warm, at least 10 minutes, before devouring. Cooled cookies can be stored airtight for up to 3 days.
- FOR TEFF COOKIES: Omit the oat flour, using 3/4 cup (100 grams) teff flour (preferably Bob's Red Mill brand) in its place.
- FOR BUCKWHEAT COOKIES: Omit the oat flour, using 3/4 cup plus 1 tablespoon buckwheat flour (100 grams) flour (preferably Bob's Red Mill brand) in its place.
- FOR MESQUITE COOKIES: Omit the oat flour, using 1 cup (130 grams) mesquite flour (preferably Zocalo brand Algarroba Flour) in its place. To measure, break up any big clumps of flour, then use the dip-and-sweep method. Be sure to sift super-clumpy mesquite flour. Since mesquite flour is prone to burning, bake these at 350° F for 8 to 12 minutes.

143. Gluten Free Cornbread Waffles

Serving: Makes two 6-inch belgian-style waffles | Prep: | Cook: | Ready in:

Ingredients

- 1/2 cup masa harina
- 1/4 cup fine/medium ground cornmeal
- 1/4 cup oat flour (gluten-free if needed)
- 1 teaspoon baking powder
- 1/2 teaspoon salt
- 1 large egg
- 3/4 cup unsweetened almond milk (or other milk)
- 2 tablespoons butter, melted and slightly cooled
- 1 1/2 tablespoons honey

Direction

- Preheat your waffle maker to just over medium heat and grease if necessary.
- Mix the dry ingredients together in a large bowl.
- Whisk the egg until pale yellow, then whisk in the milk, melted butter, and honey.
- Pour the wet into the dry and whisk until just combined. Do not over-stir.
- Let sit undisturbed for 7 minutes. The batter will thicken and puff during this time. After sitting the batter will be very thick and airy.
- Scoop half of the batter onto the hot waffle maker and gently spread around with a spatula or butter knife.
- Cook until golden brown. I like to cook over a medium heat for about 1 1/2 cycles. The resulting waffle will be golden brown and soft [but fully cooked through] to the touch, but it will firm up slightly as it cools. If your waffle maker is too hot, the exterior will become very crispy and the inside won't fully cook.
- Serve immediately with fruit topping, butter, and honey, or all three.
- To store: Let fully cool before storing in an airtight container. Keep in the fridge for 1 to 2 days and reheat in the toaster or oven, or freeze and reheat the same way.
- Notes/Substitutions: To make this dairy-free use unrefined coconut oil in place of the butter. It will lead to a mild coconut flavor but will lend the same buttery texture. If you cannot tolerate oats in your diet sub in a high quality all-purpose gluten-free flour blend only for the oat flour at a 1:1 ratio.

144. Gluten Free Poppy Seed Rhubarb Bread

Serving: Makes 1 loaf | Prep: | Cook: | Ready in:

Ingredients

- 1 cup rhubarb
- 1 cup sugar, divided
- 1/2 cup olive oil, plus some for the pan
- 1 1/3 cups white rice flour
- 1/4 cup oat flour
- 1/4 teaspoon salt
- 1 1/2 tablespoons poppy seeds
- 1 teaspoon baking powder
- 1/2 teaspoon baking soda
- 1/4 teaspoon xanthan gum
- 1/2 cup plain yogurt
- 2 eggs
- 1 teaspoon vanilla extract
- 3/4 teaspoon almond extract

Direction

- Preheat your oven to 350°F. Grease an 8.5×4.5 inch loaf pan with a small drizzle of olive oil.
- In a small bowl, toss the rhubarb with 2 Tbsp. of sugar. Set aside.
- In the bowl of a stand mixer fitted with the paddle attachment, mix the remaining sugar (1 cup minus 2 Tbsp.) with the olive oil, rice flour, oat flour, and salt. Let this go for about a minute, scraping down the sides if need be – you want the texture to be like a somewhat damp brown sugar. Once that is thoroughly combined, add the poppy seeds, baking powder, baking soda, xanthan gum, yogurt, eggs, and vanilla and almond extracts. Mix this on low-medium speed until the batter is smooth and glossy.
- Pour half of the batter into the prepared loaf pan, then top with half of the sugared rhubarb (leaving behind any juice in the bowl). Fold the remaining rhubarb into the remaining batter and pour this all into the loaf pan.
- Bake for 45-50 minutes, or until the top is a deep golden brown and a toothpick inserted comes out clean. Allow to cool in the pan before turning it out carefully. Slice and enjoy!

145. Gluten Free Strawberry Tart Bars

Serving: Serves 20 to 25 | Prep: | Cook: |Ready in:

Ingredients

- 2 cups (scant) brown sugar, plus 2 tablespoons for the strawberries
- 2 sticks (16 tablespoons) butter, melted and cooled
- 2 eggs, at room temperature
- 1 teaspoon vanilla extract
- 1 teaspoon almond extract
- 1 1/2 cups almond flour
- 1/2 cup coconut flour
- 1/2 teaspoon salt
- 1/4 cup rolled oats
- 1/4 cup chopped almonds (it's fine to substitute slivered or sliced!)
- 4 cups hulled and sliced ripe strawberries (about 1 1/4 pounds)
- 2 tablespoons cornstarch

Direction

- In a stand mixer or working vigorously by hand, mix the cooled melted butter and 2 cups brown sugar until smooth and caramel-colored. Add the eggs one at a time, mixing each in thoroughly. Add the extracts and mix to combine.
- In a small bowl, whisk together the flours and the salt to combine. Add them into the bowl with the wet ingredients and mix until incorporated.
- Scoop out 3/4 cup of the batter and put it in a separate bowl. Add the oats and the chopped almonds and stir to combine. This will be your crumble topping. Refrigerate both batters until firm, at least 1 hour.
- When the dough is close to chilled, preheat the oven to 350° F and line a 9- by 13-inch pan with parchment paper, leaving an overhang so you can lift it out of the pan later.
- In a medium bowl, mix the strawberries, cornstarch, and the remaining 2 tablespoons brown sugar. Set aside.
- Take the dough without the oats and almonds and press it into the bottom of the parchment-lined pan. It should cover the pan's bottom: Don't worry. Bake for 25 minutes, until golden-brown and baked through. If it's not fully crisp, bake for another 3 minutes and check again. This is your chance to cook the crust fully before you apply the strawberries.
- Take the crust out of the oven and distribute the sliced strawberries over top. You don't have to avoid getting the cornstarchy-juice on the crust, but don't pour spoonfuls of it on, if you can help it. Use your fingers to break the crumble top into clumps over the strawberries.
- Bake for an additional 15 to 20 minutes, until strawberries are somewhat jammy and the crumble top has cooked and browned slightly (it's okay for it to be a bit gooey!).
- Let cool, then slice into small (or large) squares. If storing, wrap in aluminum foil and keep in the refrigerator for 2 to 3 days.

146. Gluten Free Strawberry Rhubarb Almond Crisp

Serving: Serves 8 | Prep: | Cook: |Ready in:

Ingredients

- Fruit Base
- 3 1/2 cups rhubarb, cut into 1-inch pieces, leaves discarded and stringy layers trimmed from stalks
- 3 cups strawberries, stemmed and sliced
- 1/3 cup sugar
- 1/2 teaspoon almond extract
- 1 tablespoon balsamic vinegar, optional
- 2 tablespoons cornstarch
- 1 pinch kosher salt
- Topping
- 1/2 cup finely-ground almond flour, packed

- 3/4 cup quick-cooking, gluten-free, oats
- 1/2 cup dark brown sugar, packed
- 1/2 teaspoon cinnamon
- 1 pinch kosher salt
- 1/4 cup chilled butter, cut into small pieces
- 1 cup sliced almonds

Direction

- Preheat oven to 350°F. In a large bowl, mix rhubarb and strawberries with sugar. Macerate 10 minutes, then mix well with almond extract, optional balsamic vinegar, cornstarch and salt, and let sit for an additional 20 minutes.
- Combine almond flour, oats, brown sugar, cinnamon and salt in a medium bowl; cut in butter with a pastry blender or 2 knives until mixture resembles coarse meal. Stir in sliced almonds and toss until evenly distributed.
- Pour fruit into a 2-quart casserole dish or into individual oven-safe serving dishes. If using individual dishes, fill almost to the top with fruit base. Spoon the topping over the fruit. Bake at 350°F for 35 minutes or until topping is golden brown.

147. Gluten Free Sweet Potato Spice Cake With Cream Cheese Frosting

Serving: Serves 12 | Prep: | Cook: | Ready in:

Ingredients

- For the cake:
- 1 1/4 cups flavorless vegetable oil (such as soybean, corn, or safflower)
- 2 cups (400 grams) sugar
- 4 large eggs
- 1 1/2 cups plus 1 tablespoon (240 grams) white rice flour or 2 1/3 cups (240 grams) Thai white rice flour
- 3/4 cup plus 1 tablespoon (80 grams) oat flour
- 1 teaspoon baking soda
- 2 teaspoons baking powder
- 2 teaspoons ground cinnamon
- 1/2 teaspoon ground nutmeg
- 1/4 teaspoon ground cloves
- 1/2 teaspoon salt
- 3 cups (340 grams) lightly packed peeled and shredded sweet potatoes
- 1 cup (100 grams) coarsely chopped walnuts
- Cream Cheese Frosting (recipe below)
- For the cream cheese frosting:
- 8 ounces (225 grams) cream cheese
- 8 tablespoons (1 stick/115 grams) unsalted butter
- 1 1/2 cups (170 grams) confectioners' sugar
- 1/2 teaspoon pure vanilla extract

Direction

- For the cake:
- Position a rack in the lower third of the oven and preheat the oven to 350° F. Grease a 9- by 13-inch glass baking dish with vegetable oil spray or butter.
- Combine the oil, sugar, and eggs in the bowl of a stand mixer and beat on medium speed with the paddle attachment until lighter in color, about 2 minutes. Or beat with a handheld mixer on medium-high for 3 to 4 minutes.
- Add the rice and oat flours, baking soda, baking powder, cinnamon, nutmeg, cloves, salt, sweet potatoes, and walnuts and beat on low speed until smooth. Scrape the batter into the prepared dish.
- Bake for 30 minutes at 350° F, then reduce the heat to 325° F and bake for 30 minutes longer, or until a toothpick inserted in the center comes out clean. Set the pan on a rack to cool for at least 2 hours before frosting.
- To frost, use a spoon or drop dollops of frosting all over the cake, ten spread with a small spatula. Cut into 3-inch squares to serve.
- This cake keeps, covered, in the refrigerator for up to 5 days.
- Note: To make this into a layer cake, grease the sides of two 9- by 2-inch round cake pans and line the bottoms with parchment paper. Divide

the batter evenly between the pans. Bake for 30 minutes at 350° F and 20 minutes at 325° F. Fill and frost the cake with 1 1/2 batches of the Cream Cheese Frosting.
- For the cream cheese frosting:
- Warm the cream cheese and butter in a microwave oven on low until soft but not melted.
- Add the confectioners' sugar and vanilla and beat with a spoon until smooth.

148. Gluten Free, Mostly Whole Grain Chocolate Shortbread Cookies

Serving: Makes about 36 cookies | Prep: | Cook: | Ready in:

Ingredients

- 1 (11-12 ounce) bag (311-340 grams) dark chocolate chips
- 3/4 cup plus 2 tablespoons (140 grams) gluten-free oat flour
- 1/3 cup (50 grams) white rice flour
- 1/4 cup (50 grams) sugar
- 3/8 teaspoon salt (I use fine sea salt)
- 1/8 teaspoon baking soda
- 4 tablespoons (60 grams) cream cheese, softened
- 12 tablespoons (170 grams) unsalted butter, softened
- 1 tablespoon water

Direction

- Combine the chocolate chips, oat flour, rice flour, sugar, salt, and baking soda in the bowl of a food processor fitted with the steel blade. Process and pulse until the mixture feels like fine gravel, with the largest chocolate pieces no bigger than ¼ inch (some of the chocolate will be more finely ground — this is correct).
- Add the cream cheese and the butter to the bowl in several small pieces. Add the water. Process just until the butter and cream cheese are blended in and the dry ingredients look damp. Scrape the mixture together onto a sheet of wax or parchment paper and knead in any stray dry ingredients. Form a 12-inch log about 2 inches thick and wrap it well. Refrigerate for at least two hours and up to a couple of days.
- Position racks in the upper and lower thirds of the oven. Preheat the oven to 325° F for non-convection (adjust the temperature for convection according to the instructions with your oven). Line two baking sheets with parchment paper.
- Use a sharp knife to cut slices 1/3 inch thick (I mark the log at 1-inch intervals and cut three slices between each mark) and place them 1 inch apart on lined sheets
- Bake 16-20 minutes; the cookies will still be very soft but will firm up as they cool. Rotating the sheets from top to bottom and front to back about half way through the baking time. Set the pans on racks to cool and cool cookies completely before storing. Cookies keep for at least a week in an airtight container.

149. Gram's Best Oatmeal Cookies

Serving: Makes 2-3 dozen | Prep: | Cook: | Ready in:

Ingredients

- 1 cup canola oil
- 1 1/2 cups dark brown sugar
- 2 eggs
- 1 teaspoon vanilla
- 1 1/2 cups all-purpose flour
- 1 teaspoon cinnamon
- 3 cups oats
- 1 cup raisins or chocolate chips

Direction

- Beat together oil, sugar, eggs, and vanilla until creamy. If your sugar is right, it should be the color of melted dark chocolate.
- Sift together the flour, baking soda, and cinnamon. Stir in the oats and raisins/chocolate chips. Add to wet ingredients.
- Place parchment paper over your baking sheet(s). Form about 1 1/2 inch balls of dough, and bake at 350 degrees for 10-11 minutes.

150. Grandma's Ranger Cookies

Serving: Makes 3-4 dozen | Prep: | Cook: | Ready in:

Ingredients

- 1 cup margarine (2 sticks)
- 1 cup canola or vegetable oil
- 1 cup brown sugar, packed
- 1 cup white sugar
- 1 egg
- 2 teaspoons vanilla extract
- 3-1/2 cups flour
- 1 teaspoon cream of tartar
- 3/4 teaspoon baking soda
- 1/4 teaspoon salt
- 1 cup crushed walnuts
- 1 cup oats
- 1 cup Rice Krispies

Direction

- Cream margarine, oil and sugars.
- Add egg and vanilla and beat well.
- Sift in flour, cream of tartar, soda and salt.
- Add nuts, oats and Rice Krispies. Mix well.
- Drop by tablespoon onto lightly greased baking sheets. Roll each into a loose ball, and press down gently with a fork.
- Bake at 350°F for 10 minutes or until edges are lightly browned.

151. Granola

Serving: Makes 4 cups | Prep: | Cook: | Ready in:

Ingredients

- Dry ingredients
- 2 cups Rolled oats
- 1/4 cup Cashews, chopped
- a handfuls Almonds, chopped
- 4   Dried figs, cut into small pieces
- 1/4 cup Sun flower seeds
- 1/4 cup Raw cacao powder
- Wet ingredients
- 1/3 cup War m water
- 3 tablespoons Honey

Direction

- Combine all dry ingredients together in a large bowl, except the cacao powder.
- Mix the honey and water together until the honey dissolves, then add in the cacao powder, stir until it's all combined.
- Pour the honey-cacao mixture into the bowl, stir until everything is coated with the mixture.
- Line a baking tray with parchment paper, spread out the oats and bake at 200 C for 30-35 minutes, stir it once half way through.

152. Granola Clusters

Serving: Makes 2 dozen | Prep: | Cook: | Ready in:

Ingredients

- 2 large ripe bananas, mashed
- 1 teaspoon vanilla extract
- 1/2 cup maple syrup
- 2 cups rolled oats
- 2/3 cup shredded coconut
- 1/2 teaspoon salt

- 1/2 teaspoon cinnamon
- 1/4 cup dried apricots, chopped
- 1/2 cup dried cranberries
- 1 teaspoon baking powder

Direction

- Pre-heat your oven to 350 degrees, with racks in the upper third. Line two baking sheets with parchment paper or other liner (I didn't have any parchment or liners, so I just lightly greased each pan with a little olive oil and had no trouble).
- Mix syrup, vanilla, and bananas in a large bowl. In another bowl, mix oats cinnamon, baking powder, coconut, dried fruit, and salt. Add dry ingredients to the wet and mix well (I just used my hands...don't be shy).
- Mold the mixture into little balls in your hands. They may be a little loose, but that's ok: they'll firm up in the oven.
- Put baking sheets in the oven and bake until outside starts to brown, about 15 minutes. Remember, the bigger the cluster, the longer it will take to firm up.
- I found this recipe yielded about 2 dozen 2-bite clusters (a little bigger than "bite size") that were slightly crispy on the outside yet moist and chewy on the inside. Store on a cake stand with a lid (they're pretty too). Enjoy!

153. Great Graham Crackers

Serving: Makes about 3 dozen 2-inch grahams | Prep: | Cook: | Ready in:

Ingredients

- Ingredients:
- 1 3/4 cups (225 grams) graham flour
- 1/2 cup plus 1 tablespoon (55 grams) oat flour
- 1/4 cup (50 grams) sugar, plus 3 to 4 teaspoons for sprinkling
- 1/2 teaspoon salt
- 1/2 teaspoon baking powder
- 1/4 teaspoon baking soda
- 6 tablespoons (85 grams) cold unsalted butter, cut into 1/2-inch cubes
- 3 tablespoons (65 grams) honey
- 3 tablespoons milk
- 1/2 teaspoon pure vanilla extract
- Equipment:
- 2 sheets of parchment cut to fit the baking sheet
- 2 large sheet pans (about 12 x 16 inches)
- Food processor

Direction

- In a food processor fitted with the steel blade, combine the graham and oat flours, ¼ cup sugar, salt, baking powder, and baking soda. Pulse to mix thoroughly. Sprinkle the butter cubes over the flour mixture. Pulse until the mixture resembles cornmeal. In a small cup, stir the milk, honey, and vanilla together until the honey is dissolved. Drizzle the honey mixture into the bowl. Process just until the mixture gathers into a single mass.
- Divide the dough in half and shape each piece into a 6 or 7-inch flat square patty. Wrap and refrigerate it until they are very firm but supple enough to roll out, 20-30 minutes. Or keep them refrigerated up to two days; let soften slightly at room temperature before rolling.
- Position racks in the upper and lower thirds of the oven. Preheat the oven to 350 degrees. Roll one patty between the sheets of parchment paper until it is 1/8 inch thick (about 8 by 12 inches) and as even as possible from the center to the edges. (Try to avoid a thick center with thinner edges). Flip the paper and dough over once or twice to check for deep wrinkles; if necessary, peel the parchment and smooth it over the dough before continuing. Peel the top sheet of parchment off. Prick the dough all over with a fork. Sprinkle the dough evenly with 1 to 2 teaspoons of sugar. Repeat with the second patty.
- Slide one sheet of dough, with the bottom layer of parchment, onto each cookie sheet.

With a sharp knife, even up the edges of the dough and score it into squares, diamonds, or rectangles. Leave edge scraps in place (good for nibbling and to protect the rest of the grahams from burnt edges).
- Bake for 20 to 25 minutes until the grahams are golden brown with deep brown edges. Rotate the pans from upper to lower and front to back a little over halfway through the baking time to ensure even baking. Set the pans on racks to cool. Break the grahams along the score lines. Cool the grahams completely before storing. Grahams keep in an airtight container for at least 3 weeks.
- Troubleshooting: Grahams crisp up after they are completely cool unless they are under baked. If your grahams are not thoroughly crunchy when cool (especially any in the center that might be a little thicker), return them (on a parchment lined baking sheet) to a preheated 325-degree oven for about 15 minutes. Let cool and check for crunch.

154. Gussied Up Preacher Cookies

Serving: Serves 25 3-inch cookies | Prep: 0hours0mins | Cook: 0hours0mins | Ready in:

Ingredients

- vegetable shortening, cocoa powder, salt, coconut sugar, unsweetened almond milk
- 1/2 cup vegetable shortening
- 1/2 cup cocoa powder
- 1/8 teaspoon salt
- 2 cups cocnut sugar
- 1/2 cup unsweetened almond milk
- rolled oats, salted peanut butter, vanilla extract, sea salt
- 3 cups rolled oats, not instant
- 1/3 cup salted peanut butter, creamy or chunky
- 1 teaspoon vanilla extract

Direction

- Vegetable shortening, cocoa powder, salt, coconut sugar, unsweetened almond milk
- Over medium heat add ingredients into a medium pot and bring to a boil, stirring constantly.
- Once it reaches a boil, lower heat to medium-low and continue to stir for another 2-3 minutes. Drop a few drops of the mixture into cold water. It is ready if the drops solidify and congeal into solid little balls. Turn off heat.
- Rolled oats, salted peanut butter, vanilla extract, sea salt
- Add rolled oats, PB and vanilla extract into the chocolate mixture. Thoroughly combine.
- Drop heaping tablespoons of the "dough" onto a wax/parchment paper lined cookie sheet. (I like to use a 3-inch round cookie cutter to help form uniform cookies. They otherwise look like "cow pies.") Chill in the refrigerator for 15 minutes then transfer to a room temperature space to finish cooling and solidifying. Enjoy!

155. Harry's Favorite Better Than IHOP Multigrain Pancakes

Serving: Serves 4 hungry people | Prep: | Cook: | Ready in:

Ingredients

- 1 cup white whole wheat flour
- 1/2 cup old fashioned oats, whirred in a food processor till they're the consistency of flour
- 1/4 cup wheat germ
- 1/4 cup toasted walnuts or pecans, chopped fine
- 1 tablespoon baking powder
- 1/2 teaspoon kosher salt
- 1 tablespoon sugar
- 1 ripe banana, pureed into liquid
- 2 large eggs

- 1 1/2 cups milk
- 1 teaspoon vanilla extract
- butter for the griddle or frying pan (Optional-- you might not need it if you use a nonstick pan, but it definitely improves the taste.)
- warm maple syrup, confectioner's sugar and/or jam for serving

Direction

- Heat your oven to 200 (for holding the pancakes). In a large bowl, mix together the flour, oats, wheat germ, nuts, baking powder, salt and sugar.
- In a medium bowl, mix together the liquefied banana, milk and vanilla extract, and beat the eggs into the mixture till fully blended. Pour into the dry ingredients and fold gently till just blended. Add a little more milk if the batter seems thick. Let the batter sit while you and heat a griddle or large frying pan (I use a non-stick pan) over medium low heat.
- Melt about a teaspoon of butter in the pan. When the foam subsides, ladle in the batter, making the pancakes any size you like. Adjust the heat so that the bottom browns in 2-4 minutes. Flip when they're cooked on the bottom and cook the other side.
- Serve immediately or hold in the warm oven till all pancakes are cooked. Harry likes his with maple syrup. I prefer mine with piles of confectioner's sugar. The kids like strawberry jam. Your choice.

156. Healthy Homemade Granola In 30 Minutes

Serving: Serves 20 | Prep: | Cook: |Ready in:

Ingredients

- 4 cups oats
- 1 cup nuts/seeds
- 0.5 cups sugar (maple syrup, brown sugar or honey)
- 0.33 cups coconut oil
- 1 tablespoon cinnamon
- 1.5 teaspoons vanilla extract

Direction

- Pre-heat oven to 300 degrees
- Mix together the oats, nuts and cinnamon in a large bowl
- Melt the coconut oil in the microwave and add it to the bowl along with the vanilla and sugar of your choice
- Mix thoroughly, and spread out over 2 baking sheets
- Bake for about 20 minutes, or until golden and crunchy
- Optional: add dried fruit and/or dark chocolate chips after the granola cools

157. Healthy Pumpkin Crumble

Serving: Makes 1 20cm pan | Prep: | Cook: |Ready in:

Ingredients

- 400 Pumpkin puree
- 150 Steel Cut Oats
- 30 grams bran
- 50 rice flour
- 4 tablespoons tahini
- 3 tablespoons raw honey
- 3 butter
- 1 walnuts
- 5 cloves
- 4 cardamom pods
- 1 and half teaspoons cinnamon powder
- half a nutmeg, grated
- 1 teaspoon grated orange zest
- fresh juice of one big orange
- 1 pinch salt

Direction

- Preheat the oven at 180C° | 350F°. Grease your pan very well. Add the rice flour and the salt to a bowl. Divide your oats into 3 parts. We want to have three different textures of them; refined, coarse and whole.
- Crush the cloves and the break the cardamom pods to get the seeds. Put them in a good food processor with half of the walnuts and 1 part of oats and blend for a couple of minutes or as long as it gets as refined as possible. Add to the bowl.
- Put the second part of oats and the rest of the walnuts in the blender and pulse it for some seconds until they're coarsely chopped. Don't overdo this. Add them to the bowl.
- Add the rest of the oats, the bran, half of the cinnamon, the orange zest, the tahini, 2 tbsp. of honey and the butter and mix everything. Massage it with your hands so that the spices, tahini and honey are equally spreader on the dry ingredients.
- Blend the pumpkin puree with the orange juice, 1 tbsp. of honey, the grated nutmeg and the rest of the cinnamon.
- Spread the pumpkin mix into the pan and cover it with the oat mix. Even the surface but do not press the dry mix very hard because it will penetrate the pumpkin mix, absorb it and there will no crumble, just a weird cake.
- Bake in the oven for 30-40 minutes, until lightly browned on top. Serve hot with a topping.

158. Healthy Vegan Cookies

Serving: Serves 9-10 | Prep: | Cook: | Ready in:

Ingredients

- 2 cups almond flour (preferably not Bob's Red Mill)
- 1 cup dry oats
- 1/2 teaspoon salt
- 3/4 teaspoon baking soda
- 1/4 teaspoon xantham gum
- 1/4 cup unsweetened coconut flakes
- 1/4 cup unsalted dry roasted almonds, sliced
- 2 tablespoons coconut palm sugar
- 3 tablespoons vanilla flavored agave (or plain agave with dash of vanilla)
- 1/2 cup cacao chips
- 1/2 cup extra virgin olive oil

Direction

- Preheat the oven at 350 degrees Fahrenheit. Make sure it is organized so there is a rack in the middle for the tray of cookies. Put a sheet of parchment paper on a sheet pan.
- Mix the almond flour, oats, baking soda, salt, and xanthan gum in a medium-large bowl. Next, add coconut flakes, coconut palm sugar, almonds, and cacao chips and mix well. Afterwards, add the olive oil and agave; mix until mixture is completely coated.
- The mixture might seem like it doesn't hold well, but that is okay. Form 9-10 clumps, because that is how they might appear, spacing each about 2 inches apart (they will expand in width much more than height). Place on the middle rack and bake for about 15-20 minutes, or until they have a golden-brown color. They might seem undercooked if you touch them but allowing them to cool up to 10 minutes will give them a nice texture that melts in your mouth!

159. Hearty Baked Oatmeal

Serving: Serves 6 | Prep: | Cook: | Ready in:

Ingredients

- 2 large eggs
- 3/4 cup brown sugar
- 1/3 cup unsalted butter, melted and cooled slightly
- 1.5 teaspoons baking powder
- 1.5 teaspoons vanilla extract
- 3 teaspoons ground flax seed

- 1 teaspoon cinnamon
- 1 teaspoon nutmeg
- 1 pinch salt
- 1 cup 2 tablespoons milk
- 1/2 cup shredded sweetened coconut, toasted
- 3 cups rolled oats
- Toasted walnuts, cranberries, or any assortment of toppings you like

Direction

- Lightly grease an 8"x8" baking dish.
- Mix eggs and brown sugar in the bottom of the dish, whisking to remove lumps. Add melted butter and carefully whisk to combine.
- Add baking powder, vanilla, ground flax seed, cinnamon, nutmeg and salt directly to the dish and whisk well. Carefully add the milk and stir to combine.
- Add the toasted coconut and oats and carefully fold into the mixture, making sure everything is combined really well. Cover the dish with plastic wrap and refrigerate overnight.
- The next morning, preheat the oven to 350 degrees and bake the oatmeal for approximately 45 minutes, or until the edges are brown.
- Remove from oven and let cool for a few minutes. Then cut yourself a piece, top it with toasted walnuts and dried cherries, and pour some warm milk over the top. Enjoy!

160. Heidi Swanson's Baked Oatmeal

Serving: Serves 6 | Prep: 0hours15mins | Cook: 0hours45mins | Ready in:

Ingredients

- 2 cups rolled oats
- 1 cup walnuts, toasted and chopped
- 1 teaspoon baking powder
- 1 1/2 teaspoons cinnamon
- 1/2 teaspoon fine-grain salt
- 2 cups milk
- 1/3 cup maple syrup
- 1 large egg
- 3 tablespoons unsalted butter, melted and cooled slightly
- 2 teaspoons vanilla extract
- 2 bananas, sliced into 1/2-inch pieces
- 1 1/2 cups blueberries or a mix of berries

Direction

- Preheat the oven to 375 degrees. Butter the inside of a square 8-inch baking dish.
- In a bowl, combine the oats, half of the walnuts, the baking powder, cinnamon, and salt.
- In another bowl, whisk together the maple syrup, the milk, egg, half of the butter, and the vanilla.
- Spread a single layer of bananas across the bottom of the buttered baking dish. Sprinkle about two-thirds of the berries on top. Cover all that with the oat mixture and then drizzle the milk mixture over the oats. Scatter the remaining berries and walnuts over the top.
- Bake for 35 to 45 minutes, until the top is golden and the oats are set. Let cool for a few minutes. Drizzle with the remaining melted butter and serve.

161. Home Made Organic Maple Granola With Fresh Fruit

Serving: Makes 26 ounces | Prep: | Cook: | Ready in:

Ingredients

- 3 cups organic rolled oats
- 1 cup slivered almonds
- 2 cups of assorted dry fruits (raisins, figs, apricots, dates, cranberries, blueberries, etc.)
- 1/3 cup dark brown sugar
- 1/3 cup maple syrup
- 1/4 cup vegetable oil; peanut oil preferred

- 3/4 teaspoon salt
- 1 cup cashew pieces

Direction

- Preheat oven to 250°F.
- In a large bowl, combine the oats, nuts, salt and brown sugar. Add in the maple syrup and oil and mix thoroughly.
- Spread mixture thinly and evenly onto two cooking tins with sides about ½ inch high. Cook for 45 to 60 minutes stirring carefully every 15 minutes and inter-changing where the cooking tins are placed every time you stir. This will give you more even browning.
- Note: The granola is done when it has a nice tan color, not dark, and can be chewed easily. Remove trays from oven. Let granola cool; then mix in dried fruit and place in sealed plastic bags. It will keep for two weeks, unrefrigerated.

162. Homemade Cranberry Almond Granola Bars

Serving: Makes 12-16 bars | Prep: | Cook: | Ready in:

Ingredients

- 6 cups large flake oats
- 1/4 cup butter, melted
- 1 teaspoon kosher salt
- 1 cup slivered almonds
- 3/4 cup dried cranberries
- 3/4 cup brown sugar
- 1/2 cup honey
- 1/4 cup maple syrup
- 1/4 cup butter
- 2 teaspoons vanilla extract
- 1/2 teaspoon ground cinnamon
- 1/4 teaspoon ground ginger

Direction

- Preheat oven to 350°F. Cover a rimmed baking sheet with parchment paper.
- In a large bowl, toss together oats, melted butter and salt. Spread oat mixture in an even layer on the parchment covered baking sheet. Bake for 10 minutes, stir and continue to bake 5 minutes more. Remove from oven and lower temperature to 300°F. Place oats in a large bowl and toss in almonds and cranberries set aside. Cover the baking sheet once again with parchment paper set aside.
- In a medium saucepan, combine brown sugar, honey, maple syrup and butter over medium heat. Whisk continuously to combine all ingredients for about 2 minutes. Remove from heat and whisk in vanilla, cinnamon and ginger. Pour mixture over oats and almonds, tossing well to combine. Transfer to prepared baking sheet and spread into an even layer. Bake for 35 minutes until golden brown. Remove from oven and allow to cool 10 minutes before cutting into bars. Once cut, allow bars to cool completely on the baking sheet before eating.

163. Homemade Pizza Crust

Serving: Serves 1 | Prep: | Cook: | Ready in:

Ingredients

- For the Pizza Crust
- 500 grams cauliflower florets
- 20 grams flax meal
- 62.5 milliliters water
- 50 grams rolled oats (gluten-free optional)
- 1 teaspoon dried rosemary
- 1/4 teaspoon garlic powder
- 1/2 teaspoon salt
- For the Marinara Sauce
- 1 tablespoon olive oil
- 20 grams garlic, finely chopped
- 400 grams can crushed tomatoes
- 1 teaspoon red pepper flakes

- 2 tablespoons balsamic vinegar
- 1 teaspoon maple syrup
- 1 teaspoon dried oregano
- 1 teaspoon salt
- 1/2 teaspoon pepper

Direction

- For the Pizza Crust
- Line a baking sheet with parchment paper.
- Whisk together flax meal and water in a bowl. Leave for 5 minutes.
- Steam cauliflower until fall-apart tender. Let it cool then squeeze out as much of the moisture through a fine cheesecloth.
- Grind rolled oats, dried rosemary, garlic powder, and salt in a food processor to a flour-like texture.
- Combine the pressed cauliflower and flax meal mixture. Stir well.
- Stir in the oat mixture.
- Form a ball and put it on top of the lined baking sheet.
- Press it down to a circle. Lay a sheet of parchment paper on top and roll it flat to about ¼ inch thick using a rolling pin.
- Bake for 15 minutes at 230C/450F.
- For the Marinara Sauce
- Sautee garlic in olive oil.
- Add all remaining ingredients and simmer for 10 minutes.
- Puree in a blender.

164. Honey Granola Tart

Serving: Makes 8 pieces | Prep: | Cook: |Ready in:

Ingredients

- For the crust
- 1 cup brown rice flour
- 1/2 cup oat flour
- 2 tablespoons confectioners sugar
- 1/2 teaspoon sea salt
- 12 tablespoons unsalted butter, plus 1 tablespoon
- For the tart
- 1/4 cup pecans
- 1/4 cup sliced almonds
- 3 tablespoons sprouted quinoa
- 3 tablespoons hulled buckwheat groats
- 1/4 cup pepitas (hulled pumpkin seeds)
- 1 cup old-fashioned oatmeal
- 1 cup ricotta
- 1/2 cup honey, plus 2 tablespoons
- 1/2 teaspoon vanilla extract
- 1/4 teaspoon teaspoon salt

Direction

- Preheat the oven to 375°F. In a large mixing bowl combine the rice and oat flours, salt, and sugar. Cube 12 tablespoons of butter and, just as you would with biscuits, cut in the butter until the crust looks cornmeal-ish -- you know how that goes. and doesn't it depend on your mood as to how far you take this step?
- Using an eight-inch tart pan with a removable bottom, press in the crust starting with the sides and working to the middle. Press it in as evenly as you can.
- Bake in a preheated 375? F oven for 30 minutes.
- While the crust is baking, combine the ricotta, honey, and vanilla. Don't combine it too vigorously -- I sort of like it swirly.
- At the end of the thirty minutes remove the crust. It will be puffy. Let the crust settle, collapse, drop, whatever you want to call it, and then gently smear on the ricotta-honey mix. Top with the granola, gently press the granola down, and put the tart back into the oven.
- Reduce the heat to 350? F and bake the tart another 25 minutes.
- While the tart is baking, heat the remaining 2 tablespoons of honey and 1 tablespoon of butter in the microwave. Swirl them together. When the timer goes off, drizzle the honey butter over the tart and then put it back into the oven for another 10 minutes.

- When the tart is done, cool it to room temp and then put it in the fridge for at least 2 hours or overnight. I would cover it if I was leaving it in the fridge overnight.

165. Honey Oat Whole Wheat Loaf

Serving: Makes one 9-inch loaf | Prep: | Cook: | Ready in:

Ingredients

- 2 cups (10 3/4 ounces) whole wheat flour
- 1 cup (4 3/4 ounces) all-purpose flour
- 1 cup (31/4 ounces) oats, plus more for finishing
- 2 teaspoons (8 grams) salt
- 2 1/2 teaspoons (7 grams) instant yeast
- 1 1/4 cups (9 1/2 ounces) warm water
- 1/4 cup (3 ounces) honey
- 4 tablespoons (2 ounces) unsalted butter, melted

Direction

- In the bowl of an electric mixer fitted with a dough hook, mix the flours, oats, salt, and yeast to combine. Add the water, honey, and butter and mix on low speed until the mixture forms a ball around the hook. (This can also be done by hand in a large bowl using a wooden spoon).
- Raise speed to medium and mix until the dough is smooth and elastic, 5 minutes more. (This can also be done by hand on a clean surface for 10 to 12 minutes).
- Transfer the dough to a lightly greased medium bowl and let rise until doubled in size, about 1 1/2 to 2 hours. Preheat the oven to 375° F.
- Shape the dough into an oblong shape by pressing it out into a rectangle about 1-inch thick, then folding it over onto itself to expel excess air. Seal the final fold using the heel of your hand, then gently roll into an oblong loaf. Place the dough, seal side down, into a lightly greased 9-inch loaf pan.
- Let the dough rise inside the pan until nearly double in size, 1 1/2 to 2 hours. Brush the surface with water and sprinkle with more oats.
- Bake the loaf until golden brown and crusty (and until the internal temperature reads about 195° F), 45 minutes to 1 hour. Cool completely before slicing and serving.

166. Honey Vanilla Almond Granola

Serving: Makes 16 cups | Prep: | Cook: | Ready in:

Ingredients

- 10 cups old fashioned oats
- 3 cups sliced almonds
- 1 cup packed brown sugar
- 1/2 cup coconut oil
- 1/2 cup honey
- 1/2 cup water
- 1 teaspoon vanilla extract

Direction

- Heat oven to 250 degrees. Spray 2 cookie pans with cooking spray. In a large bowl, mix oats and almonds.
- In a saucepan, heat brown sugar, oil, honey and water over medium-high heat 3 to 5 minutes, stirring constantly, until brown sugar is melted. Remove from heat. Stir in vanilla extract. Pour over oats and almond mixture; stir until well coated. Spread mixture evenly in pans.
- Bake 1 hour until golden brown (oven times vary), gently mixing granola halfway through baking. Cool completely in pans, about 1 hour. Break into pieces. Store in a tightly covered container.

167. Honey Oat Crunchies

Serving: Makes 24 | Prep: | Cook: | Ready in:

Ingredients

- 2 cups gluten free oats
- 1 cup macadamia nut flour
- 1/2 cup desiccated coconut
- 2 teaspoons cinnamon
- 2 tablespoons citrus peel
- 1/2 cup raw honey
- 1/4 cup coconut oil
- 1 teaspoon bicarb
- 1 teaspoon vanilla extract

Direction

- Preheat the oven to 180°C. Grease a 20cm square baking tin and line with baking paper. Mix the oats, macadamia flour, coconut, cinnamon and citrus peel together in a bowl.
- Put the honey and coconut oil in a small saucepan and stir over a medium heat until the coconut oil has melted. Remove from the heat and stir in the bicarb and vanilla.
- Pour the hot mixture into the dry ingredients and mix well. Tip the mixture into the prepared tin and gently flatten into an even layer.
- Bake the crunchies for 25-30 minutes. Set aside until completely cold. Cut into squares and serve.

168. Hoppin' John Fritters

Serving: Serves 4 | Prep: | Cook: | Ready in:

Ingredients

- Hoppin' John
- 2 cups dried black-eyed peas
- 6 cups chicken or vegetable stock
- 1 celeriac, peeled and diced
- 2 carrots, peeled and diced
- 1 large onion, diced
- 2 tablespoons olive oil
- 2 tablespoons apple cider vinegar
- 1 bay leaf
- salt and pepper
- Hoppin' John Fritters
- 2 cups cooked Hoppin' John
- 1/2 cup oat flour or quick or whole oats ground in a food processor
- 1 egg, lightly beaten
- corn meal for dredging
- canola oil for frying
- 1 tablespoon pureed chipotle in adobo
- 1/4 cup mayonnaise
- 1 tablespoon apple cider vinegar

Direction

- Hoppin' John
- In a large stock pot, sauté the onions, celeriac, and carrots in olive oil. When softened add beans and stock to the pan, and bring to a boil. Reduce heat to a simmer, and cook for 45 – 50 minutes. Add liquid as necessary. Beans are done when tender. Remove from heat, and season with salt, pepper, and cider vinegar. Serve over rice.
- Hoppin' John Fritters
- Use a fine mesh strainer to strain excess liquid from the beans. Lightly mash the beans, and then stir oats and egg into the beans. If the mixture looks too soupy, add a few more tablespoons of oats. Spread about a half cup of cornmeal onto a plate. Set the plate and bean mixture next to the stove while the oil heats.
- Heat a 1/2 inch of oil, in a cast iron pan for frying. When the oil is shimmering, drop about a 1/4 cup of the bean mixture onto the cornmeal. Carefully flip and transfer to the skillet. Fry about 3 fritters at a time, being careful not to overcrowd the pan. Drain on rack or paper towels.
- Whisk together the mayonnaise, apple cider vinegar, and chipotle in a small bowl. Taste and adjust chipotle or vinegar if necessary.

Serve each fritter topped with a dollop of the aioli.

169. How To Drink Your Way To A Better Night's Sleep

Serving: Makes 3 | Prep: | Cook: | Ready in:

Ingredients

- 1 3/4 cups water
- 1 cup oats
- 2 tablespoons brown sugar
- 1 piece medium banana, peeled and sliced into thin rounds
- 2-3 tablespoons tablespoons peanut butter
- 1/2 cup blueberries

Direction

- Add the water to a medium pot and head over medium-high heat until it boils.
- Add the oats and cook for about 5 minutes (water should be absorbed and oatmeal tender); stir intermittently.
- Add the brown sugar and stir.
- Transfer oatmeal to a bowl and top with the banana, blueberries, and peanut butter. Serve immediately.

170. Iced Oatmeal Pie Bars

Serving: Makes 9 medium bars | Prep: | Cook: | Ready in:

Ingredients

- For the bars
- 1/2 cup (4 ounces) butter
- 1 teaspoon cinnamon
- 1/2 teaspoon nutmeg
- 1/4 teaspoon ginger
- 1/4 teaspoon cloves
- 1 egg
- 1 cup (7 1/2 ounces) brown sugar, lightly packed
- 2 tablespoons molasses
- 2 teaspoons vanilla extract
- 1/2 teaspoon salt
- 1 cup (3 1/8 ounces) quick-cooking oats
- 3/4 cup (3 1/8 ounces) all-purpose flour
- For the frosting
- 1/2 cup (4 ounces) butter, softened
- 1 1/4 cups (5 ounces) confectioners' sugar
- 7 ounces marshmallow cream (fluff)
- 1 teaspoon vanilla extract
- 1/2 teaspoon salt

Direction

- In a large skillet or saucepan, melt the butter over medium heat. Swirl it constantly until the butter begins to brown and dark solids appear--it will start to quickly smell nutty. Remove it from the heat and whisk in all the spices, then set aside to let cool to room temperature.
- Preheat the oven to 350 degrees F. Butter an 8" x 8" baking pan (I like to line it with parchment for good measure).
- Add the egg, brown sugar, molasses, vanilla, and salt to the cooled butter and beat until light in color and well-mixed.
- Fold in the oats and the flour. Pour the batter into your prepared pan and bake for 25 minutes. Remove from the oven and let cool while you prepare your frosting.
- Beat the softened butter until fluffy, then add the confectioners' sugar and keep beating until pale in color.
- Add the marshmallow cream, vanilla, and salt and beat until light and fluffy.
- Spread over the bars, cut into squares, and serve!

171. Indian Spiced Porridge

Serving: Serves 4 | Prep: | Cook: | Ready in:

Ingredients

- 7 ounces porridge oats
- 3 cups skimmed milk
- 3 cups water
- 2 bananas
- 1 tablespoon sugar
- 1/2 teaspoon ground cinnamon
- 1/4 teaspoon ground cardamom
- 2 tablespoons orange juice

Direction

- Put the oats, milk, and water in a large saucepan. Bring to the boil and simmer for 5 minutes, stirring occasionally.
- Mash the bananas, then add them to the porridge along with the rest of the ingredients.

172. Irish Oats In Vermont

Serving: Serves 2 | Prep: | Cook: |Ready in:

Ingredients

- 1/2 cup steel cut oats
- 2 cups apple cider
- 1/2 teaspoon Chinese 5 spice
- 1 granny smith apple
- 1/2 cup grated extra sharp Vermont cheddar cheese
- 2 tablespoons real maple syrup (preferable grade B)
- a drizzle of cream

Direction

- Bring the cider to a boil and stir in the oats and the Chinese 5 spice. Reduce the heat and simmer.
- While the oats are simmering - peel, core and dice the apple. After about 15 minutes, stir the apple into the oats.
- Simmer and stir until the oats are done, about a half an hour total. Serve into two bowls and top each with a tbs. of maple syrup and 1/4 C of the cheese. You might pop it in the microwave for just a few seconds to help the cheese melt.
- Drizzle a bit of cream over and enjoy!!

173. Irish Soda Bread With Flax Seeds

Serving: Makes 1 medium loaf | Prep: | Cook: |Ready in:

Ingredients

- 2 cups wholemeal flour
- 1/2 rolled oats
- 1 teaspoon baking soda
- 1 teaspoon salt
- 4 tablespoons flaxseed
- 1 cup buttermilk
- 1 tablespoon honey

Direction

- Preheat your oven to 400°F (200°C). Prepare a baking sheet covered with baking paper and sprinkle a little whole meal flour.
- Mix the flour, oats, flaxseed, baking soda and salt. Form a small pit in the center and add the buttermilk and honey. Knead by hand. When dough is smooth (it is normal that it remains sticky) form a ball.
- Place the ball on your cooktop. Using a large knife, draw a fairly deep cross. Sprinkle the bread with a little whole meal flour. Bake for 45 minutes at 400°F (200°C).

174. Jasmine Tea Poached Pear Crumble

Serving: Serves 2 | Prep: | Cook: |Ready in:

Ingredients

- 3 pears, cored and chopped
- 1 tablespoon jasmine tea buds
- 1 cup water
- 2 tablespoons sugar
- 2 tablespoons flour
- 2 tablespoons unsalted butter
- 1/3 cup oats
- 1 pinch salt
- 1 pinch cinnamon
- 1 pinch ground ginger

Direction

- Preheat the oven to 350 degrees and grease a small tart dish. Set aside.
- To make the crumble topping, cream the flour and butter together with your fingers until it resembles coarse breadcrumbs. Add the oats, salt, cinnamon, and ginger and mix well.
- Remove the pears from the tea mixture and add to the tart dish, pour the remaining tea over the top, and top with the crumble. Dot the top of the crumble with the some butter and bake for 7-10 minutes until the top is golden brown.

175. LLBT Lemon Lime Souffle Blueberry Tart

Serving: Serves 1 tart 9" | Prep: | Cook: | Ready in:

Ingredients

- Tart Crust
- 1/2 cup unsalted butter softened (1 stick)
- 1/3 cup confectioner sugar
- 1 egg, lightly beaten
- 1 cup all purpose flour
- 1/2 cup toasted oat flour (toast oat flakes, cool, grind)
- Pinch of salt
- 9" tart pan
- Tart filling
- 1 cup sugar
- 2 eggs seperated
- 2 tablespoons all purpose flour
- 1 1/2 tablespoons lemon juice
- 1 1/2 tablespoons lime juice
- 1 tablespoon sugar
- 5 to 6 ounces wild blueberry jam

Direction

- Tart Crust
- Put the butter and sugar and beat until well combined. Then add the egg blending well.
- In a separate bowl whisk the flour, toasted oat flour, and salt. On low speed slowly add the dry ingredients, scraping sides of bowl as needed. Combing well.
- Place the dough on some plastic wrap forming a round. Wrap tight placing in the fridge for an hour or so.
- When ready to bake take the dough out and on a floured surface roll out to about a 1/8th inch or so. I like rolling my dough between the plastic wrap, it makes it easy for transfer and clean up. I use a 9" tart pan or spring form pan. Roll the dough out larger than the baking vessel. Gently transfer to pan and fitting the bottom and side. Cut away excess from the top, and prick the dough all over with a fork. Place in the fridge to chill (at least 30 minutes).
- Preheat oven to 325 degrees. I like to use a tart weight or some dry rice over foil to help with shrinkage. Bake for about 20 min. with weight and 5 without. Or until golden. Cool
- Tart filling
- Preheat the oven to 375 degrees. Set a bowl over simmering water whisk the sugar, egg yolks, and flour, lemon and lime juice. Whisk constantly so the eggs incorporate but not curdle. Whisk until thick, the coloring will also change, about 8 to 10 mins. Strain through a mesh sieve to an electric mixer bowl. Beat cream on high speed to thicken some more and cool about 6 minutes.
- In a separate bowl beat the eggs whites to form soft peaks then slowly add the 1 T of sugar. Beat until stiff peaks.

- Now in 3 batches fold the whites into the cream mixture very carefully so the mixture remains fluffy.
- Take the tart shell spoon the blueberry jam on the bottom. Add the soufflé mixture filling just to the top. Bake for about 20 25 minutes.

176. Lemon And Toasted Almond Risotto

Serving: Serves 4 to 6 | Prep: | Cook: | Ready in:

Ingredients

- 1/3 cup raw almonds, coarsely chopped (Measure before chopping; and feel free to use more, to taste.)
- 2 tablespoons olive oil
- 1 cup finely chopped shallots
- 2 cloves of garlic, coarsely chopped
- About 2 tablespoons chopped parsley stems (if green and fresh)
- Salt and pepper to taste
- 1 cup Arborio rice
- 1/2 cup Sauvignon Blanc (plus a glass for you to enjoy while stirring the pot!)
- 3 to 4 cups light vegetable broth (best to use homemade -- see note below**)
- 1/4 cup finely chopped parsley leaves
- Juice and zest of two small Meyer lemons (or one medium regular lemon)
- 1 cup cooked whole oats (or "oat groats," as they're often called), in their cooking liquid (up to about 1/4 cup of liquid), optional but recommended

Direction

- Heat the oil in a wide heavy pot. (I use my enameled cast iron braising pan for this.) Add the chopped almonds and cook just until fragrant, stirring all the while. Remove immediately, once most of them have started to turn light brown. Work quickly, as they can go from light brown to dark almost instantly.
- Add the shallots, and stir to coat with the fragrant oil. Sweat them, covered, over medium low heat for about five minutes, stirring after 2 minutes. Add the garlic and a good pinch of salt and cook, uncovered, for about thirty seconds, stirring.
- Turn the heat up to medium and add the rice, stirring constantly to mix it thoroughly with the aromatics and oil.
- Add the parsley stems and the wine (and take a sip of the glass you poured for yourself). Let it cook down for a minute or so, and then add about one half cup of the stock, stirring constantly. Once the stock is mostly absorbed, add another half cup or so of stock, stirring all the while. Continue to do this (adding more stock once most but not all of the stock you just added has been absorbed) until you have used about 3 cups of the stock. Test a grain of rice. Is it firm but tender? If not, add more stock, one half cup at a time, and continue to stir.
- When the rice is al dente, add the cooked whole oats and their cooking liquid and cook for about 30 seconds, to heat them through. (If you made the oats well in advance, and they are cold, you will need a few minutes to warm them up.) Stir in the lemon juice and zest, as well as the almonds, and give it a good stir. Test for salt and correct (and add pepper, if you like). Add the parsley and gently toss.
- Serve immediately. Enjoy!! ;o)
- ** I make a quick vegetable stock for this using the green tops of 2 leeks, a small carrot, a stalk of celery and the stems from the parsley chopped for this dish, covering with about 6 cups of water and simmering for 30 to 40 minutes.
- To make oat groats, cover with at least two inches of cold water and bring to a boil. Turn the heat down and simmer for about ten minutes. Add about a cup of water, bring it back up to the boil, and then turn off the heat. Cover and let sit for at least 2 hours. Four to six hours, or overnight, is even better. Remove the lid, bring to a boil and simmer for another 20 to 30 minutes, until soft but still chewy. You

can also cook them on the stove for 45 minutes to an hour, adding water as necessary to keep the oats covered, if you prefer. Let them sit for at least fifteen minutes before using. ;o)

177. Lemon Curd Tart (V + GF)

Serving: Serves 10 | Prep: | Cook: | Ready in:

Ingredients

- the crust
- 1/2 cup brown rice
- 1 cup oat flakes
- 1 teaspoon psyllium husk
- 1 teaspoon baking powder
- 1 pinch salt
- 1 tablespoon flax seeds, ground
- 1/4 cup coconut sugar
- 1/4 cup coconut oil
- the filling
- 1/2 cup raw cashews
- 2/3 cup fresh lemon juice
- 1/3 cup water
- 2/3 cup maple syrup
- 2 tablespoons corn starch + 2 tbsp water
- some lemon zest
- 1/4 cup almond flakes

Direction

- The crust
- Preheat oven at 350° F / 175 ° C.
- In a high-speed blender grind brown rice, oat flakes and sugar with psyllium, baking powder and salt. Add it to a bowl, combine with flax seeds mixture and oil and mix everything with a fork and then with your hands. Add some cold water until you can manage the dough.
- Prepare you cake pan – I used a removable bottom once covered at the base with some parchment paper – and press the crust evenly, creating borders too. Drill the dough with the fork and bake for 20-25 minutes and let completely cool.
- The filling
- Soak cashews for 4 hours with a drop of lemon juice.
- Rinse and drain cashews and blend them with lemon juice, water and maple syrup until smooth. Pour the mixture in a saucepan and bring to boil. Lower the heat and add the corn starch mixture whisking to prevent lumps. It will take 1-2 minutes to thicken.
- Let it cool until room temperature, add some grated lemon zest, whisk very well and pour the curd into the crust. Sprinkle with almond flakes and reserve in fridge.

178. MAPLE OATMEAL NUT GRANOLA BARS: THE PRETTY FEED

Serving: Makes 20 bars | Prep: | Cook: | Ready in:

Ingredients

- 3 1/2 cups oats
- 2 1/2 tablespoons coconut oil
- 2 tablespoons brown sugar
- 1/4 cup honey
- 1/4 cup maple syrup
- 1 teaspoon vanilla extract
- 1 teaspoon cinnamon
- 2 cups mixed nuts, dried fruit and seeds (pecans, walnuts, pumpkin seeds, almonds, goji berries, sunflower seeds, cranberries, raisins, etc)

Direction

- On a sheet pan lined with parchment paper, toast the oats for 15 minutes on 350.
- While the oats are baking, heat the coconut oil, cinnamon, vanilla, honey, maple syrup, and brown sugar in a saucepan until it comes to a boil and stir it until it's well mixed.

- Place all the seeds and fruits, and toasted oats in a large bowl and pour the syrup mixture over it. Mix everything up until it's all evenly covered with the syrup.
- Then pack it down (firmly) to desired thickness on a sheet pan covered with parchment paper (same one you used to toast the granola). Bake on 350 for 20 mins. Remove from the oven and cut desired size bars before it cools and hardens. Then place in the refrigerator for at least an hour to allow it to set properly!

179. Mama Yoder's Chocolate Chip Cookies

Serving: Makes 48 | Prep: | Cook: | Ready in:

Ingredients

- Ingredients to cream
- 1/2 cup Unsalted Butter, softened
- 1/2 cup Shortening
- 1 Egg
- 1 teaspoon Vanilla
- 1 teaspoon Baking Soda
- 1 teaspoon Salt
- 1 cup Granulated Sugar
- 1/2 cup Brown Sugar
- Dry Ingredients
- 1 and 1/2 cups Flour
- 1 and 1/2 cups Quick Oats
- 12 ounces Semi-Sweet Chocolate Chips

Direction

- Preheat oven to 350 degrees.
- Add all of the ingredients to cream and beat until smooth. A few tiny lumps of shortening are alright.
- Stir in flour and beat until smooth.
- Stir in quick oats and semi-sweet chocolate chips. Stir until both are incorporated.
- Using a medium cookie scoop, scoop the cookie dough into balls on the cookie sheet. Press each ball down with your fingers so that they are slightly smushed.
- Bake for 13 minutes at 350 degrees. Make sure you don't let them brown too much on the edges. I am typically able to bake two cookie sheets at once. You may need to leave the top or bottom cookie sheet in 1 minute longer depending on where the heat is coming from in your oven.

180. Mango Oat Pancakes

Serving: Makes 8 | Prep: | Cook: | Ready in:

Ingredients

- Honey Lime Syrup
- 1/2 cup honey
- 1/3 cup water
- 2 tablespoons juice of 1 lime
- Pancakes
- 1 cup whole milk
- 2/3 cup rolled oats
- 1 1/4 cups flour
- 1 tablespoon sugar
- 2 teaspoons baking powder
- 1 teaspoon salt
- 4 tablespoons butter, melted and slightly cooled
- 4 tablespoons butter, melted and slightly cooled
- 2 eggs
- 1 teaspoon vanilla
- 2 ripe mangoes, peeled, pitted, and sliced into strips
- shredded coconut for serving (optional)

Direction

- To make the syrup, combine the honey, water, and lime juice in a small saucepan. Bring to a boil, stirring often, then reduce heat and simmer for about 10 minutes (syrup will still be on the thinner side). Remove syrup from heat and cool slightly before serving (you can

also make the syrup up to a few days ahead and store in a sealed container in the refrigerator).
- For the pancakes, combine the milk and the oats in a bowl and set aside to soak while you prepare the rest of the batter.
- In a large bowl, stir together the flour, sugar, baking powder, and salt. In a separate bowl, mix together the eggs, melted butter, and vanilla. Add to the flour mixture, followed by the milk/oat mixture, mixing until well incorporated.
- Serve pancakes topped with honey lime syrup and a sprinkle of shredded coconut if desired.

181. Mango Smoothie Bowl

Serving: Serves 2 | Prep: | Cook: | Ready in:

Ingredients

- 1 mango
- 1 banana
- 2 nectarine peaches
- 2 passion fruits
- 2 tablespoons rolled oats
- 1 lime
- handful of blueberries
- cacao nibs (optional)
- glueten-free granola

Direction

- Wash and dry fruits. Peel and cut mango into chunks and place in a blender. Save a few mango slices for topping. Peel banana and nectarine peaches, cut in chunks and add to blender. Cut 1 passion fruit in half, extract juice and add to blender. Save one passion fruit for topping. Add rolled oats and juice of 1 lime to blender, then blend until smooth.
- Transfer blended smoothie into bowls. Decorate with mango slices, blueberries, juice of a passion fruit, cacao nibs (optional) and some gluten-free granola. Serve.

182. Maple Blueberry Granola

Serving: Makes 4 1/2 cups | Prep: | Cook: | Ready in:

Ingredients

- 3 cups old fashioned rolled oats
- 1/3 cup maple syrup (preferably Grade B)
- 1 tablespoon honey
- 1/3 cup olive oil
- 1 teaspoon vanilla
- 1 teaspoon fleur de sel or flaky sea salt
- 1/2 cup raw pepitas
- 1/3 cup ground flax seeds
- 3/4 cup walnuts, roughly chopped
- 1/2 cup dried blueberries

Direction

- Preheat the oven to 350 degrees. Spread the oats on a rimmed baking sheet and bake for 10 minutes. Remove from oven and set aside. Keep the oven on.
- In a large bowl, whisk together the syrup, honey, olive oil, vanilla and fleur de sel. Stir in the oats and mix to coat. Add the pepitas, ground flax seeds and walnuts and gently mix.
- Spread the mixture on the rimmed baking sheet and bake for 18 minutes. Stir the granola halfway through the baking time, being sure to get the corners. Remove from the oven and let cool. Mix in the dried blueberries. Store the granola in an airtight container within easy reach for snacking.

183. Maple Coconut Spice Granola

Serving: Makes about 11-12 cups | Prep: | Cook: | Ready in:

Ingredients

- 6 cups gluten-free rolled oats
- 1 1/2 cups raw almonds
- 1/2 cup unsweetened coconut flakes
- 1 cup unsweetened shredded coconut
- 2/3 cup melted coconut oil
- 1/4 cup pure maple syrup
- 1/4 cup brown sugar
- 1 teaspoon sea salt
- 1 teaspoon ground cinnamon
- 1/2 teaspoon ground nutmeg
- 1/4 teaspoon ground ginger

Direction

- Preheat oven to 350 F.
- In a large bowl, combine oats, almonds, both kinds of coconut, coconut oil, and maple syrup, stir well.
- When the granola is thoroughly saturated, add the brown sugar on top and continue to stir.
- Season with salt, add cinnamon, nutmeg, and ginger, and spread the granola evenly onto 2 baking sheets both lined with parchment paper.
- Bake in the oven for 25-30 minutes making sure to stir the granola evenly every 10 minutes.
- Let granola cool and transfer to an airtight container. Store for up to two weeks.

184. Maple Espresso Baked Oatmeal

Serving: Serves 6 to 8 | Prep: | Cook: | Ready in:

Ingredients

- 2 1/2 cups rolled oats (I use Bob's Red Mill)
- 2 teaspoons baking powder
- 1 teaspoon kosher salt
- 1 tablespoon powdered instant espresso
- 2 ounces unsalted butter (1/2 stick)
- 2/3 cup grade B maple syrup
- 3 eggs, room temperature
- 2/3 cup whole milk
- 1 cup chopped pecans
- 3/4 cup dried cherries, roughly chopped if they're very large

Direction

- Melt butter in a small skillet over medium heat. Cook it until it is brown and smells nutty. Set aside to cool.
- In a large bowl, mix together oats, baking powder, salt, and powdered espresso.
- In a medium bowl, mix together syrup, milk and eggs. Whisk well until well-blended. Stir in melted butter and whisk until blended. Pour into oat mixture and stir well. Let it sit for about 10 minutes, stirring occasionally, while the oven is heating and you're preparing the pan you're using.
- Heat oven to 350. Butter a loaf pan, or line a 12-cup muffin tin with foil liners and butter the liners.
- Stir nuts and cherries into oat mixture until well mixed. Scoop mixture in half-cup measurements into your muffin tin, or spoon into your prepared loaf pan. Press down on tops to compact somewhat.
- Bake at 350 for 35 to 50 minutes (a loaf pan will take longer), until a tester comes out clean.
- Serve in a bowl with milk, yogurt, or crème fraîche. You can refrigerate leftovers and reheat them in the microwave.

185. Maple Mulberry Quinoa Oatmeal Bowl

Serving: Serves 1 | Prep: | Cook: | Ready in:

Ingredients

- 1/4 cup oats
- 1/4 cup quinoa
- 1 pinch salt

- 1 1/2 cups liquid (milk of choice/water)
- 1/4 teaspoon vanilla extract
- 1/2 teaspoon cinnamon
- 2 tablespoons maple syrup (or to taste)
- 1 bunch berries of choice
- 1/8 teaspoon orange zest
- Splash milk of choice (optional)

Direction

- In a pot on the stove, combine the oats, quinoa, salt, and 1 cup of liquid. Bring to a gentle simmer, and cook on low heat while stirring. Continue to cook so that the grains absorb the liquid, and begin to plump up.
- After about 5 minutes, most of the liquid will be gone, but the quinoa will still be hard. Add the rest of the liquid, vanilla, cinnamon, and maple syrup. Continue cooking, stirring occasionally, for about 5 minutes.
- You'll know the grains are done when the liquid is gone and the quinoa looks like a little spiral. You can cook more or less, depending on your preferred tenderness. Turn off the heat and toss in the berries, giving them a gentle stir, just enough so that the heat up and become a bit jammy.
- Transfer all to a bowl or dish. Top with orange zest, extra berries, a splash of milk, and/or maple syrup. Enjoy!

186. Maple Oatmeal Pie

Serving: Serves 8 | Prep: | Cook: | Ready in:

Ingredients

- 1 crust for a 9" pie
- 4 eggs
- 1/2 cup sugar
- 2 tablespoons flour
- 1/4 teaspoon cinnamon
- 1/2 teaspoon kosher salt
- 1/4 cup pure Grade B maple syrup
- 3/4 cup light corn syrup
- 2 tablespoons butter, melted
- 1 cup quick-cook oats

Direction

- Preheat oven to 350F.
- Place pie crust into a glass pie tin.
- In a large bowl, whisk together eggs, sugar, flour, cinnamon, and salt.
- Whisk together maple syrup, corn syrup, and butter; stir into egg mixture.
- Stir in oats, then pour mixture into prepared pie crust.
- Bake for 45 minutes until golden and puffed; filling will sink as it cools.

187. Maple Pecan Granola

Serving: Makes 4 cups | Prep: | Cook: | Ready in:

Ingredients

- 3 tablespoons coconut oil
- 1/4 cup maple syrup
- 1 dash salt
- 1/8 teaspoon cinnamon
- 4 cups raw oats
- 1/2 cup shredded, unsweetened coconut
- 1/4 cup pecans, coarsely chopped

Direction

- Preheat the oven to 350°.
- Melt the oil. In a small bowl, combine the oil with the maple syrup, salt and cinnamon.
- Put the oats, coconut and pecans into a large bowl. Pour the oil mixture over the oat mixture. Stir well to combine.
- Pour the granola onto a large baking sheet and spread it out evenly.
- Bake for about 35 minutes until golden brown, stirring occasionally so all the granola bakes evenly.
- Remove from the oven and let the granola cool thoroughly before transferring to an airtight

container or ziploc bag. Enjoy plain, with milk or on ice cream or yogurt.

188. Maple Quinoa Granola

Serving: Makes 5 to 6 cups | Prep: 0hours7mins | Cook: 1hours0mins | Ready in:

Ingredients

- 2 cups whole rolled oats
- 1/3 cup pre-rinsed, uncooked quinoa
- 1/2 cup raw walnuts, in pieces or coarsely chopped
- 1/3 cup raw almonds, coarsely chopped
- 1/3 cup raw sunflower seeds
- 1/3 cup unsweetened coconut flakes (raw)
- 1/4 cup white raisins
- 1/4 cup dried sweetened cranberries
- 3 tablespoons split hemp seeds (optional)
- 1/3 cup coconut oil
- 1/3 cup grade B maple syrup
- 1 dash cinnamon
- 1 dash nutmeg

Direction

- Preheat your oven to 225°F.
- Mix all dry ingredients (excluding cinnamon and nutmeg) in a great big mixing bowl.
- In a small saucepan over really low heat (or just in a bowl if your coconut oil is liquid), combine oil, syrup, and a dash each of the spices. You only need to get it up to a temperature that melts the coconut oil, then turn it off immediately. Pour your syrup/oil over the mixing bowl, then stir it all up until you don't see any more dry oats. Mix it up good.
- Spread the mix onto a cookie sheet lined with parchment paper. Flatten it out so it's even; it should take up the whole sheet. Bake at 225° F for 60 minutes.
- Let cool completely. When cooled, lift the ends of the parchment and let it crumble to the center. I leave the big chunks big; they'll break up as you pour everything into your jar. You can also just grab them and eat them.
- Because of the coconut oil here, this needs to be kept in an airtight container in the fridge, or safely below 70°, otherwise it risks losing its crispy crunchy.

189. Maple Walnut Steelcut Oatmeal With Peach Compote

Serving: Serves 2 | Prep: | Cook: | Ready in:

Ingredients

- For the oatmeal:
- 1 cup steelcut oats
- 2 cups water
- 1 tablespoon butter
- 1.5 teaspoons maple syrup
- 1 teaspoon walnut oil
- 1/8 teaspoon salt
- 1/8 cup whole milk or cream, for finishing
- For the peach compote:
- 2 cups fresh peaches, peeled, sliced, and halved, or 2 cups frozen peach slices
- 1 tablespoon butter
- 2 tablespoons maple syrup
- 1/2 teaspoon cinnamon
- 1/2 cup water
- splash white wine or lemon juice

Direction

- For the oatmeal:
- In a small pot, bring water and salt to a boil. Add oats, stir to incorporate, and turn heat down to low. Let oatmeal simmer, stirring regularly, for about 25 minutes, until water is absorbed and remaining liquid is thick, as with grits or polenta. While oatmeal is cooking, make peach compote.
- For the peach compote:

- Combine all ingredients in a small sauté pan. Simmer over medium heat until liquid is reduced and syrupy, about 10-15 minutes.
- Serve oatmeal in deep, comfort-food bowls, with a drizzle of cream and peach compote.

190. Maple Grilled Nectarines & Almond Oat Crumb (gluten Free)

Serving: Serves 4 | Prep: 0hours10mins | Cook: 0hours15mins | Ready in:

Ingredients

- For the grilled nectarines:
- 4 nectarines
- 20 grams unsalted butter
- 2 tablespoons maple syrup
- For the crumb:
- 50 grams ground almonds
- 25 grams unsalted butter, cold and cut into cubes
- 1 1/2 tablespoons oats
- 1/4 teaspoon ground cinnamon
- 1 tablespoon demerara or brown sugar
- 2 teaspoons pumpkin seeds (optional)
- A small pinch of salt

Direction

- Add ground almonds, oats, sugar, and butter to a bowl. Break up the butter into the dry mixture using the tips of your fingers until it resembles coarse breadcrumbs.
- Toss in the cinnamon powder, pumpkin seeds if using and salt into the almond mix.
- Spread the crumb out evenly on a lined baking tray and bake in a preheated 180 C/360 F oven for 12-15 minutes, or until lightly golden. Remove and set aside.
- Halve the nectarines and gently remove the stones. Heat a griddle pan or a regular pan and toss in the butter and maple syrup. Place the nectarines cut side down on the pan and turn the heat down. Let them cook for 8-10 minutes or until they soften. If your nectarines were very ripe, keep an eye out so they don't go mushy.
- To serve: place a nectarine half face up in a bowl, and top with ice cream and a handful of crumbs.

191. Maple, Almond, And Cranberry Granola

Serving: Makes 6 cups | Prep: | Cook: | Ready in:

Ingredients

- 3 cups rolled oats
- 1/2 cup wheat germ
- 1/4 cup 2 tablespoons pure maple syrup
- 1/4 cup vegetable oil
- 1 teaspoon ground cinnamon
- 1/2 teaspoon kosher salt
- 1 1/2 cups sliced almonds
- 1/4 cup sweetened shredded coconut
- 1/2 cup dried cranberries

Direction

- Preheat the oven to 350°F. Spray a large rimmed baking sheet with nonstick cooking spray. Toss together the oats, wheat germ, maple syrup, vegetable oil, cinnamon, salt, almonds, and coconut and arrange in an even layer on the prepared baking sheet. Bake for 30 to 40 minutes, stirring occasionally, until golden brown. Remove from the oven and stir in the cranberries. Store in an airtight container for up to 1 month.

192. Maple, Buckwheat & Nut Brittle

Serving: Makes about 3/4 pound brittle | Prep: | Cook: | Ready in:

Ingredients

- 4 teaspoons (20g) coconut oil
- 1/2 cup (140g) maple syrup
- 1 teaspoon vanilla extract
- 1/4 teaspoon kosher salt
- 1/2 cup (80g) raw buckwheat groats
- scant 1/2 cups (45g) roughly chopped walnuts
- scant 1/2 cups (60g) roughly chopped pecans
- scant 1/2 cups (50g) roughly chopped cashews
- 1/3 cup (40g) rolled oats
- 1 pinch flaky salt

Direction

- Preheat the oven to 350° F. Line a baking sheet pan with a silicone mat or piece of parchment.
- Combine the coconut oil, maple syrup, vanilla, and salt in a small saucepan. Set over medium heat and bring to a boil. Immediately remove from the heat and stir in the buckwheat, nuts, and oats. Pour this mixture onto the prepared sheet tray. Use an offset spatula to spread out until everything is, more or less, in a single layer. Sprinkle with flaky salt.
- Bake for about 20 minutes, until deeply browned and caramelized. Remove from the oven. Use the offset spatula to encourage any maple syrup that's tried to run away to join its friends again.
- Let cool completely on the sheet pan until firm and set. Break into pieces with a knife or by hand.

193. Marbled Jam Cake

Serving: Serves 8 | Prep: | Cook: | Ready in:

Ingredients

- 1/3 cup oat flour (40g)
- 1/3 cup buckwheat flour (40g)
- 1/3 cup all-purpose flour (40g)
- 1 teaspoon baking powder
- 1/2 teaspoon baking soda
- 1/4 teaspoon salt (omit if you are using salted butter)
- 1/3 cup sugar (67g)
- large pinches grated nutmeg or spice of your choice
- 4 tablespoons unsalted butter, cold and cut into small cubes
- 1/4 cup quick oats (20g) or rolled oats (the latter will remain chewy in the completed cake)
- 1/2 cup plain yogurt (if you only have greek style, you'll need to increase the amount of milk)
- 1/8 to 1/4 cups whole milk (milk and yogurt can be interchanged, or replaced by buttermilk)
- 1 teaspoon vanilla extract (optional)
- 1/2 to 2/3 cups simple, runny, fruit-based jam or preserves, preferably with pieces of fruit

Direction

- Mix the flours, baking soda, baking powder, salt, spice and sugar together with a whisk in a medium bowl.
- Add the butter, and squeeze the cubes into the flour with your fingers, as you might with a pastry dough, until you have a mealy consistency.
- Add the yogurt, a splash of milk and vanilla extract. Stir to completely combine--it should be like thick cake batter, not watery but not as stiff as a muffin or biscuit dough. If you need to thin it, use the greater amount of milk.
- Use a few turns of a wooden spoon to fold in the rolled oats.
- Pour into a buttered 9" pie plate (a round cake tin works, too). The batter will rise

considerably, so don't go for anything smaller unless it has high sides.
- Drop 3-5 generous dollops of your jam on top of the batter.
- Use a table knife to drag the jam strategically throughout the batter. Resist the urge to stir and blend. Use a few (ok, maybe several) carefully-planned drags to marbleize the jam into the batter, starting in the dollop of jam and moving the knife (or the pie plate) in simple arcs. Add smaller spoonfuls and streaks as you see fit.
- Bake in a 350 degree (preheated) oven for 35-40 minutes. The center should be firm and the jam fairly well hidden under the golden, risen cake.
- Let cool at least 1 hour. Yes, the cake will fall in places where the jam had been hot and bubbly.
- Slice and serve wedges with whipped cream or ice cream, or eat with a big spoon.

194. Marian Burros' Cowboy Cookies

Serving: Makes 30 two-bite cookies | Prep: | Cook: | Ready in:

Ingredients

- 1 cup all-purpose flour
- 1 teaspoon baking powder
- 1 teaspoon baking soda
- 1 teaspoon cinnamon
- 1/3 teaspoon salt
- 1 stick butter, at room temperature
- 1/2 cup granulated sugar
- 1/2 cup packed light-brown sugar
- 1 egg
- 1 teaspoon vanilla
- 1 cup semisweet chocolate chips
- 1 cup old-fashioned rolled oats
- 2/3 cup cup unsweetened flake coconut/coconut chips
- 2/3 cup chopped pecans

Direction

- Heat oven to 350 degrees.
- Mix flour, baking powder, baking soda, cinnamon and salt in bowl.
- In a large bowl, beat butter with an electric mixer at medium speed until smooth and creamy. Gradually beat in sugars, and combine thoroughly.
- Add egg, beat into batter. Beat in vanilla.
- Stir in flour mixture until just combined. Stir in chocolate chips, oats, coconut and pecans.
- For each cookie, drop a heaping tablespoon of dough onto ungreased baking sheets, spacing 3 inches apart.
- Bake for 13 to 15 minutes, until edges are lightly browned; rotate sheets halfway through. Remove cookies from rack to cool.

195. Masala Chai Tea Oatmeal

Serving: Serves 4 | Prep: | Cook: | Ready in:

Ingredients

- 2 cups whole milk
- 2 cups water
- 1/4 cup black tea
- 2 inch chunk of ginger, roughly chopped
- 2 teaspoons black peppercorns
- 2 teaspoons whole cloves
- 1 cinnamon stick
- 1/4-1/2 cups sugar (to taste)
- 1 dash salt
- 1 cup oats
- 5 cardamom pods

Direction

- Simmer tea, spices, sugar, milk and water and let steep for five minutes or until desired strength.

- Strain spices and reserve liquid chai. Return chai to pan, add oats and a pinch of salt. Simmer oatmeal until desired consistency.

196. Maya's Chocolate Fudge Sheet Cake

Serving: Serves 12 | Prep: | Cook: | Ready in:

Ingredients

- For the chocolate sheet cake:
- 2 cups (400 grams) sugar
- 1 1/3 cups (200 grams) white rice flour
- 1/2 cup (50 grams) oat flour (gluten-free oat flour if gluten is an issue)
- 2/3 cup (60 grams) natural unsweetened cocoa powder
- 1/2 teaspoon salt
- 1/4 teaspoon xanthum gum
- 1 1/2 teaspoons baking powder
- 3/4 teaspoon baking soda
- 2 large eggs
- 1 cup milk
- 2 teaspoons pure vanilla extract
- 1/2 cup neutral flavored vegetable oil (such as corn, safflower, or soybean)
- 1 cup boiling water
- For the milk chocolate frosting:
- 1 cup heavy cream
- 17 1/2 ounces (500 grams) milk chocolate or 55% to 62% dark chocolate, coarsely chopped
- 1/4 teaspoon salt, plus more to taste
- 1/2 pound (225 grams/2 sticks) unsalted butter, very soft

Direction

- Position a rack in the lower third of the oven and preheat the oven to 350° F. Grease a 9- by 13-inch metal or glass baking pan.
- Put the sugar, rice flour, oat flour, cocoa powder, salt, xanthan gum, baking powder, and baking soda in the bowl of the stand mixer and mix with the paddle attachment until well combined. Add the eggs, milk, and vanilla and beat on medium speed for 2 minutes. Add the oil and beat until smooth. Stir in the hot water until well incorporated. The batter will be thin.
- Scrape the batter into the pan and bake for 30 to 35 minutes in the metal pan or a little longer in glass, until the cake pulls away slightly from the edges of the pan and a toothpick inserted near the center comes out almost clean. Set the pan on a rack to cool completely before frosting or storing.
- Make the frosting: Put the cream, chocolate, and salt in a medium stainless steel bowl. Bring an inch of water to a simmer in a wide skillet.
- Turn off the heat and set the bowl of chocolate in the water. Let it rest for 15 minutes, gently shaking the bowl several times to submerge the chocolate in the cream.
- When the chocolate is melted, start whisking at one edge and continue whisking until all of the chocolate is incorporated and the mixture is smooth.
- Add the butter in chunks and whisk once or twice to break them up; let the mixture rest for 5 minute to finish melting the butter before whisking it smooth. Taste and adjust salt if necessary. Set aside, without mixing or disturbing, until needed.
- If the frosting is stiff by the time you need it, set the bowl in a pan of hot water to soften it, stirring occasionally until smooth and just pourable. Scrape the frosting over the cake and spread it evenly. Let set at room temperature, then cover and refrigerate the cake or keep it at room temperature—it's great either way. The cake keeps for at least 3 days at room temperature and 5 days in the refrigerator.

197. Mookies (Muffin Top Cookies)

Serving: Makes about a dozen cookies | Prep: | Cook: | Ready in:

Ingredients

- 1/2 cup unsalted butter
- 1 cup sugar
- 1 egg
- 1/3 cup milk
- 1 teaspoon vanilla extract
- 2 cups all-purpose flour
- 1 cup oats
- 2 teaspoons baking powder
- 1/2 teaspoon kosher salt
- 3 cups corn flakes
- 1/2 cup rice crispies
- 1/2 cup chocolate chips
- 1 cup chopped pecans

Direction

- Heat the oven to 350°F. Beat butter and sugar together until fluffy. Add egg and mix well. Add milk and vanilla and mix well.
- In a separate bowl, combine flour, oats, baking powder, and salt. Add dry ingredients to wet ingredients and mix until just combined. Stir in the cereals, nuts, and chocolate chips.
- Scoop dough into 2 inch balls on a cookie sheet. Bake for 20 to 25 minutes, until the tops are golden brown. Sadly, cookies need to cool before eating. They are definitely better after they cool than fresh from the oven.

198. Morning Person Zucchini Bread

Serving: Makes 1 loaf | Prep: 0hours40mins | Cook: 1hours0mins | Ready in:

Ingredients

- 2/3 cup olive oil (143 grams), plus more for the pan
- 1 1/3 cups white whole-wheat flour (170 grams), plus more for the pan
- 2 1/3 cups grated zucchini (from about 11 ounces zucchini)
- 1/3 cup sugar (67 grams)
- 1/3 cup brown sugar (71 grams)
- 2 large eggs
- 1/2 teaspoon baking powder
- 1/2 teaspoon baking soda
- 3/4 teaspoon kosher salt
- 2/3 cup walnuts (75 grams)
- 1/3 cup golden raisins (53 grams)
- 1/3 cup oats (33 grams), plus more for topping

Direction

- Preheat the oven to 350° F. Grease an 8 1/2- by 4 1/2-inch loaf pan with some oil. Add some flour and tap around to distribute evenly. Gather the zucchini in a kitchen linen or paper towel and squeeze over the sink to get rid of any excess moisture.
- Combine the sugars, eggs, and oil in a large bowl. Whisk until smooth. Add the zucchini to the bowl and use a rubber spatula to combine. Add the baking powder, baking soda, and salt. Stir to combine. Add the flour, walnuts, raisins, and oats. Stir to combine.
- Pour the batter into prepared pan. Sprinkle oats on top. Bake for about 1 hour until a thin knife inserted in the center comes out clean. Let cool in the pan for 15 or so minutes before turning onto a wire rack. Cool completely before slicing and serving.

199. Muesli Bread With Raisins, Apricot And Almonds

Serving: Makes 1 | Prep: | Cook: | Ready in:

Ingredients

- 700 grams Wholemeal flour
- 160 grams Wheat flour
- 50 grams Porridge oats
- 1.75 ounces Lukewarm water
- 1 Envelope dry yeast
- 2 Tbs sugar
- 1 Tbs salt
- 85 grams Dried apricots
- 45 grams Almonds
- 55 grams Raisins

Direction

- Take a large bowl, dissolve yeast and sugar in the water. Mix the different flour and porridge oats in another bowl. Stir in 200 grams (7 ounces) of the flour at the time little by little, beating well after each addition. Add the almonds, apricots and raisins. When the dough has pulled together, turn it out onto a lightly floured surface and knead until smooth and elastic. This takes about 5 minutes.
- Lightly flour a large bowl, place the dough in the bowl. Cover with a damp cloth and let rise in a warm place (I usually put it on the bathroom floor) until ca. doubled in volume, about 55 minutes.
- Deflate the dough and turn it out onto a lightly floured surface. Place the dough into a lightly greased 9x5 inch loaf pan (or whatever pan shape you like). Cover the loaves with a damp cloth and let rise until doubled in volume, about 40 minutes.
- Preheat oven to 190 degrees C (375 degrees F).
- Brush some egg on top of the bread and bake for 35 minutes.

200. Multigrain Marmalade Muffins

Serving: Makes 16 | Prep: | Cook: | Ready in:

Ingredients

- 1/2 cup whole wheat flour
- 1/2 cup oat flour [ground oats]
- 1/2 cup spelt flour
- 1/2 cup buckwheat flour
- 1 teaspoon baking powder
- 1/2 teaspoon baking soda
- 1/2 teaspoon kosher salt
- 1 cup buttermilk
- 1/2 cup greek yogurt
- 2 ounces unsalted butter, room temperature
- 1 tablespoon honey
- 8 ounces marmalade
- 1 egg

Direction

- Preheat the oven to 350 degrees. Line two 12-cup muffin tins with liners [16].
- In a medium bowl, place the whole wheat flour, oat flour, spelt four, buckwheat flour, baking powder, baking soda and kosher salt [all dry ingredients]. Whisk thoroughly to aerate and combine.
- In a small bowl, whisk together the buttermilk and yogurt.
- In a large bowl, beat together the butter, honey and half of the marmalade [4oz] for about three minutes. Scrape down the sides of the bowl with a spatula and add the egg and beat until mixed in thoroughly. Add the last 4oz of the marmalade and beat until combined, about 1 minute. Scrape down sides of the bowl.
- Add a third of the flour mixture on low speed and mix until just combined. Add half of the dairy mixture, mix again until just combined. Repeat with another third of the flour, milk, and flour, each time beating only until just barely combined.
- Scoop batter into muffin tins with an ice cream scoop or spoon, about halfway up. Bake 35-40 minutes, until golden brown. Remove to a rack to cool.
- Serve warm right out of the oven or toasted the next day.

201. Muscovado Baked Beans

Serving: Serves 4-6 | Prep: | Cook: |Ready in:

Ingredients

- Baked Beans
- 1 splash olive oil
- 1 onion, finely chopped
- 2 large cloves of garlic, crushed
- 2 teaspoons paprika
- 1 can chopped tomatoes
- 10 ounces dried haricot beans, soaked and cooked as per packet instructions
- 3 tablespoons dark muscovado sugar
- 2 tablespoons ketchup
- 1 tablespoon dijon mustard
- 150 milliliters beer
- a few sprigs fresh thyme
- Salt and freshly ground pepper
- Crumble Topping
- 4 ounces butter
- 4 ounces flour
- 3 ounces porridge oats
- 4 ounces cheddar cheese

Direction

- Pre-heat the oven to 200degreesC/350degreesF.
- Heat olive oil in a heavy based pan and sauté the onion and garlic till soft.
- Add paprika, beans and tomatoes. Stir well then add the sugar, ketchup and mustard.
- Add beer to thin the sauce a little.
- Season with thyme, a few grinds of black pepper and a hefty pinch of salt.
- Allow to simmer gently for around 20 minutes to allow the flavors to combine. Add a little water if too thick.
- For the crumble: Rub the butter into the flour with your fingertips until the mixture resembles breadcrumbs, then stir in the oats and cheese.
- To assemble: Put the beans into an ovenproof dish and top with the crumble mixture.
- Bake in the oven for 20 minutes until golden and bubbling.

202. My Coffee Group's Favorite Bircher Muesli

Serving: Serves 4 | Prep: | Cook: |Ready in:

Ingredients

- 1 1/4 cups old-fashioned oats (not quick cooking)
- 2/3 cup milk of your choice
- 2/3 cup Greek yogurt (I use non-fat)
- 1 apple, peeled, then grated or diced finely
- 1/4 cup organic cane sugar
- 1/4 cup golden raisins, or other dried fruit (I sometimes omit this in summer when there's so much fresh fruit around)
- 1 to 2 cups chopped fresh fruit -- I love bananas and strawberries, blueberries, or pears, depending on the season. I also love to add in persimmons.
- 1/2 cup toasted almonds, slivered or sliced (you can use the pre-toasted ones, or toast them carefully in a pan over medium heat or on a baking sheet for about 10 minutes in a 350° F oven)

Direction

- The evening before you want to serve the muesli: In a medium to large bowl, mix together the oats, milk, yogurt, sugar, grated apple, and dried fruit (if using). Cover, then refrigerate overnight.
- In the morning, remove the bowl from the refrigerator. Add a little more milk if it's gotten too thick. Add the fresh fruit, and top with the nuts.

203. Nekisia Davis' Olive Oil & Maple Granola

Serving: Makes about 7 cups | Prep: 0hours10mins | Cook: 0hours45mins | Ready in:

Ingredients

- 3 cups old-fashioned rolled oats
- 1 cup hulled raw pumpkin seeds
- 1 cup hulled raw sunflower seeds
- 1 cup unsweetened coconut chips
- 1 1/4 cups raw pecans, left whole or coarsely chopped
- 3/4 cup pure maple syrup
- 1/2 cup extra-virgin olive oil
- 1/2 cup packed light brown sugar
- 1 pinch coarse salt, to taste

Direction

- Heat oven to 300°F.
- Place oats, pumpkin seeds, sunflower seeds, coconut, pecans, syrup, olive oil, sugar, and 1 teaspoon salt in a large bowl and mix until well combined. Spread granola mixture in an even layer on a rimmed baking sheet. Transfer to oven and bake, stirring every 10 to 15 minutes, until granola is toasted, about 45 minutes.
- Remove granola from oven and season with more salt to taste. Let cool completely before serving or storing in an airtight container for up to 1 month.

204. No Bake Banana Oatmeal Cookies

Serving: Serves 12 | Prep: | Cook: |Ready in:

Ingredients

- 240 grams ripe bananas, cut into chunk
- 150 grams vegan chocolate chips
- 60 milliliters coconut oil
- 30 grams chia seeds
- 7,5 grams cocoa powder
- 200 grams quick-cooking oats
- 10 milliliters vanilla extract
- 15 milliliters maple syrup

Direction

- Combine bananas, chocolate chips, coconut oil, chia seeds, cocoa powder and maple syrup in a sauce pan. Simmer over low heat until bananas are fully tender, about 5 minutes.
- Mash the bananas using a potato masher and continue heating for another 5 minutes.
- Turn off the heat and stir in the vanilla.
- Fold in the oats.
- Spoon onto a baking sheet lined with parchment paper.
- Leave in the chiller for an hour to set.

205. No Bake Chocolate, Oatmeal, Peanut Butter Cookies

Serving: Makes 30 cookies | Prep: | Cook: |Ready in:

Ingredients

- 1/2 cup butter
- 1 3/4 cups sugar
- 1/2 cup low-fat milk
- 4 tablespoons unsweetened cocoa powder
- 1/2 cup peanut butter (preferably natural, creamy)
- 3 cups quick oats
- 2 teaspoons vanilla

Direction

- Combine the butter, sugar, milk, and cocoa powder in a pot on the stove on medium heat
- Bring the mixture to a boil, stirring occasionally
- Once it boils, hold the boil for a minute and a half

- Remove from heat and stir in the peanut butter, oats, and vanilla
- Drop the mixture in rounded tablespoons onto wax paper or a cookie sheet
- Allow the cookies to fully cool and harden before storing or stacking

206. No Bake Cookies

Serving: Makes 12 | Prep: 0hours5mins | Cook: 0hours6mins | Ready in:

Ingredients

- 6 tablespoons (85 grams) unsalted butter, at room temperature
- 1/4 cup (57 grams) whole milk
- 1/2 cup (100 grams) granulated sugar
- 3 tablespoons (16 grams) Dutch-process cocoa powder
- 1/2 teaspoon kosher salt
- 1/2 cup (132 grams) sweetened, creamy peanut butter, like Skippy's
- 4 ounces (113 grams, about 3/4 cup) semi-sweet or dark chocolate chips, or chopped-up bar (50-65% cacao)
- 1 teaspoon pure vanilla extract
- 2 cups (176 grams) quick-cooking oats
- Flaky sea salt, like Maldon

Direction

- Line a plate or baking sheet with parchment paper or a silicone mat, and place a timer set for one minute or a clock with second hands nearby.
- In a medium saucepan over medium-low heat, melt the butter. Add the milk, sugar, cocoa powder, and salt, and whisk together. Continue whisking until the sugar dissolves and the contents of the pan come to a rolling simmer throughout (not just at the sides). At this point, use your timer or clock to let the mixture bubble, uninterrupted, for exactly one minute.
- When the timer rings, immediately cut the heat and add the peanut butter, chocolate chips, vanilla, and oats. Stir with a wooden spoon until the chocolate and peanut butter melt and everything's fully combined.
- Use a 2-tablespoon scoop (or two spoons) to make little mounded cookies on the wax paper. If you like these flatter, use the back of your scoop to gently press them down at this stage. Sprinkle the middle of each with a small pinch of flaky salt, and let sit out on the countertop for about an hour or stick in the fridge until they've firmed up.

207. No Bake Peanut Butter Dog Treats

Serving: Serves 3 | Prep: | Cook: | Ready in:

Ingredients

- 1/2 cup unsweetened peanut butter
- 1/2 cup unsweetened applesauce
- 1 tablespoon coconut oil
- 1/4 cup blueberries
- 2 cups oats

Direction

- Add the wet ingredients and mix thoroughly.
- Drop in the oats; stir to combine.
- Form tablespoon-size balls and dust with more oats.
- Refrigerate for 1 hour.
- Enjoy!

208. Nordic Oats With Pumpkin Seed Oil & Booster Topping

Serving: Serves 4 | Prep: | Cook: | Ready in:

Ingredients

- 1 cup steel cut oats
- 1 teaspoon sea salt
- 1 cup walnuts
- 1/2 cup unsweetened coconut flakes or chips
- 1/3 cup pumpkin seeds
- 6 to 8 dried figs, sliced
- Birch syrup
- Pumpkin seed oil
- Buttermilk, well-shaken

Direction

- Make the oats: In a large pot, bring oats, salt, and 4 cups water to a boil, reduce to medium, and cook, uncovered, for 25 minutes, stirring once or twice. Lower temperature nearing end of cooking time to avoid splatters, if necessary.
- Make the Booster Topping: In a large skillet, add walnuts, coconut, and pumpkin seeds. Toast over medium for 1 to 2 minutes, until fragrant and beginning to brown (watch carefully to avoid burning coconut). Transfer to a bowl and cool before storing in an airtight container or jar in the pantry or refrigerator for up to 2 months.
- To serve: Divide cooked oats evenly between 4 bowls. Top with Booster Topping, dried figs, and a drizzle of birch syrup and pumpkin seed oil. Serve with buttermilk.

209. Oat Breakfast Cookies

Serving: Serves 20 | Prep: | Cook: | Ready in:

Ingredients

- 190 grams gluten free rolled oats
- 130 grams almond butter
- 110 grams maple syrup (or honey)
- 15 grams pumpkin seeds
- 30 grams dried cranberries, sweetened
- 30 grams pistachios
- 1 teaspoon cinnamon

Direction

- Add the oats and cinnamon to a large bowl and mix until combined.
- Add the almond butter and maple syrup to a saucepan and heat over a medium heat until melted and fully combined, stirring regularly.
- Divide the mixture into small balls (it should make around 20), then flatten and place in the refrigerator to set (about 30 minutes) before serving.

210. Oat Gnocchi With Shaved Asparagus & Brown Butter Vinaigrette

Serving: Serves 4 as a light main course | Prep: 6hours0mins | Cook: 1hours0mins | Ready in:

Ingredients

- Neutral oil
- 1 cup steel-cut oats
- 1/4 teaspoon salt
- 4 cups water
- 4 ounces melty cheese, such as Gruyère, cheddar, or manchego, grated (optional)
- 1/4 cup oat flour, cornmeal, or wheat flour (see Author Notes for tips)
- 1/4 cup extra-virgin olive oil
- 2 tablespoons white wine or cider vinegar
- 2 lemons, zest and juice (about 2 oz juice)
- 1 orange, zest
- 4 tablespoons unsalted butter
- 1 small shallot, minced (a tiny yellow onion works in a pinch)
- 1/2 pound asparagus, trimmed and washed
- 3 ounces spinach, washed
- 1/2 cup pecans (or another nut like almonds), toasted and roughly chopped

Direction

- In a larger pot than seems necessary, heat a glug of neutral oil over medium heat (just enough to coat the bottom of the pan). Add the oats and briefly toast, 30 to 60 seconds. Add the salt and water and bring to a boil, then reduce to a simmer. Cook, stirring regularly, until the oatmeal is tender and thickened, about 20 minutes. Add the grated cheese, if using, and stir to distribute evenly.

- Spread the oatmeal into a small sheet pan (such as a quarter sheet pan) or similar-size baking dish—the smaller the container, the thicker the oat gnocchi will be. Refrigerate until fully cool and thick (at least 4 hours or ideally overnight).
- To make the brown butter vinaigrette, combine the olive oil, vinegar, lemon zest, lemon juice, orange zest, and a big pinch of salt in a bowl. Add the minced shallot to another, heatproof bowl. In a small frying pan, heat the butter over medium heat and until brown, swirling regularly. (As the butter cooks, its milk proteins will fall to the bottom of the pan, where they'll caramelize.) Remove from the heat and pour over the shallot and let sit 3 minutes to soften. Add the shallot-butter mixture to the lemon-olive oil mixture and whisk to combine.
- Using a sharp knife, vegetable peeler, or mandolin, shave the asparagus into thin ribbons. Combine the asparagus with the spinach and pecans and set aside.
- Remove the set oatmeal from the fridge and pop out of the baking dish. Cut the oatmeal into wide planks or squares. Dredge the pieces in the oat flour (or cornmeal or wheat flour).
- In a large frying pan, heat a large glug of neutral oil over medium-high heat. Add the oat gnocchi and pan-fry until golden brown; if the pan looks dry, add a bit more oil along the way. Flip and brown the other sides evenly, adjusting the heat of the pan as needed. Depending on the shape, you may have to brown them in batches. The all-ready browned fritters can be held warm in a low oven while the others brown.
- To serve, place the oat gnocchi on a serving platter or individual plates. Dress the asparagus salad in some warm vinaigrette with several turns of black pepper and salt to taste. (Note: For the leftover vinaigrette, store in the fridge, then simply rewarm and dress again on your next salad.) Heap the salad on top of the oat gnocchi and serve immediately.

211. Oat Porridge Bread

Serving: Makes 2 loaves | Prep: 168hours0mins | Cook: 1hours30mins | Ready in:

Ingredients

- Starter and Leaven
- 625 grams white bread flour
- 625 grams whole wheat bread flour
- Slightly warm water
- Oat Porridge Bread
- 500 grams high-extraction wheat flour
- 500 grams medium-strong wheat flour
- 70 grams wheat germ
- 750 grams water
- 150 grams leaven
- 25 grams fine sea salt
- 500 grams cooked oat porridge, cooled
- 200 grams almonds, toasted and coarsely chopped (optional)
- 50 grams almond oil (optional)
- Coarsely chopped oat flakes (rolled oats) for coating (optional)

Direction

- Starter and Leaven
- Mix the flours to make 1250 grams of 50/50 flour blend. Use this blend to feed your culture and develop your starter.
- To make your starter, in a medium bowl, place 300 grams of slightly warm (80 to 85° F, 26 to 29° C) water. Add 315 grams of flour blend (reserve the remaining flour blend), and mix with your hand or a wooden spoon to combine until the mixture is free of any dry bits. Cover the mixture with a clean, dry kitchen towel or cheesecloth and let stand at warm room

temperature until bubbles start to form around the sides and on the surface, about 2 days. It's important to maintain a warm temperature. Let stand another day to allow fermentation to progress a bit. More bubbles should form. This is your starter. It will smell acidic and slightly funky. At this stage it's time to train your starter into a leaven by feeding it fresh flour and water at regular intervals.

- Feed the starter: Transfer 75 grams of the starter to a clean bowl and discard the remainder of the starter. To the 75 grams of starter, add 150 grams of the 50/50 flour blend and 150 grams warm (80 to 85°F, 26 to 29°C) water. Mix to combine; it should have the consistency of pancake batter. Repeat this feeding process once every 24 hours at the same time of day, always transferring 75 grams of the starter to a clean bowl and discarding the remainder, then adding the flour and water and re-covering the bowl with a clean, dry kitchen towel after each feeding and letting the mixture stand at warm room temperature. The batter should start to rise and fall consistently throughout the day after a few days of feedings. As the starter develops, the smell will change from ripe and sour to sweet and pleasantly fermented, like yogurt. Once this sweet lactic character is established and the fermentation (the regular rise and fall of the batter) is predictable, a few days to one week, it's time to make the leaven from this mature starter.
- Leaven is the portion of prefermented flour and water that will go into your final dough and raise the whole mass during the bulk (first) and final rises. Two days before you want to make bread, feed the matured starter twice daily, once in the morning and once in the evening (the process described above) to increase fermentation activity. When you are ready to make the dough, discard all but 1 tablespoon of the matured starter. To the remaining 1 tablespoon, add 200 grams of the 50/50 flour blend and 200 grams warm (80 to 85°F, 26 to 29°C) water. This is your leaven. Cover and let rest at moderate room temperature for 4 to 6 hours.
- To test the leaven's readiness, drop a spoonful into a bowl of room temperature water. If it sinks, it is not ready and needs more time to ripen. When it floats on the surface or close to it, it's ready to use to make the dough.
- To maintain the leaven for regular use, continue feeding daily as described above. To save leaven for long periods without use, add enough flour to make a dry paste and keep covered in the refrigerator. When you want to use it again, keep at warm room temperature for at least 2 days and do three to four feedings to refresh and reduce the acid load that builds up while it is stored in the refrigerator.
- Oat Porridge Bread
- To make the dough/premix, in a large mixing bowl, combine the flours and wheat germ. In a second, large mixing bowl, add 700 grams of water. Add the leaven to the water and stir to disperse. Add the flour mixture to the liquid-leaven mixture and stir to combine until no dry bits remain. Cover and let the premix rest for at least 30 minutes and up to 4 hours to hydrate during this rest period, taking care to keep the mixture where it is at warm room temperature. After autolyse (or the rest), add the salt and the remaining 50 grams of slightly warm water, folding the dough on top of itself to incorporate.
- For the bulk rise, transfer the dough to a medium bowl and keep covered to maintain a warm dough temperature of 80 to 85° F (26 to 29° C) to accomplish the first rising time, 3 to 4 hours. During the bulk rise, the dough is developed by folding and turning it in the container. Fold the dough every 30 minutes for the first 2 1/2 hours of bulk rising. To do a fold, dip one hand in water, grab the underside of the dough, stretch it out, and fold it back over itself. Rotate the container one-quarter turn and repeat three to four times. When you are folding the dough, note its temperature to the touch and how the dough is becoming aerated and elastic. Fold in the

cooked oat porridge, almonds, and almond oil gently by hand after the first two series of turns, about 1 hour into the bulk rise. After 3 hours and six foldings, the dough should feel aerated, billowy, and softer. You will see a 20 to 30 percent increase in volume. If not, continue bulk rising for 30 minutes to 1 hour longer.

- When the dough is 20 to 30 percent increase in volume, billowy, and elastic, remove it from the container with a dough spatula. We don't "punch" the dough down tode-gas at Tartine. We strengthen the dough by using gentle folds and turns. As flavor develops during the first rising, it is key to preserve that flavorful gas built up within the dough until the bread is baked. Lightly flour the top surface of the dough and cut into two pieces using the dough spatula. Work each piece gently into a round by drawing the spatula around the side of the dough in a circular motion. Surface tension builds as the dough anchors to the surface while you rotate and work it. Again, take care to work the dough gently to preserve the flavorful gasses that have formed during fermentation. When well-shaped, the dough should have a taut, smooth surface.

- For the bench rest, lightly flour the tops of the rounds, cover with a kitchen towel, and let rest on the work surface for 20 to 30 minutes. Line two medium baskets or bowls with clean, dry kitchen towels and dust generously with a 50/50 mixture of any wheat and rice flours. Starchy rice flour (whether white or brown) is more absorbent than wheat flour and keeps the dough from sticking to the cloth-lined rising basket. Tapioca flour can also be used.

- For the final shaping, slip the dough spatula under each piece of dough and flip it, floured-side down. Pull the bottom of the dough up to fold into one-third of the round. Pull each side and fold over the center to elongate the dough vertically. Fold the top down to the center and then fold the bottom up over the top fold-down, leaving the seam underneath. Let the dough rest for a few minutes, seam-side down, so that the seam seals.

- For the final rising, transfer the dough to the floured baskets, flipping the dough over so that the seam-side is facing up and centered. Coat the loaf with the cracked oat flakes by rolling the smooth side of the dough in the coating before transferring it to the floured rising baskets, placing the dough coated-side down, seam-side up. Cover with a clean, dry kitchen towel and let rise at warm room temperature for 3 to 5 hours or overnight in the refrigerator.

- Twenty minutes before you are ready to bake the bread, preheat the oven to 500°F (260°C), adjust the oven rack to its lowest position, and place a 9 ½-in/24-cm round cast-iron Dutch oven, 11-inch oval cast-iron Dutch oven, or any other heavy ovenproof pot with a tight-fitting lid into the oven to preheat (with its lid on). Carefully transfer one dough round into the pre-heated Dutch oven, tipping it out of the basket into the pot so it is now seam-side down. Score the top of the dough with a razor blade or cut with scissors. Cover the pot and return to the oven. After 20 minutes, reduce the oven temperature to 450°F (230°C). Bake another 10 minutes, then carefully remove the lid (a cloud of steam will be released). Continue to bake for another 20 to 25 minutes, until the crust is a deep golden brown. When it's done, turn the baked loaf out onto a wire rack to cool. To bake the second loaf, raise the oven temperature to 500°F (260°C), wipe out the Dutch oven with a dry kitchen towel, and reheat with the lid on for 15 minutes. Repeat the baking procedure as with the first loaf.

212. Oat Streusel Jam Bars

Serving: Makes 9x9-inch pan | Prep: 0hours20mins | Cook: 1hours0mins | Ready in:

Ingredients

- 3 cups rolled oats, divided
- 3/4 cup brown sugar

- 2 1/2 teaspoons kosher salt
- 1 cup unsalted butter, roughly chopped, plus more for greasing
- 1 (13-ounce) jar blackberry jam (about 1 heaping cup)

Direction

- Add 2 1/4 cups rolled oats to a food processor. Blend until a fine flour forms. Add the brown sugar and salt and pulse to combine. Scatter the butter evenly on top and pulse until a shaggy dough just starts to form. Add the remaining oats and pulse a couple times to incorporate.
- Remove 1 1/4 (loosely packed!) cups of streusel. Spread out the clumps (clumps are good!) on a plate and stick in the freezer to firm.
- Meanwhile, preheat the oven to 350° F. Arrange a baking rack in the bottom third of the oven. Line a 9- by 9-inch baking pan with parchment. The easiest way to do this is cut a roughly 12- by 12-inch square. Now cut slits inward from each corner—this will help the paper fold into place. Smear a bit of butter inside the pan. Place the parchment inside and smooth out with your hands.
- Press the remaining oat streusel into the lined pan, forming an even layer. Spread the jam on top. Take the streusel from the freezer—it should be very firm—and sprinkle on top.
- Bake—on a rack toward the bottom of the oven—for 50 minutes, rotating halfway through. Let cool for at least 30 minutes in the pan, then use the parchment to remove from the pan, and transfer to a rack to cool completely. Cut into 16 or 12 or 9 pieces, depending on how big or little you like your jam bars.
- These freeze well. I like to wrap them individually and grab on my way out the door.

213. Oat And Flax Pancakes With Spiced Apple Compote

Serving: Serves 6 | Prep: | Cook: | Ready in:

Ingredients

- For the Spiced Apple Compote:
- 3 apples, cored and chopped
- 1 tablespoon lemon juice or cider vinegar
- 1/4 cup water
- 2 teaspoons cinnamon
- 5 whole cloves
- 1/2 teaspoon kosher salt
- 2 tablespoons raisins
- 2 tablespoons maple syrup, preferably grade B
- Oat and Flax Pancakes:
- 1 cup oat flour
- 1/2 cup cold milled flaxseed
- 1/2 cup potato starch
- 1 tablespoon baking powder
- 1/2 teaspoon cinnamon
- 1/4 teaspoon kosher salt
- 3 large eggs
- 2 cups buttermilk (or 2 cups almond milk with 1 tsp lemon juice)
- butter or avocado oil, for cooking
- 2% Greek yogurt, to serve
- apple compote, to serve
- grade B maple syrup, to serve

Direction

- For the Spiced Apple Compote:
- Place all ingredients in a small-medium pot, cover and bring to a gentle boil. Once bubbling, reduce heat to low and tilt lid. Continue to simmer for 20-30 minutes, until apples are soft and liquid has reduced to a syrup.
- While the apples simmer, prepare the pancakes:
- Oat and Flax Pancakes:
- In a medium bowl, whisk together oat flour, ground flaxseed, potato starch, baking powder, and cinnamon.

- In a separate large bowl, beat eggs with whisk. Next, add sugar and oil and whisk well to make fluffy. Finally, add buttermilk or almond milk-lemon mixture. Whisk until frothy.
- Pour dry ingredients into the large bowl with the wet ingredients and mix until just combined (do NOT over mix- a few flour clumps are fine). Don't worry if the batter seems thin.
- Heat a large pan or skillet over medium heat for five minutes (yes, five minutes) to ensure thorough heating. In the meantime, let the batter stand. The ground flaxseed will congeal and cause the batter to thicken a bit.
- Pour 1 teaspoon grape seed oil in the pan and swirl to cover. Grab a 1/4 cup measure or ladle and use it to scoop drops of batter into the pan. Once each drop of batter is bubbling (about 2 minutes), flip and cook for another minute or two.
- Serve pancakes immediately or place in a 200F degree oven on a cooling rack placed on top of a baking sheet. Top pancakes with apple compote, yogurt and a drizzle of maple syrup.

214. Oat And Wheat Sandwich Bread

Serving: Makes 2 loaves | Prep: | Cook: | Ready in:

Ingredients

- 1/2 cup bulgur wheat
- 1/2 cup oats
- 1 tablespoon salt
- 1 tablespoon dry yeast (or three packets)
- 1 cup whole wheat flour
- 4 tablespoons honey
- 4 tablespoons canola oil or melted butter
- 3-4 cups white flour

Direction

- Combine the bulgur, oats, and salt with 1 1/2 cups of boiling water in a medium bowl.
- Cover the bowl with foil and let it stand for 30-45 minutes until the water is absorbed and the mixture is no longer hot.
- Meanwhile, in the bowl of a stand mixer, combine 1/2 cup warm water with the yeast and a bit of honey. Let it sit for a few minutes and then stir in the whole wheat flour. Let the mixture rest for 30-45 minutes or so, while the grains cool.
- Once the grains are cool and the flour mixture has proofed for about 30-45 minutes, add the grains to the flour.
- Mix till combined. Add the honey, oil, and 3 cups of white flour and use the dough hook to mix for about five minutes, adding flour as needed until the dough is smooth and no longer sticking to the bowl.
- Place the dough in a large bowl coated with cooking spray, turning to coat the top. Cover and let it rise in a warm place for about two hours or until doubled in size. Punch the dough down and divide it in half. Use a rolling pin or the palms of your hands to flatten each half into a rough oval shape about 8 inches wide in the center. Then, just roll the oval up jelly-roll style (lengthwise) and place each one, seam sides down, in a 9-inch loaf pan coated with cooking spray.
- Let the loaves rise for about an hour longer.
- About 15 minutes before baking time, preheat the oven to 350*. Bake the loaves for about 45 minutes, till they are golden and sound kind of hollow when you tap them. Cool the loaves on wire racks (this is important; they will get soggy if you let them cool in the pans) for at least 1/2 hour before serving. You can also wrap the loaves well in foil after they have cooled thoroughly and freeze for up to a month.

215. Oat And Chocolate Chip Cookies

Serving: Makes 12 | Prep: | Cook: | Ready in:

Ingredients

- 1 cup plain flour
- 100 grams dark chocolate, chopped
- 1 teaspoon vanilla extract
- 1 egg
- 1 1/4 cups oats
- 1/2 teaspoon baking soda
- 1/2 teaspoon baking powder
- 1/2 cup caster sugar
- 1/2 cup butter
- 1/2 cup soft light brown sugar

Direction

- Preheat the oven to 180 degrees C and line a baking tray with grease proof paper
- Mix together butter and sugars with a hand mixer until thoroughly mixed
- Add egg and stir in thoroughly.
- Meanwhile in another bowl mix flour, oats and baking powders together. Now stir in the chocolate
- Mix together the dry and wet ingredients thoroughly
- Roll into 2cm balls and space about 5cm apart
- Bake for about 8 to 10 minutes in the preheated oven until golden and crispy on outside but still gooey on inside
- Leave to cool for at least two minutes.
- Eat warm!

216.   Oat Scrambled Eggs

Serving: Serves 1 | Prep: | Cook: |Ready in:

Ingredients

- 2 eggs
- 3 tablespoons oats (rolled, porridge oats)
- 2 tablespoons milk of your choice (cow's, almond, rice, oat)
- 1 teaspoon coconut oil
- 1 teaspoon toasted pumpkin seeds

Direction

- Heat a non-stick pan on medium heat and toast pumpkin seeds. When done set aside. Lower the heat to low-medium and add coconut oil.
- Crack eggs into a bowl, add oats, milk, good pinch of salt and pepper. Whisk until smooth. Pour the egg mixture into the pan. You should hear a nice sizzle. Don't touch the eggs just yet, let the eggs brown slightly on the oil for up to a minute - these are the good bits. Stir the eggs and cook for another minute or two stirring constantly until they are cooked through.
- Serve with cucumber slices and your favorite greens sprinkled with toasted pumpkin seeds.

217.   Oatmeal Cherry Berry Cookies

Serving: Makes 24 | Prep: | Cook: |Ready in:

Ingredients

- .5 cups Butter
- .66 cups Light Brown Sugar
- 1 Egg
- 1 teaspoon Grated Orange Zest
- .75 cups All-Purpose Flour
- .5 teaspoons Baking Soda
- 1 tablespoon Ground Cardamom
- .25 teaspoons Salt
- 1.5 cups Rolled Oats
- .75 cups Dried Mixed Berries and/or Dried Cherries
- .5 cups Walnuts

Direction

- Preheat oven to 350 F. Prepare two baking sheets with parchment paper.
- In a medium bowl, whisk together the flour, baking soda, cardamom, and salt.

- In a large bowl, cream the butter, sugar, egg, and zest together till smooth.
- Add flour mixture to the wet mixture. Mix together until combined.
- Add the oats, berries, cherries and walnuts. Mix together until fairly evenly distributed.
- Scoop heaping tablespoon sized cookies onto baking sheets.
- Bake for 10-12 minutes until just set and slightly golden top.

218. Oatmeal Cookies

Serving: Makes about 50 cookies | Prep: | Cook: | Ready in:

Ingredients

- 2 cups dark raisins
- 2 cups all-purpose flour
- 1 cup unsalted butter, browned
- 2 cups light brown sugar
- 2 large eggs
- 1 teaspoon vanilla extract
- 2 cups old-fashioned rolled oats
- 1 teaspoon baking soda
- 1 1/4 teaspoons kosher salt
- 1/2 teaspoon ground cinnamon
- Optional, white/turbinado sugar, for rolling

Direction

- EDIT No.1: Feel free to reduce the sugar amount to 1 and 1/2 cups if you want your cookies less sweet. I think they are better the way they are.
- EDIT No.2: Since I wrote this recipe, I have tweaked it to make an even better version. Try the original, or make the following adjustments for the "Suped Up" version: Substitute light for dark brown sugar. Add 1 tsp "espresso powder" or very finely ground coffee to the dry mixture. Cut the rolled oats amount to 1 cup and add another 1 cup of oat bran (if you do not have access to oat bran, add 1 cup of rolled oats in a food processor, and pulse about 10 to 12 times). Overall, the changes will result in a cookie with deeper flavor, chewier texture, and ultimately, better cookie. Hint: They will also pair excellently with coffee.
- Preheat your oven to 350 degrees Fahrenheit. Line two baking sheet with parchment paper.
- To make the raisin paste: Toss raisins with 1/4 cup of the flour. Grind in a food processor with a blade attachment for 20-30 seconds until the raisins form a very thick paste and come together in a ball. If you don't have a food processor, you can use a blender or meat grinder to form the raisin paste.
- Brown the butter in a sauté pan, making sure it does not burn. It is better to take the time and stay with the butter, than walk away from the pan. When you begin to see the bottom of the pan becoming browned, remove from heat. Add sugar, vanilla extract, and browned butter to a bowl and mix using a hand mixer or in a stand mixer; on medium speed. If it looks separated, it's okay. Mix for about 5 minutes to incorporate some air into the batter. Add eggs, and continue to mix on a medium speed. At this time the mixture should almost immediately come together. When the mixture appears homogeneous, add raisin paste and mix until thoroughly combined.
- In a separate bowl, combine the remaining 1 3/4 cups of flour, oatmeal, baking soda, salt, and cinnamon. Mix the dry ingredients into the wet mixture in 2 additions, until there is no flour visible.
- Roll small pieces of dough into balls slightly smaller than a ping pong ball, about 38mm. If using, roll the balls in a dish of sugar, this will make them extra crunchy when baked. Place balls on the lined baking sheet, making sure they are about 2 inches apart. Using the buttery side of the butter wrapper, flatten each dough ball slightly to allow for even baking.
- Bake for 12-15 minutes, until the cookies are crinkly on top and just begin to turn golden brown. Another good way of testing is to lift a corner of the cookie, if it bends slightly and

reforms when let go, they are ready. Allow to cool for 5 minutes on the baking sheet, before transferring cookies to a cooling rack. Store in an airtight container for up to 1 and a half weeks.

219. Oatmeal Cookies With Sea Salt And Olive Oil

Serving: Serves 24 | Prep: | Cook: | Ready in:

Ingredients

- 1/4 cup and 3 tbsp. Bertolli Extra Light Tasting Olive Oil
- 1   Large egg
- 1 teaspoon Vanilla extract
- 2 tablespoons Hot water
- 2 tablespoons Honey
- 1/2 cup Sugar
- 1 cup All-purpose flour
- 1/2 teaspoon Cinnamon
- 1/4 teaspoon Salt
- 1 cup Rolled oats
- 1/2 cup Almond meal
- 1/2 teaspoon Baking soda
- 2/3 cup Chocolate chips
- 1-2 teaspoons Coarse sea salt for sprinkling
- Bertolli Extra Light Tasting Olive Oil Spray

Direction

- Preheat the oven to 325°.
- In a large bowl, mix the egg, vanilla, water, honey and sugar. While mixer is still on low, slowly pour in olive oil. In a separate bowl, sift the flour, cinnamon, salt, oats, almond flour and baking soda together. Gradually add the dry mixture to the wet mixture and stir until well combined. Lightly mix in the chocolate chips until just incorporated.
- Prep cookie sheet by spraying with Bertolli Extra Light Tasting Olive Oil. Drop about 2 tablespoons of the dough onto the cookie sheets, leaving at least an inch of space between them. Sprinkle cookies lightly with sea salt before baking. Bake for 12-15 minutes, or until the edges of the cookies start to turn golden brown.

220. Oatmeal Currant Bread

Serving: Makes 1 loaf | Prep: | Cook: | Ready in:

Ingredients

- 150 grams stiff levain (sourdough starter that has a ratio of 2:1 of flour:water)
- 200 grams bread flour
- 50 grams whole rye flour
- 100 grams high-gluten flour
- 150 grams rolled oats (I prefer thick rolled oats, not quick-cooking)
- 350 grams room temperature water
- 15 grams salt (I use kosher, non-iodized)
- 80 grams zante currants
- 80 grams whole shelled hazelnuts, toasted

Direction

- This bread will have 600g flour and 400g water altogether -- a 66% bread. 50g of water comes from the levain; the other 350g is what you've added. Similarly, the flours are made up of 100g that the levain contributes, and 500g that you've added on top of that.
- Dissolve the starter in the water; you should get a milky, slightly viscous liquid.
- Add bread flour, rye flour, high-gluten flour, rolled oats, and salt. Stir until it is a shaggy ball. Cover the bowl with a damp towel and let it sit for 30 minutes. (This is the autolyze.)
- Knead the dough either by hand until it is well kneaded; or in a stand mixer with a dough hook for about 6 minutes on 3-speed.
- When the dough has come together, add the currants and hazelnuts. Either knead them in by hand, or in the stand mixer on low speed for about a minute.

- Let the dough rise for its first fermentation in a dough bucket or a covered bowl. I let it rise at room temperature for up to 12 hours, allowing the flavors to develop. You can speed it up with a light-bulb warmed oven or placing the dough bowl in a larger bowl of warm water.
- When the dough has at least doubled in volume (I've gotten it to triple), remove it from the bucket and form it into a loaf. Typically I use a boule shape, which is essentially a round loaf about the size of a soccer ball, and bake it directly on a stone. If you prefer to use a bread pan, that would work as well.
- Let the bread rise for its final fermentation for around 2 hours.
- Bake the bread in an oven preheated to 450F. If you have no baking stone but still want a free-form bread, you can use a preheated baking sheet.
- After 35 minutes check the bread. An instant-read thermometer should tell you it is at 195-200F. If it's not, let the bread bake for another 5-10 minutes.
- Let it cool. Then hide it where only you can find it. Else it will disappear miraculously.

221. Oatmeal Ice Cream With Toasted Walnuts

Serving: Serves 1, on a bad day | Prep: | Cook: | Ready in:

Ingredients

- 3/4 cup granulated sugar
- 4 large egg yolks
- 3 1/4 cups homogenized milk
- 1 cup heavy cream
- 1/2 cup rolled oats
- 1 vanilla bean pod, without seeds
- Good pinch of kosher salt
- 1/2 cup   walnuts

Direction

- Preheat oven to 350F. Evenly scatter oats on a baking pan lined with parchment and bake until golden brown and fragrant -- anywhere from 5 to 10 minutes, depending on the oven. Stir them around once in a while to prevent any burning. Any burnt oats will make your ice cream taste bitter.
- Using the same tray you used for your oats, toast your walnuts for 5-7 minutes, stirring once or twice to prevent burning. Cool, chop roughly, and set aside.
- Seed the vanilla bean. Save the pod for your milk and cream. Save the seeds for a project on another day. (I like to make vanilla sugar with my seeds. With your hands, rub the seeds into a huge amount of granulated sugar and keep on hand for baking. Perfect for vanilla crème brûlée, anglaise or plain vanilla ice cream!)
- Combine the vanilla bean pod, a generous pinch of salt, homogenized milk, and heavy cream in a medium pot over medium-high heat. Once the mixture is hot, add your freshly toasted oats to the milk and let them steep 15-20 minutes over medium heat. Taste the milk to ensure the oats have steeped good flavor into your ice cream base.
- Over a bowl, strain the milk and oat mixture with a strainer lined with cheesecloth (or a thin towel) and squeeze (channel your inner hulk) the milk and cream from the oats. You may want to wait for the oats in the cheesecloth to cool before wringing it out. ;)
- Re-measure the milk mixture to ensure you will have 3 3/4 cups of milk as the oats will soak up liquid. You're looking for 3 3/4 cups of total liquid -- the recipe is overcompensating for what the oats will absorb. Top as needed with milk or cream. Put the milk mixture back on the burner to reheat.
- Whisk the egg yolks and sugar together. Once the milk is hot, add about 1 cup of the steeped milk to the yolk and sugar mixture, while whisking vigorously. Repeat this step with 1 more cup of steeped milk. Return custard to the remaining milk in the stock pot and heat through just to eliminate any grit from the

sugar, then cook until the mixture coats the back of a spoon.
- Strain the ice cream through a strainer into a container that fits in your fridge. Cover with lid or plastic wrap and chill for 3 hours, or until thoroughly cool.
- Pour base into ice cream maker and spin until gorgeous and thick. Pour into storage canisters, folding in toasted walnuts as you go. Line the top of the canister with parchment paper and freeze through for at least 4 hours.

222. Oatmeal Pancakes

Serving: Serves 2 | Prep: | Cook: |Ready in:

Ingredients

- 1 cup rolled oats*
- 2 tablespoons bran
- 2 tablespoons wheat germ
- 1/2 teaspoon baking soda
- 2/3 cup buttermilk**

Direction

- Mix dry ingredients.
- Add buttermilk. Let stand 5 minutes (to allow oats to absorb the buttermilk).
- Brown pancakes in a hot buttered skillet. (They can be a little difficult to flip the first time, but if they break just shmoosh them back together! Don't worry, they'll still form a pancake in the end!)
- Top with your choice: maple syrup, honey, preserves (shown here with blackberry puree).
- NOTES: *Quick or regular both work - regular oats makes for a heavier, chewier pancake, while quick oats soaks in the buttermilk more easily, making it easier to form. **If you haven't any buttermilk, put 2 tsp. white vinegar in a liquid measuring cup, fill with milk to 2/3 cup, let sit 5 minutes.

223. Oatmeal Pancakes With Caramelized Bacon And Herbed Crème Fraiche

Serving: Serves 5 | Prep: | Cook: |Ready in:

Ingredients

- 3/4 cup rolled oats
- 1/2 cup flour
- 1 1/4 cups buttermilk
- 1/2 teaspoon salt
- 2 tablespoons olive oil
- 1 teaspoon baking soda
- 1 egg
- 5 bacon slces (1/8 inch thick)
- 2 teaspoons turbinado sugar
- 6 ounces crème fraiche
- 1 teaspoon finely minced mint
- 1 teaspoon finely minced parsley
- 1 tablespoon finely minced chives
- Vegetable oil for frying

Direction

- Preheat the oven to 325°F. Line a baking sheet with parchment paper. Place the bacon slices on the sheet in a single layer and sprinkle with sugar. Bake for about 25-30 minutes, until the bacon is caramelized. Let the bacon cool completely (the bacon will crisp as it cools), and then cut in halves.
- In a small bowl, mix the crème fraiche with mint, parsley and chives.
- In a food processor, grind the oats until powdery. Add the flour, salt, olive oil, baking soda, egg and buttermilk and process into smooth batter. Let the batter rest for about 15 minutes.
- Heat a lightly oiled cast iron pan or griddle over medium high heat. Pour about ¼ cup of batter onto the griddle, and flatten with a spatula into a 4-5 inch round. Brown for about 2 minutes on each side.

- Arrange the pancakes on a plate and top with herbed crème fraiche. Serve with the bacon and additional crème fraiche on the side.

224. Oatmeal Raisin Cookie Porridge

Serving: Serves 3-4 | Prep: | Cook: | Ready in:

Ingredients

- 2 cups water
- 2 cups milk
- 1 cup steel cut oats
- 1/4 teaspoon salt
- 1 cinnamon stick
- 1/4 cup raisins
- 1/4 cup unsweetened shredded coconut
- Agave nectar (or honey or maple syrup) to taste

Direction

- Pour the water and milk into a medium saucepan and bring to a simmer over medium heat.
- Slowly pour the oats into the simmering liquid, stirring to distribute the oats. Add the salt, cinnamon stick, raisins and coconut and stir again.
- When the porridge begins to thicken slightly (anywhere from 1-5 minutes), turn the heat to low and simmer uncovered for 30 minutes, stirring occasionally, until the oats are tender but chewy and the liquid is absorbed. Remove cinnamon stick and discard.
- Ladle porridge into bowls and serve with a hefty drizzle of agave nectar or other sweetener to taste.

225. Oatmeal Raisin Cookies

Serving: Makes 2 dozen | Prep: | Cook: | Ready in:

Ingredients

- 1/2 cup plus 6 tablespoons butter, softened
- 3/4 cup firmly packed brown sugar
- 1/2 cup granulated sugar
- 2 eggs
- 1 teaspoon vanilla extract
- 1 1/2 cups all-purpose flour
- 1 teaspoon baking soda
- 1/4 teaspoon ground nutmeg
- 1/2 teaspoon salt
- 3 cups rolled oats
- 1 cup raisins

Direction

- Preheat the oven to 350° F.
- Cream together the butter and sugars until very light and fluffy.
- Add the eggs, one at a time, mixing well with each one.
- Add the vanilla and mix well.
- Whisk together the flour, baking soda, nutmeg, and salt. Add to the wet ingredients a little bit at a time and beat until it just comes together.
- Add the oats and raisins and stir until just combined and thoroughly distributed.
- Scoop the dough onto a parchment-lined baking sheet using a 1/3- or 1/4-cup scoop. Leave a few inches between each as they will spread.
- Bake for about 20 minutes, or until golden brown on the edges and still quite soft in the center. Let cool for a few minutes, then transfer to a wire rack to finish cooling.

226. Oatmeal Scotchies

Serving: Makes 42 | Prep: | Cook: | Ready in:

Ingredients

- 1 cup plus 2 tablespoons old-fashioned oats
- 1 cup (8 ounces) unsalted butter, at room temperature
- 1/2 cup cane sugar
- 1/2 cup packed dark brown sugar
- 1/2 cup packed light brown sugar
- 1 extra-large egg, at room temperature
- 1 teaspoon vanilla extract
- 1/2 cup cake flour
- 1/2 cup all-purpose flour
- 1 1/2 teaspoons baking soda
- 1 teaspoon kosher salt
- 1 teaspoon sea salt flakes
- 1 cup butterscotch chips

Direction

- Heat the oven to 350° F and line a couple of half sheet pans with parchment paper.
- On another sheet pan, spread the oats and toast lightly, for approximately 5 minutes. Once they've cooled, grind 2 tablespoons of the oats into a fine powder.
- In a stand mixer, use the paddle attachment to mix the butter very briefly, 5 to 10 seconds, on medium speed. Add the sugars and beat until the butter mixture is pale in color, about 4 minutes. Scrape the sides and bottom of the bowl.
- In a small bowl, crack the egg and add the vanilla. In a different and larger bowl, whisk together the powdered and whole oats, flours, baking soda, and salts. Add the butterscotch chips and stir lightly.
- On medium speed, add the egg and vanilla to the butter mixture and beat very briefly, about 5 seconds. Scrape the sides and bottom of the bowl. Mix again on medium speed for another 20 seconds, until well-combined. Then add the dry ingredients all at once and mix on low for approximately 30 seconds; the batter will come together in a shaggy sort of way. Do not over-mix. With a bowl scraper, mix the rest of the dough together by hand.
- Scoop out the dough with an ice cream scoop (technically, a 3/4-ounce or 1 and 1/2 tablespoon scoop) and place on the prepared cookie sheets, with a good amount of space between each. Each half-sheet pan should take no more than 8 cookies. (They'll spread.) Bake for 8 minutes. Then rotate the pan, and in the process, tap it against the counter or the oven to deflate the cookies. Bake for another 4 to 6 minutes, or until the edges are a deep golden color and the cookies are beginning to crisp and brown. Let the cookies cool on the pan. Repeat with the remaining dough. Store in an airtight container for up to 3 days.

227. Oatmeal Vanilla Sandwiches

Serving: Makes approx.15 sandwiches | Prep: | Cook: | Ready in:

Ingredients

- 1/3 cup coconut oil
- 1/2 cup dark brown sugar
- 1 tablespoon golden ground flax seed
- 3 tablespoons water
- 2 tablespoons honey
- 1 1/3 cups oat flour
- 1/2 teaspoon baking soda
- 1/2 teaspoon salt
- 3/4 cup dark chocolate chips
- 2 quarts high quality or homemade vanilla ice cream

Direction

- In a mixer fitted with paddle attachment, cream the dark brown sugar and coconut oil together for about 5 minutes. During this time prepare the tbs. of flax with the 3 tbs. of water until the mixture congeals and becomes egg like.

- Then, add the flax "egg," honey and peanut butter to the mixer and allow it to mix for another 5 minutes.
- During this time whisk together the oat flour, baking soda, and sea salt. Slowly add the dry mixture to the wet ingredients and combine until it is well blended. Throw in the chocolate chips and knead them into the dough.
- Now place all of the prepared dough into the refrigerator for about an hour. Preheat the oven to 350°F. Line two baking sheets with parchment paper.
- When the dough is chilled, roll it into about thirty 1 1/2 inch balls and space them about an inch apart on the trays. Bake the cookies for 8-10 minutes and then cool them to room temperature. At this point, place them into the freezer until they harden (30-60 minutes).
- Finally scoop a generous amount of ice cream onto fifteen of the cookies and place the remaining cookies on top as "lids." Place the cookies back into the freezer and they can be served anytime.

228. Oatmeal And Carrots Pancakes Served With Avocado Cream And Poached Peaches

Serving: Makes 12 medium size pancakes | Prep: | Cook: | Ready in:

Ingredients

- For the pancakes
- • 1 full cup old fashioned whole grain rolled oats
- • 1 1/4 cup whole milk
- • 2 extra large eggs (separated)
- • 2 large carrots (peeled, grated on the large side of the grater and juice squeezed slightly out)
- • 2 tablespoons sugar
- • Zest of 1 lemon
- • 1 teaspoon pure vanilla extract
- • 1/4 teaspoon cinnamon
- • 1/4 kosher salt
- About 3 tablespoons canola oil + 2 tablespoons butter for frying pancakes
- For the Avocado cream
- • 1 large Hass avocado (cut in half, seeded and the flash scooped out)
- • 2 tablespoons sweetened condensed milk
- • 2 tablespoons sour cream
- • 1/4 teaspoon sea salt
- • Juice of half a lime
- • Zest of 1 lime
- • 1 teaspoon pure vanilla extract
- For the Poached Peaches:
- • 1 large or 2 medium ripe but firm peaches (blanched for 30-40 seconds and peeled)
- • 1 cup freshly squeezed orange juice
- • 1 tablespoon light brown sugar
- • 1 cinnamon stick
- • 1 tablespoon cold butter

Direction

- To make the pancakes: In medium size sauce pan scold the milk, mix in oats, tightly cover and let stand until all of the milk is absorbed and cooled to room temperature. Add carrots, lemon zest, vanilla and egg yolks. Mix well to combine.
- In a medium bowl beat, with a hand mixer, egg whites with the salt and 1/2 teaspoon lemon juice until soft picks form; then slowly add the sugar, while continuing beating until stiff and shiny.
- Gently fold in the meringue to the oats and carrot mixture.
- Heat 1 tablespoon oil and 1/2 tablespoon butter in large heavy-bottomed, nonstick skillet over medium heat until shimmering.
- Drop 3 or 4 heaping tablespoonful batter in pan. Fry until golden brown, about 1-2 minutes per side. Transfer pancakes to a large plate lined with paper towels. When necessary, add more oil and butter to skillet and fry remaining batter.
- To make the Avocado Cream: In a medium bowl combine all ingredients and beat with a

hand mixer until smooth and fluffy. Transfer to a serving dish.
- To make poached peaches: In a medium sauce pan simmer orange juice, brown sugar and cinnamon stick until reduced approximately in half, add the peaches and simmer for 3-4 minutes.
- With a slotted spoon transfer peaches to a serving dish, add 1 tablespoon butter to the sauce pan, turn of the flame and stir in the butter. Pour over peaches.
- Serve the pancakes immediately. For every day breakfast serve with sour cream, maple syrup, or crème fraîche.
- Notes: These pancakes can be made also with other vegetables such as parsnips, zucchini, celery root and in the autumn with pumpkin or butternut squash. A savory variation with salt, freshly ground black pepper and herbs of your choice, and served with Tzatziki dip, would be equally delicious.

229. Oatmeal And Lavender Shortbread With Whipped Goat Cheese And Lemon Coulis

Serving: Serves 4-6 | Prep: | Cook: | Ready in:

Ingredients

- For the cookies
- 1 ¼ cups rolled oats, gently toasted
- 8 tablespoons (1 stick) butter, softened
- 1/2 cup all purpose flour
- 1/4 cup sugar
- 1 teaspoon salt (I like my shortbreads on the salty side, if you do not start with 1/2 tsp)
- 3/4 tablespoon dry lavender flowers
- For the whipped goat cheese and couils
- 4 ounces goat cheese, at room temperature
- 3 tablespoons creme fraiche
- Juice and zest of one lemon
- 1/2 cup good quality extra virgin olive oil
- 1/4 cup brown sugar

- A pinch of salt

Direction

- Preheat the oven to 325°F convection (or 350°F regular bake). Toast the oats for about 10 minutes. Let the oats cool completely and then process in a food processor, until powdery.
- Beat the butter with sugar until creamy. Stir in the oats, flour, salt and lavender. Mix on low speed until the dough comes together. Scrape the dough out onto a work surface and pat it into a log 1 1/4 inches in diameter. Wrap up the log in plastic wrap and refrigerate until very firm, about 2 hours.
- Preheat the oven to 325°F convection (or 350°F regular bake). Slice the dough into 1/4-inch-thick slices and arrange on baking sheet lined with parchment paper. Prick the top of the shortbreads with a fork. Bake for about 20 minutes, or until golden (somehow, for a lot of cookies in my oven I found 22 minutes to be the magic number). Slide the parchment onto a wire rack and let the shortbreads cool. (The shortbreads can be kept in an airtight container for about a week.)
- To make the whipped goat cheese, beat the goat cheese and crème fraiche until light and fluffy (if needed add a bit more crème fraiche).
- To make the coulis, in a small bowl (or mini-blender) combine the lemon juice, lemon zest, brown sugar, olive oil and salt. Blend until emulsified. Refrigerate for about an hour or two.
- Remove the coulis from the refrigerator and mix well. Place 4-5 cookies on a plate next to a scoop of whipped goat cheese. Top generously with the coulis and serve.

230. Oatmeal With Stewed Fruit And Almonds

Serving: Serves 4 to 6 | Prep: | Cook: | Ready in:

Ingredients

- Oatmeal
- 4 cups whole milk
- 4 cups water
- 2 cups steel-cut oats
- 1/4 teaspoon kosher salt
- 3/4 cup packed brown sugar
- 2 teaspoons orange zest
- 1/2 teaspoon ground cinnamon
- 1/4 teaspoon ground nutmeg
- Fruit
- 3 red plums, pitted and cut into 1/2-inch slices
- 3/4 cup water
- 1/2 cup granulated sugar
- 1/2 cup fresh blueberries
- 1 teaspoon pure vanilla extract
- 1/2 cup sliced almonds, toasted

Direction

- Oatmeal
- Combine the milk, water, oats, and salt in a medium saucepan over high heat. Bring the mixture to a boil, then reduce the heat to low and simmer for about 30 minutes, stirring occasionally, until the mixture thickens and the oats have absorbed the liquid. Stir in the brown sugar, orange zest, cinnamon, and nutmeg.
- Fruit
- Combine the plums, water, and sugar in a medium skillet over medium-high heat. Bring to a boil, then reduce the heat to low and simmer for 5 to 6 minutes, until the fruit is softened and the liquid has thickened slightly. Stir in the blueberries and vanilla extract.
- Spoon the oatmeal into bowls and top with the stewed fruit and some of their juices. Sprinkle the almonds over the top and serve.

231. Oatmeal With Cinnamon And Apples

Serving: Serves 1 | Prep: | Cook: | Ready in:

Ingredients

- 1/2 cup wheat free quick oats
- 1/2 organic gala apple, cored and diced
- 1 tablespoon ground flaxseed
- 1 tablespoon ground pumpkin seeds
- 1 teaspoon cinnamon
- drizzle organic maple syrup
- water

Direction

- Put oats in microwave safe bowl and add water until the water line is just above the oatmeal. Put in microwave for 90 seconds.
- Remove from microwave (careful, it's hot!) and add in diced apples, flax and pumpkin seeds and cinnamon. Stir.
- Drizzle with maple syrup.

232. Oaty Brown Sugar Soda Bread

Serving: Makes 1 loaf | Prep: | Cook: | Ready in:

Ingredients

- 2 1/2 cups (400 grams) whole-wheat flour
- 1 cup (120 grams) rolled oats
- 2 tablespoons dark brown sugar
- 1 1/2 teaspoons baking soda
- 1 teaspoon kosher salt
- 2 1/4 cups (423 grams) whole-milk kefir

Direction

- Preheat the oven to 400° F. Line a 4-quart (or close enough!) Dutch oven with parchment. It doesn't need to fit perfectly.
- Combine the flour, oats, sugar, baking soda, and salt in a large bowl. Break up the brown sugar with your fingers to get rid of any lumps. Whisk everything together until smooth. Switch to a rubber spatula or wooden spoon and slowly add the kefir, stirring as you

do, just until a cohesive dough forms. It will be sticky.
- Scrape the dough into the Dutch oven and spread to even out. Use a small serrated knife to cut an X, about 1/2 inch deep, in the center. Cover the pot and get it in the oven.
- Bake for 40 minutes. Remove the lid and bake for another 5. The bread should be springy to the touch. Cool in the pot until you can grab the bread without burning yourself. Transfer to a rack to cool.

233. Olive Oil Braised Broccoli Rabe

Serving: Serves 4 to 6 | Prep: | Cook: | Ready in:

Ingredients

- For the broccoli rabe:
- 1 1/4 cups extra-virgin olive oil
- 3 cloves garlic, thinly sliced
- 1 small hot red chile, seeded and thinly sliced
- 1 medium lemon, thinly sliced into rings
- 2 bunches broccoli rabe, cleaned and hard, woody parts of stems removed
- Salt
- Freshly ground black pepper
- Ricotta and baguette, for serving
- For the pine nut crumble:
- 1/2 cup all-purpose flour
- 1/4 cup old-fashioned rolled oats
- 4 tablespoons unsalted butter, cool
- 1/4 cup pine nuts
- 2 teaspoons freshly grated lemon zest
- 1 tablespoon finely chopped fresh parsley
- 1/4 teaspoon crushed red pepper
- Salt
- Freshly ground pepper

Direction

- For the broccoli rabe:
- In a large saucepan over medium heat, combine the oil, garlic, chile, and lemon and cook for 5 minutes, until the oil is shimmering and everything is just beginning to get hot and sizzle.
- Add the broccoli rabe and stir to coat.
- Cover the pot and cook over medium-low heat for 25 minutes. Stir the broccoli rabe, recover the pot, and cook for another 25 minutes.
- Remove the pot from the heat and season with salt and pepper. Serve the rabe topped with the pine nut crumble (see below) and topped with dollops of ricotta cheese. Or, spread ricotta on baguette, then top it with broccoli rabe and crumble.
- For the pine nut crumble:
- Preheat the oven to 350° F. In a medium bowl, combine the flour, oats, butter, pine nuts, lemon zest, parsley, and crushed red pepper. Season with salt and pepper, then use your fingers to combine until large chunks form.
- Spread the mixture onto the sheet pan and bake until browned and fragrant, 15 to 20 minutes, mixing halfway through to prevent burning. Set aside until ready to use. Store leftovers in an airtight container in the refrigerator for up to 1 week.

234. Ooey Gooey Magic Cookies

Serving: Serves 35 cookies | Prep: | Cook: | Ready in:

Ingredients

- 2 1/4 cups almond flour
- 1/4 cup ground flax-seed meal
- 1 1/4 teaspoons baking powder
- 3/4 teaspoon baking soda
- 1 teaspoon cinnamon
- 1/2 teaspoon nutmeg
- 1/4 teaspoon ground cloves
- 1/4 teaspoon salt
- 1/2 cup butter (1 stick room temperature butter)
- 2 eggs

- 1/4 cup molasses
- 1/4 cup low fat greek yogurt
- 1 tablespoon lemon zest (zest about one lemon)
- 1 tablespoon freshly grated ginger
- 1 teaspoon vanilla extract
- 1 1/2 cups old fashioned oats
- 1 cup raisins
- 1 cup dried cranberries
- 2 cups chooped pecans, walnuts, slivered almonds
- 1 cup dark chocolate chips
- 1 cup unsweetened shredded coconut

Direction

- Line your baking sheets with parchment paper. Whisk the flour, baking powder, baking soda, cinnamon, nutmeg, cloves and salt in a medium bowl.
- Beat the butter and brown sugar in a large bowl with a mixer on medium speed until light and fluffy, a few minutes. Then beat in the eggs one at a time, fully incorporating each before adding the next. Add the molasses, yogurt, ginger, lemon zest and vanilla and beat until smooth. Reduce the mixer speed to low and add in the flour mixture slowly to make a sticky batter. Fold in the oats, raisins, cranberries, nuts, chocolate chips and coconut.
- Drop rounded tablespoons on the baking sheets and chill for 30 minutes to make the batter stiffer. Preheat the oven to 375 degrees.
- Once cookies have chilled, bake them for 10-12 minutes, until the cookies are golden brown but still soft. They need to cool for a little before messing with them because they are ooey and gooey!

235. Our Best Açaí Bowl

Serving: Makes 1 acai bowl | Prep: 0hours3mins | Cook: 0hours7mins | Ready in:

Ingredients

- Açaí Base
- 1/4 cup nutless, seedless granola, such as Purely Elizabeth Original (see note)
- 1 packet frozen, unsweetened açaí puree (such as Sambazon), broken into thirds
- 1 frozen banana, cut into thirds
- 1/4 cup frozen strawberries
- 1/4 cup extra-creamy dairy-free milk, such as Oatly barista
- Toppings
- 1 ripe banana, sliced
- 1/2 kiwi, sliced
- 2 fresh strawberries, thinly sliced
- 1/4 cup fresh blueberries
- 1 tablespoon unsweetened, shredded coconut
- 1/2 teaspoon bee pollen
- 1 tablespoon honey

Direction

- Line the bottom of a serving bowl with the granola. Combine açaí, frozen banana, frozen strawberries, and oat milk in a high-powered blender, and blend on High, plunging contents as needed, until the texture of ice cream.
- Plop blender contents onto granola in bowl; smooth and level surface with the back of a spoon. Artfully top with sliced bananas, strawberries, and kiwi. Sprinkle with blueberries, shredded coconut, and bee pollen, and zig-zag with honey.

236. Overnight Banana Oats

Serving: Serves 1 | Prep: 0hours0mins | Cook: 0hours0mins | Ready in:

Ingredients

- 1/2 cup rolled oats
- 1/2 banana (chopped)
- 1/2 cup milk (I use soy or almond milk)
- 1/4 cup greek yoghurt
- 1 teaspoon chia seeds
- 1 pinch cinnamon

- 1 tablespoon seed/nut/fruit mix (optional)
- 1 tablespoon shredded coconut (optional)

Direction

- Mix together oats, banana, milk, yoghurt, chia seeds and cinnamon in a bowl or jar.
- Cover and place in fridge overnight.
- Top with seed/nut/fruit mix, shredded coconut and extra cinnamon before eating in the morning.

237. Overnight Oatmeal Cold Prep

Serving: Serves 2 | Prep: | Cook: | Ready in:

Ingredients

- 2 cups Steel-cut oats
- 1 cup Milk or almond milk (will try soy milk soon)
- 1 tablespoon Cinnamon
- 1 cup Berries (raspberries, blueberries, blackberries, or strawberries)

Direction

- Mix the oats with milk.
- Store for at least 5 hours or overnight in a refrigerator.
- Mix in your berries and cinnamon. Be sure to mix it evenly.
- Add more milk if you like.

238. Overnight Oatmeal Pancakes

Serving: Serves 4 to 6 | Prep: 8hours10mins | Cook: 0hours6mins | Ready in:

Ingredients

- 2 cups rolled oats
- 2 cups buttermilk, shaken
- 1/2 cup whole wheat flour
- 2 tablespoons brown sugar, packed
- 1 teaspoon baking powder
- 1 teaspoon baking soda
- 1/2 teaspoon salt
- 2 eggs, lightly beaten
- 1/2 cup coconut oil, or any oil (or butter), melted but not hot
- 1 splash Oil or non-stick spray for greasing the pan
- 1 splash Maple syrup, yogurt, berries, or bananas, for serving

Direction

- The night before, mix the oats and buttermilk together in a large bowl. Cover tightly with plastic wrap and stick in the fridge. If you're feeling especially efficient, mix the dry ingredients in a smaller bowl and set aside on the counter.
- The next morning, take the oat mixture out of the fridge. If you haven't already, mix the dry ingredients together with a whisk or fork until incorporated. Add the eggs and oil to the oat mixture, stir together, then add the dry ingredients. Mix until fully incorporated, but be careful not to over mix. Batter will be very thick.
- Grease a griddle or large pan with and set it over medium-high heat. When you flick water at the skillet and it sizzles, it's ready. Pour batter onto the hot pan (I used a 1/3 cup measure, but feel free to adjust if you want larger or smaller pancakes). If desired, sprinkle on sliced bananas, berries (fresh or frozen), nuts, or chocolate chips. When the top of the batter bubbles, the edges begin to set, and the bottom is bronzed, flip pancakes. They're done when the underside is done and they don't squish when pressed lightly with your finger.
- Serve with maple syrup, a dollop of yogurt, and two cups of coffee.

239. Overnight Oatmeal With Rhubarb Cherry Compote

Serving: Serves 4 | Prep: 0hours0mins | Cook: 0hours0mins | Ready in:

Ingredients

- Overnight Oats
- 1 cup Steel Cut Oats, rinsed in cold water
- 1 cup Cooked Quinoa, cooled
- 1 1/2 cups Almond Milk
- 1/2 cup Greek Yogurt
- 1 teaspoon Cinnamon
- 1/4 cup Maple Syrup, or to taste
- Pinch Sea Salt
- Hemp Hearts (optional)
- Unsweetened Coconut, shredded (optional)
- Greek Yogurt (optional)
- Rhubarb-Cherry Compote
- 4 cups Rhubarb, sliced into 1 inch cubes
- 1 tablespoon Vanilla
- 1/4 cup Maple Syrup
- 2 cups Unsweetened Cherries, canned or frozen

Direction

- For the Overnight Oats: Add oats and quinoa to a bowl. Add almond milk, yogurt, cinnamon and maple syrup. Mix until combined. Cover and refrigerate overnight, at least 8 hours.
- For the Compote: Preheat oven to 350*Combine the rhubarb, vanilla and maple syrup. Mix until the rhubarb is evenly coated. Place on a baking sheet and bake for 15-20 minutes or until the rhubarb is softened. Remove from the oven and cool until room temperature. Mix in cherries and refrigerate. This can be served hot or cold.
- To serve, place oats in 4 bowls. Top with compote and optional hemp hearts, coconut and yogurt.

240. Overnight Swiss Style Muesli

Serving: Serves 1 | Prep: | Cook: | Ready in:

Ingredients

- 0.25 cups steel-cut oats
- 1 tablespoon shredded unsweetened coconut flakes
- 1 tablespoon raisins or cranberries
- 1 tablespoon flax seeds
- 0.3 cups blueberries (frozen or fresh)
- 1 teaspoon cinnamon
- 1 cup kefir (plain)
- 1 teaspoon honey
- 10 roasted unsalted almonds, chopped

Direction

- Mix all dry ingredients and the blueberries in a breakfast bowl or over-sized coffee mug.
- Add 1c of plain kefir and mix well. Good substitutes for kefir are a thin plain yogurt or a 50:50 mix of plain Greek yogurt and milk (or almond or soy, etc.).
- Cover with plastic wrap and set in fridge overnight.
- In the morning, take out of fridge to warm a little (15min or so). Then drizzle with honey and enjoy.
- For more depth of flavor, steel-cut oats and coconut flakes can be lightly toasted and then cooled prior to mixing.

241. PB&J Granola

Serving: Serves 6 | Prep: | Cook: | Ready in:

Ingredients

- 3 cups old-fashioned rolled oats
- 3/4 cup flax seed meal

- 1 teaspoon ground cinnamon
- 1 cup salted peanuts
- 1 cup cashews or nut of your choice
- 1 cup creamy peanut butter
- 1/2 cup honey
- 1/2 cup fresh or frozen strawberries
- 2 tablespoons melted coconut oil
- 1 cup dried blueberries

Direction

- Preheat oven to 300°F. Line baking sheet with parchment paper & set aside.
- In a large bowl, combine the oats, flax, cinnamon, and nuts. Stir to combine.
- In a small saucepan, melt the peanut butter and honey together over medium heat. Add strawberries and lightly simmer until soft. Mash strawberries into the PB mix until only small bits remain. Pour over oat mixture along with the coconut oil. Gently mix. Pour mixture over the prepared baking sheet. Bake for 40 minutes, stirring halfway through.
- Remove from oven and add dried blueberries. Allow to cool, uncovered for about 30 minutes. The granola will become more crunchy as it cools.

242. Peach Blueberry Baked Oatmeal

Serving: Serves 4-6 | Prep: | Cook: |Ready in:

Ingredients

- 2 cups old fashioned rolled oats
- 2 teaspoons ground cinnamon
- 1 teaspoon baking soda
- 1/2 teaspoon kosher salt
- 1/2 cup almonds
- 1 teaspoon vanilla bean paste
- 1/3 cup pure maple syrup
- 2 tablespoons canola oil
- 2 cups almond milk
- 2 cups blueberries
- 3 large peaches, pitted and sliced

Direction

- Preheat oven to 350 degrees F. Place most of the blueberries and peaches in the bottom of an 8 inch square baking dish. Reserve a few of each for the top.
- In a large bowl, stir together the oats, cinnamon, and baking powder. Add vanilla bean paste, maple syrup, almond milk, and oil. Stir to combine. Stir in the almonds.
- Pour oat mixture over the fruit in the pan. Spread into an even layer. Top decoratively with the reserved blueberries and peaches.
- Bake for 30-40 minutes until the fruit is bubbling and the liquid has been absorbed. Serve immediately. Oatmeal may also be stored in an airtight container in the refrigerator for up to 4 days. Serve cold or reheat in the microwave in 30 second increments until warm.

243. Peach Cobbler Cake

Serving: Makes one 9-inch four-layer cake | Prep: 1hours15mins | Cook: 1hours15mins |Ready in:

Ingredients

- CAKE
- 4 cups (482 g) all purpose flour
- 2 cups (227 g) fine cornmeal
- 1 tablespoon (12 g) baking powder
- 1 teaspoon (6 g) baking soda
- 1/2 teaspoon (2 g) fine sea salt
- 1 cup (198 g) vegetable oil (or other neutral oil)
- 1/2 cup (113 g) unsalted butter, melted
- 2 cups (425 g) dark brown sugar
- 6 large (340 g) eggs
- 2 teaspoons (10 g) vanilla extract
- 2 cups (454 g) plain full-fat yogurt
- EXTRA CLUMPY STRUSEL
- 1 cup (120 g) all purpose flour

- 1/2 cup (106 g) light brown sugar
- 3/4 cup (75 g) old fashioned oats
- 1/4 teaspoon (2 g) ground cinnamon
- 10 tablespoons (142 g) cold unsalted butter, cut into 1/2 inch cubes
- FILLING + FINISHING
- 3 medium (about 467 g) peaches, thinly sliced
- 1 lemon, juiced
- 1/3 cup (66 g) granulated sugar
- 1/4 teaspoon almond extract
- 12 ounces (341 g) mascarpone cheese
- 1 cup (113 g) powdered sugar
- 1 1/2 cups (341 g) heavy cream
- 1 1/2 teaspoons (7 g) vanilla extract

Direction

- Make the cake: preheat the oven to 350°F. Grease and flour two 9 inch cake pans (the pans should be at least 2 inches tall).
- In a medium bowl, whisk the flour, cornmeal, baking powder, baking soda, and salt together to combine.
- In a large bowl, whisk the oil, melted butter, and brown sugar well to combine. Add the eggs one at a time and mix well to combine. Stir in the vanilla.
- Add about half of the flour mixture to the egg mixture, and whisk well to combine. Add all of the yogurt, and whisk to combine. Finally, mix in the remaining flour mixture. Scrape the bowl well to be sure it's all well incorporated, but don't overmix.
- Divide the batter evenly between the two prepared pans. Bake the cakes until a toothpick inserted into the center comes out clean and the cake is golden brown, 45-55 minutes.
- Cool the cakes for 15 minutes inside the pans, then invert onto a cooling rack to cool completely.
- Make the streusel: line a baking sheet with parchment paper. In a medium bowl, whisk the flour, brown sugar, oats, salt, and cinnamon to combine.
- Add the cubed cold butter and mix (with your hands or a pastry cutter) until the mixture forms moist clumps.
- Crumble the streusel onto the prepared baking sheet and bake until evenly golden brown (it will spread a bit and come together – don't worry!), 15-20 minutes. Cool completely, then use your hands to break it up into large crumbles.
- Prepare the filling: in a medium bowl, toss the peaches, lemon juice, sugar, and almond extract to combine.
- In the bowl of an electric mixer fitted with the whisk attachment, mix the mascarpone and powdered sugar to combine. Add the cream and continue to whip until the mixture becomes thick, like medium-peak whipped cream. Mix in the vanilla extract. Reserve in the refrigerator until ready to use.
- To assemble the cake, use a serrated knife to cut the domed tops off of both cakes, then to cut each into two even layers. You'll have four layers total.
- Place one layer on a platter or cake stand, and scoop ¼ of the whipped cream onto it. Top with ¼ of the peaches (I use a slotted spoon to be sure I don't bring too much juice along with the fruit), and crumble ¼ of the streusel over the peaches.
- Place another cake layer on top, and repeat the process, continuing to pile the layer cake high until you've used up all of the ingredients.
- The cake is best served within 4 hours – refrigerate until ready to serve. If you want to make it further in advance, you can prepare all the components, but wait to build it until closer to serving time!

244. Peach Crostata With Spiced Crumble

Serving: Serves 6 | Prep: | Cook: | Ready in:

Ingredients

- For the Pie Crust
- 2 cups all purpose flour
- 1 tablespoon sugar
- 3/4 teaspoon salt
- 1/2 cup shortening (I prefer non-hydrogenated)
- 1/2 cup butter
- 2 tablespoons cold water
- 2 tablespoons cold vodka
- 1 egg
- For the peach filling and streusel topping
- 4 cups fresh or frozen peaches, peeled and sliced
- 3/4 cup flour
- 1/2 cup sugar
- 1/2 teaspoon salt
- 1 teaspoon ground ginger
- 1 egg, beaten
- 1/4 cup plus 1 Tbsp. brown sugar
- 1/4 cup oats
- 3 tablespoons butter, melted

Direction

- For the Pie Crust
- This recipe works well in a food processor, but you can use a pastry cutter to mix by hand.
- Cut the butter and shortening into small cubes and place them in the freezer for 10-20 minutes.
- Mix the flour, sugar, and salt together.
- Mix the water and vodka and place in the freezer. Put the mixing bowl or food processor bowl and the dry ingredients in the freezer for 10-15 minutes or until all ingredients are very cold.
- Take ingredients out of the freezer and add half of the dry ingredients and all of the butter and shortening and pulse until the fat is in tiny chunks.
- Add the rest of the flour and pulse two or three more times until just combined.
- Mix the beaten egg into the water and vodka mixture. Pulse in the liquids until the dough just starts to come together when pressed between your fingers. The mixture will still be crumbly.
- Press dough together into a thick flat disk and cover with plastic wrap and place in the fridge for 30 minutes to one hour, or up to 24 hours. Or you may freeze for up to one month.
- Take the dough out of the fridge and split into two disks. Cover the extra disk and place back in the fridge if you are using both crusts, or freeze for later use.
- Roll the dough out in between two sheets of wax paper or lightly greased parchment paper and put back in the fridge until you are ready to fill.
- For the peach filling and streusel topping
- Preheat the oven to 350 degrees.
- Place the peaches in a bowl and add 1/2 cup flour, sugar, salt, and 1/2 teaspoon ground ginger. Stir to combine.
- To make the streusel topping, in a separate bowl combine the remaining 1/4 cup flour, oats, brown sugar, remaining 1/2 tsp. ground ginger, and melted butter.
- Remove the pie crust from the fridge and place on a sheet pan. Remove the top layer of parchment paper from the crust and top with the peach filling. Pile it in the center so that there is a two-inch rim all around the edge of the crust.
- Fold the edges of the crust toward the center of the crostata. Egg wash the edges of the crust with the beaten egg.
- Bake at 350 degrees for 35-45 minutes or until the crust is golden brown.
- Let cool for at least 20 minutes before slicing.

245. Peach Smoothie Popsicles

Serving: Makes 6 | Prep: | Cook: | Ready in:

Ingredients

- 5 nectarine peaches, or regular peaches
- 1 tablespoon rolled oats
- 3 tablespoons natural soy yogurt

- 1/2 lime, juice
- 1/4 cup water, or as needed
- blueberries to top
- granola

Direction

- Wash and dry peaches. Optionally you can peel them, or just cut into slices, removing the core. Add peach slices to blender.
- Add rolled oats, soy yogurt (or regular yogurt), juice of half a lime and a bit of water. Blend until smooth.
- Transfer smoothie into Popsicle molds and fill to about half. Add a handful of granola to each Popsicle mold, then top with the rest of the smoothie. Stir in about a spoon of soy yogurt to create delicate white swirls. Add a pops holder into each mold and place into the freezer for at least 2 hours, or overnight.
- When the popsicles are frozen, remove from freezer. If your pops are not coming out of the mold, try running water over the mold and gently move them around until they give in and you can get them out of the mold. Serve.

246. Peach Sundaes With Cardamom Gingersnap Topping

Serving: Serves 8 | Prep: | Cook: | Ready in:

Ingredients

- 1/2 cup instant oats
- 1/2 cup coarsely chopped gingersnap cookies
- 1 tablespoon canola oil
- 1 tablespoon packed brown sugar
- 1 tablespoon honey
- 1/2 teaspoon ground cinnamon
- 1/2 teaspoon ground cardamom
- 1/8 teaspoon salt
- 1/4 teaspoon vanilla extract
- 1/4 cup shredded coconut
- 1/4 cup golden raisins
- 1/4 cup butter
- 1/4 cup packed brown sugar
- 6 peaches, pitted and cut into slices
- 2 tablespoons lemon juice
- 4 cups vanilla bean ice cream

Direction

- To prepare the cardamom gingersnap topping, heat oven to 325F. Combine oats and gingersnap cookies in a large bowl. Place canola oil, 1 tablespoon brown sugar, honey, cinnamon, cardamom, salt, and vanilla extra in a small saucepan and heat over medium heat until mixture is boiling and sugar is dissolved, about 3 minutes. Pour hot sugar mixture into the bowl with the oats and mix well. Spread topping evenly onto a parchment paper lined cookie sheet and bake at 325F for 10 minutes; add coconut, stir, and bake an additional 5 to 8 minutes, or until coconut is golden brown, stirring occasionally. Cool completely, about 15 minutes, and stir in raisins.
- Meanwhile prepare the peaches. Heat butter and 1/4 cup brown sugar over medium heat in a large skillet until butter has melted. Add in peaches and cook for 12 to 15 minutes, stirring occasionally, or until fruit is soft. Stir in lemon juice.
- To assemble the sundaes, scoop 1/2 cup of ice cream into each bowl and top evenly with caramelized peaches and the desired amount of cardamom gingersnap topping. Makes 8 servings.

247. Peach And Plum Muesli Oatmeal

Serving: Makes 15 cups | Prep: | Cook: | Ready in:

Ingredients

- 15 peaches, chopped
- 5 plums, chopped
- 2 cups steel cut oats
- 2 cups rolled oats

- 1.5 cups chopped nuts (I used half brazil nuts and half walnuts)
- 1 cup pumpkin seeds
- 1 cup chia or hemp seeds (beware, chia will make the oatmeal sticky, but still delicious!)

Direction

- Heat peaches and plums in large pot (I use a 5 L pot), on medium heat
- Once juices have been released from the fruit (about 5-10 minutes), add steel cut oats
- Once steel cut oats have cooked for about 10 minutes, add rolled oats, nuts, pumpkin seeds, and chia/hemp seeds
- Cook for another 5 minutes, then take off the heat

248. Peaches And Cream Smoothie Bowl

Serving: Serves 2 | Prep: | Cook: | Ready in:

Ingredients

- 1/2 cup almond milk
- 1 teaspoon chia seeds
- 1 cup frozen bananas
- 1 frozen banana, cut into 1-inch pieces
- 1 tablespoon almond butter
- 1 teaspoon honey
- 1/2 teaspoon grated fresh ginger
- 1/2 teaspoon cinnamon
- sliced fresh peaches
- fresh figs, quartered
- chopped pistachios
- mint
- 1/4 cup chopped walnuts
- 2 tablespoons almond flour
- 2 tablespoons old-fashioned oats
- 2 tablespoons light brown sugar
- 2 tablespoons melted coconut oil
- 1/8 teaspoon kosher salt

Direction

- In a blender, add the almond milk, chia seeds, peaches, banana, almond butter, honey, ginger and cinnamon. Blend until the mixture is thick and creamy. Transfer to a bowl and let it set in the freezer while you prepare the toppings.
- Or the oat crumble: Pre-heat the oven to 375 degrees. Line a baking sheet with parchment paper and set aside. In a small bowl combine the walnuts, almond flour, oats, brown sugar, coconut oil and salt until everything is evenly coated. Spread the oat mixture on the prepared baking sheet and bake, stirring occasionally, until golden, 10-12 minutes. Let cool. Note: The crumble can be made ahead of time and will keep for 3 weeks in an airtight container.
- To serve, top with the peaches, figs, pistachios, mint and oat crumble.

249. Peanut Butter & Jelly Overnight Oats

Serving: Serves 2 | Prep: | Cook: | Ready in:

Ingredients

- 1 cup old-fashioned rolled oats
- 0.25 cups peanut butter + more for serving
- 2 tablespoons chia seeds
- 2 tablespoons pure maple syrup + more for serving
- 1.5 cups vanilla almond, soy or coconut milk
- Pinch coarse salt
- 0.25 cups strawberry fruit preserves
- 0.5 cups fresh strawberries, sliced
- 0.25 cups slivered almonds

Direction

- In a medium mixing bowl, whisk together oats, peanut butter, chia seeds, pure maple syrup, milk and salt. Transfer to a jar with a lid and refrigerate overnight. Stir in fruit preserves, more peanut butter and more maple syrup, to taste, and top with fresh strawberries and slivered almonds.

250. Peanut Butter Blondie Brownies

Serving: Makes 9 brownies | Prep: | Cook: |Ready in:

Ingredients

- 1 cup gluten-free oat flour
- 8 medjool dates
- 3/4 cup water
- 1/4 cup unsweetened cocoa powder
- 1/2 teaspoon vanilla bean powder
- 1 teaspoon baking powder
- 1/2 teaspoon baking soda
- 1/4 cup dark chocolate chips
- water, as needed to thin brownie batter
- 1 cup peanut flour
- 1 cup chickpeas, drained and rinsed
- 1 1/2 cups unsweetened applesauce

Direction

- Preheat oven to 350. Line an 8x8 baking dish with parchment paper. In a large bowl combine oat flour, cocoa, baking powder + baking soda, and vanilla bean powder. Pour in date puree. Mix together until evenly combined. Fold in chocolate chips and stir. Set aside.
- In food processor combine chickpeas and applesauce. In a bowl, place peanut flour and pour in applesauce mixture. Stir until evenly combined. Pour peanut batter into baking dish, spread evenly throughout. Bake for 15 minutes.
- Remove from oven. Spread brownie mixture on top of the blondie layer in the baking dish. Bake for 20 minutes.

251. Peanut Butter Chocolate Balls

Serving: Makes 10 balls | Prep: | Cook: |Ready in:

Ingredients

- 3/4 cup rolled oats
- 3/4 cup dates
- 1/4 cup peanut butter
- 2 tablespoons coca powder
- dash teaspoons vanilla extract

Direction

- 1) Half a cup of rolled oats
- 2) 3/4 cup of dates
- 3) 1/4 cup of peanut butter
- 4) 2 tablespoons of cocoa powder
- 5) A dash of vanilla extract.
- Blend in a high-powered blender. Spoon out, roll, and refrigerate for ideal firmness. Then eat!

252. Peanut Butter Chocolate Chunk Cookies

Serving: Makes 18 | Prep: | Cook: |Ready in:

Ingredients

- 1/2 cup unsalted butter at room temp
- 1/2 cup creamy peanut butter
- 1 cup brown sugar
- 1/2 cup sugar
- 1 large egg
- 1 teaspoon vanilla
- 1 cup all-purpose flour
- 1 cup old-fashioned oats
- 3/4 teaspoon baking soda
- 1/2 teaspoon salt
- 6 ounces milk or semisweet chocolate
- 1 cup chopped peanuts, optional

Direction

- Preheat the oven to 350 degrees and line two baking sheets with parchment paper or silicone baking mats. In a large bowl or the bowl of a stand mixer, cream together the butter and the peanut butter until well combined and smooth, about 2 minutes. Add the sugars and beat together an additional 1-2 minutes. Scrape the sides of the bowl and add the egg and vanilla. Beat briefly just to combine. In a separate smaller bowl, stir together the flour, oats, baking soda, and salt. Add to the butter mixture and beat just until combined. Add the chocolate and stir together.
- Scoop 3 tablespoon sized mounds of dough (I use a large cookie scoop) 2" apart on the baking sheet. Roll in the chopped peanuts, if desired. Bake in the preheated oven for about 12 minutes, or just until the edges have set and the top is beginning to crack. The center may seem underdone. Allow to cool on a cooling rack prior to eating. Enjoy within 2 days or freeze up to 2 months.

253. Peanut Butter Granola

Serving: Makes 7-8 cups | Prep: | Cook: | Ready in:

Ingredients

- 3 1/2 cups rolled oats
- 1/4 cup ground flax seed
- 1/4 cup toasted oat bran (or toasted wheat germ)
- 1 cup roasted, salted peanuts
- 1/2 cup roasted pepitas (shelled pumpkin seeds)
- 1 cup raisins
- 1/2 cup dried cranberries
- 1/3 cup almond flour or garbanzo flour
- 1/2 teaspoon salt
- 1 cup natural peanut butter
- 1/3 cup canola oil
- 1/2 cup maple syrup
- 1/2 cup honey
- 1 teaspoon vanilla
- 1 egg white

Direction

- Preheat the oven to 275 degrees F. Line two baking sheets with parchment paper and set aside.
- In a large mixing bowl, combine the dry ingredients (oats through salt).
- In a smaller mixing bowl, combine the wet ingredients (using a whisk really helps here).
- Stir the wet into the dry until all of the dry ingredients are well coated. It takes a few minutes of stirring, but trust me, it coats the dry ingredients perfectly.
- Spread the granola evenly between the two prepared pans and smooth to an even layer. Bake for 50-60 minutes, stirring and patting back down to a single layer, halfway through.
- Remove from the oven and let cool completely-like 1 or 2 hours. Break into large clusters.

254. Peanut Butter Oatmeal Raisin Cookies

Serving: Serves 7 | Prep: | Cook: | Ready in:

Ingredients

- 1 cup peanut butter, cinnamon raisin or creamy
- 1 cup old fashioned rolled oats
- 1 large egg
- 1 teaspoon baking soda
- 1/3 cup packed light brown sugar
- 1/3 cup pure maple syrup
- 1 teaspoon ground cinnamon
- 1/3 cup raisins

Direction

- Preheat oven to 350 degrees F. Line a baking sheet with parchment.

- In a medium bowl, stir together peanut butter, oats, egg, baking soda, brown sugar, maple syrup, cinnamon, and raisins until well combined.
- Using a regular sized ice cream scoop, scoop batter onto prepared cookie sheet.
- Bake for about 15 minutes, until golden brown and set on top. Cool completely on the sheet or serve warm. Cookies may be stored in an airtight container at room temperature for up to 3 days or frozen, wrapped in parchment and foil and placed in a zipper bag for up to 3 months. Thaw at room temperature about an hour or in the microwave about 30 seconds.

255. Pear Crumble

Serving: Makes 2 8 -inch casseroles, 1 9x13 casserole | Prep: | Cook: | Ready in:

Ingredients

- Crumble Topping
- 1 3/4 cups old fashioned rolled oats
- 1/2 cup brown sugar
- 1/3 cup all purpose flour (whole wheat if you have it)
- 1/2 - 3/4 teaspoons ground cinnamon
- 4-5 tablespoons pear butter
- Fruit
- 4 pounds firm but ripe Anjou pears
- 1/2 cup maple syrup
- 2 tablespoons lemon juice
- a few dashes ground ginger, according to your preference
- 2 tablespoons all purpose flour

Direction

- Core and chop pears into bite sized pieces. (You can peel if you like, but I prefer the rustic aspect of leaving the peel on)
- Pour syrup and juice over pears and toss gently to coat. Sprinkle with flour and ginger. Toss again. Place pears in two 8 or 9 inch round, 3-4 inch deep casseroles, or equivalent.
- Preheat oven to 350
- In a medium bowl combine oats, brown sugar, flour and cinnamon. Mix well.
- Add pear butter to dry ingredients and combine (your hands work best). Mix until the topping is evenly moist but try not to over-mix.
- Sprinkle the topping evenly over the pears.
- Bake until the pears are softened and topping is golden, about 45 - 50 minutes. If the topping beings to brown too early cover with foil.
- Let rest at least 10 minutes before serving. I love it with a scoop of vanilla ice cream!

256. Pear Crumble Pie

Serving: Serves 1 pie (serves three, if you live with roommates like mine) | Prep: | Cook: | Ready in:

Ingredients

- Pie crust
- 1 1/4 cups all-purpose flour, plus more for rolling out the dough
- 1/2 teaspoon salt
- 1/2 cup unsalted butter, cut into 1/2 inch pieces, kept very cold
- ice water
- Pear filing and crumble topping
- 7-8 ripe pears (I like using bosc, but any variety will work. use 8 if, like me, you are prone to eating slices as you cut!)
- 1 cup light brown sugar
- 2 tablespoons unsalted butter, cut into tiny little bits
- 1 cup all purpose flour
- 1 cup rolled oats (either 1 minute or the regular variety are fine, but definitely don't use steel-cut oats, which are delicious in their own right, but don't belong here!)
- 1 cup pecans, toasted and cooled
- 1/2 teaspoon ground cardamom

- 1/2 teaspoon ground cinnamon
- 1/4 teaspoon ground cloves
- 1/2 teaspoon salt
- 1/2 cup unsalted butter, softened

Direction

- Whisk together flour and salt (I just use my pastry blender, so I don't have to dirty another utensil...as if one more fork would be the end of the world!). Drop butter pieces all over the flour, and cut in with pastry blender until the dough looks quite ragged. The butter should be in many different pieces, some almost completely incorporated into the flour, some about the size of your fingernail.
- Add ice water in two tablespoon increments, scattering it all over the dough, and stirring thoroughly with a spatula after each addition, until the dough almost comes together, but is still fairly dry. I usually find I need about five tablespoons, sometimes six, but my house is quite dry.
- Gather dough together in a cohesive ball on the countertop, flatten it into a disc, wrap it in plastic wrap, and refrigerate it for one hour.
- Meanwhile, peel pears, halve them, and core them (melon baller works well). Then, slice them to 1/4 inch thickness, vertically from stem to bottom. You want them to be really thin and long, so that the pie stays together as you cut it. I find that if my fruit pieces are too short or too thick, they slip and slid around as I cut.
- Toss the pears with 1/2 cup of the light brown sugar, 1/4 cup flour, and the little bits of unsalted butter (2 Tablespoons), and set aside.
- Make the crumble topping. In a food processor, add the rolled oats, 3/4 cup flour, remaining 1/2 cup brown sugar, pecans, salt, cardamom, cinnamon, and cloves. Process until the pecans are in tiny, barley-sized pieces, and the oats are ground, but still have some texture (about 30-45 seconds). Add the 1/2 cup of softened butter in several pieces, and pulse about ten times, or until the butter is fully incorporated into the dry ingredients. If the topping seems too wet, add another couple tablespoons of flour, and continue pulsing.
- Preheat the oven to 400 F. Roll out chilled pie dough, and lay it in a pie dish. I like to crimp my edges with my fingers in the old fashioned way, but you can do whatever you like.
- Lay the pears into the dish so that all the pieces lie flat. This way, you'll get more pears into your pie, and the pie will be nicely mounded on top, even after it comes out of the oven. Pour any liquid gathered at the bottom of the bowl over the top of the pears.
- Cover the entire top of the pears with the crumble topping, making sure there are some big chunks of buttery goodness among the smaller crumbles.
- Bake at 400 F for 30 minutes, then turn the oven temperature down to 325 F, and continue baking for another 45 minutes, checking frequently to make sure the top is not getting too brown (if it does, cover with foil). You may need to bake it longer, even. I find that baking time can vary wildly, depending on the oven I'm using.
- When the top is browned all over, remove the pie from the oven and allow it to cool at room temperature for at least one hour, preferably two, before serving. Serve by itself, or with a side of vanilla, cinnamon, butter pecan, or caramel ice cream.

257. Pear Rosemary Galette

Serving: Makes 1 approx. 8-inch galette | Prep: | Cook: | Ready in:

Ingredients

- 1/4 cup tapioca starch
- 1/4 cup oat flour (make sure it's from certified gluten-free oats)
- 1/2 cup millet flour
- 1/2 teaspoon xanthan gum
- 1 pinch salt
- 1/3 cup cold butter

- 2 tablespoons ice water (more or less as needed)
- 2 cups seckel pears, sliced
- 2 tablespoons sugar
- 2 sprigs rosemary

Direction

- Remove rosemary leaves from the sprig. Combine with pears and sugar in a large bowl. Set aside.
- Stir together oat flour, millet flour, tapioca starch, xanthan gum, and salt.
- Prepare a cup of ice water.
- Cut the butter into chunks then incorporate it into the flour. If you don't have a pastry cutter (I don't!) just use a fork. You're done when the butter is evenly blended and you have mostly small pea size chunks of flour/butter.
- Using a tablespoon, gradually add cold water, just until the dough comes together. For me, 2 T was exactly enough.
- Refrigerate the dough for 20-30 min. Preheat oven to 350 degrees.
- Roll out the dough to somewhere between 1/4 and 1/8 inch thickness using your preferred method. I rolled it out between two sheets of floured wax paper.
- Sprinkle cornmeal (if you have it) on a baking sheet and transfer the rolled out dough to the baking sheet.
- Spoon the pear mixture into the center of the dough and gather the edges up around the fruit however works best. You could pinch it together or fold small sections over.
- Bake at 350 degrees until golden, about 30 minutes.

258. Pearsauce Streusel Bundt Cake

Serving: Serves 10-12 | Prep: | Cook: | Ready in:

Ingredients

- Pearsauce
- 4 Bosc pears, peeled, cored, and chopped into 1/2 inch pieces
- 1/c cups water
- 1/4 cup maple syrup
- 4 strips orange peel
- Streusel Filling
- 1/2 cup chopped almonds
- 1/4 cup white whole wheat flour
- 1/4 cup mesquite powder (or oats)
- 1 teaspoon cinnamon
- 1/4 teaspoon salt
- 3 tablespoons maple syrup
- 1 tablespoon melted coconut oil or butter

Direction

- Preheat oven to 350F and butter and flour a Bundt pan. Pear sauce: Place all ingredients in a saucepan and cook over medium heat until the pears are soft. Cool slightly and then blend in a blender. Reserve 1 c. for the cake and reserve the rest.
- Streusel Filling: Mix the almonds, white whole wheat flour, mesquite powder/oats, cinnamon, and salt together in a small bowl. Add the maple syrup and the oil/butter and mix until crumbly. Reserve for use later.
- Cake dry ingredients: 1 2/3 white whole wheat flour, 1 tsp. baking powder, 1 tsp. baking soda, 1 tsp. cinnamon, 1/2 tsp. nutmeg, 1/2 tsp. salt. Combine all in a medium bowl and reserve. Wet ingredients1/4 c. coconut oil/butter, melted1 c. pearsauce1/4 c. maple syrup1/2 c. milk/coconut milk2 tsp. apple cider vinegar. In a large mixing bowl combine all of the wet ingredients and then quickly mix in the dry ingredients and mix until fully incorporated but DON'T over-mix. Pour half the batter into the prepared Bundt pan. Evenly pour the streusel mixture onto the top of the cake batter. Pour the rest of the cake batter on top of the streusel and smooth over to cover streusel. Bake for 25-30 minutes until a toothpick comes out clean. I served it plain but it would be lovely with some ice cream or freshly whipped cream or crème fraiche. On

further thought a cream cheese frosting would be great slathered on the top for a little added decadence.

259. Perfectly Sweet Seed Bars

Serving: Makes 12 bars | Prep: | Cook: |Ready in:

Ingredients

- 1 cup walnuts
- 1 1/2 cups rolled oats, divided
- 1 scant cups shredded unsweetened coconut
- 1/4 cup flax seeds
- 1/4 cup chia seeds
- 1/2 cup raw pumpkin seeds
- 1/2 cup raw sunflower seeds
- 1/2 teaspoon ground cardamom
- 3 tablespoons melted coconut oil (plus more for greasing pan)
- 1/2 teaspoon coarse sea salt
- 1/4 cup light agave nectar (can sub honey or brown rice syrup, but sweetness will vary)
- 2 tablespoons maple syrup
- 1 teaspoon vanilla extract

Direction

- Preheat the oven to 350 degrees F. Prepare an 8x8 baking pan by lining the bottom with parchment paper and rubbing coconut oil or cooking spray along the bottom and sides, dabbing underneath the parchment paper too so it sticks.
- In the bowl of a food processor, add the walnuts, 1 cup of rolled oats, and coconut. Pulse until a fine crumble forms, less than a minute.
- Transfer the walnut crumble to a mixing bowl and add the remaining ingredients. Stir with a spatula to combine. Transfer to the baking pan and press the mixture down with your fingers, making sure the mixture is firm and even.
- Bake for 25 minutes until the edges form a golden crust. I rotate after half the time to ensure even baking. Cool completely, then slice and serve.

260. Pomegranate And Plum Yogurt Parfaits

Serving: Serves 4 | Prep: | Cook: |Ready in:

Ingredients

- 1 pomegranate
- 2 1/4 cups Greek Yogurt
- 1 cup Rolled oats
- 3 tablespoons Sunflower Seeds
- 4 Ripe Plums Chopped

Direction

- Pick 4 pretty water glasses– presentation is everything with simple dishes like these!
- Remove pomegranate seeds by halving the fruit and banging each piece over a bowl with a wooden spoon. The seeds should fall right out!
- In each glass place a layer of yogurt, chopped plums, oats and sunflower seeds, followed by more yogurt, plums, oats and seeds. Leave for 5-10 minutes or even overnight to allow the flavors to mingle. Drizzle with honey if you prefer.

261. Porridge In Pink With Raspberries & Greek Yogurt From Maria Speck

Serving: Serves 4 to 6 | Prep: 12hours0mins | Cook: 0hours15mins |Ready in:

Ingredients

- Steel-Cut Oats
- 1 cup steel-cut oats (gluten-free if desired)

- 1/4 cup dried cranberries or cherries
- 1 (2-inch) cinnamon stick (optional)
- 1 1/2 cups boiling water
- Porridge
- 1 cup whole or low-fat milk
- 1 cup water
- 1 1/2 cups fresh or frozen raspberries (no need to thaw if frozen), plus any berries you like for garnish
- 1/4 cup dried barberries, sour cherries, or cranberries
- 1 to 2 tablespoons turbinado sugar, plus extra for sprinkling
- Pinch of fine sea salt
- 1 to 1 1/2 cups whole or low-fat Greek yogurt
- about 2 tablespoons chopped lightly toasted shelled pistachios
- Ground cinnamon, for sprinkling

Direction

- Start the steel-cut oats the night before: Add the oats, cranberries, and cinnamon stick to a heavy 4-quart saucepan. Pour over the boiling water, stir once, cover, and let sit at room temperature overnight (or chill, covered, for up to 2 days).
- The next morning, make the porridge. Add the milk, water, raspberries, barberries, 1 tablespoon of the sugar, and the salt to the saucepan with the oats. Partially cover and bring to a boil over medium-high heat, stirring occasionally. Uncover, decrease the heat to maintain a steady but gentle bubble, and cook, stirring occasionally, until the oats are creamy but still slightly chewy, about 7 minutes.
- To finish, remove the cinnamon stick (if you haven't used one, add 1 teaspoon ground cinnamon). Taste for sweetness and add the remaining tablespoon of sugar if you like. Divide the oatmeal among four to six bowls. Top each with about 1/4 cup of the yogurt and 1 teaspoon of the pistachios. Garnish with raspberries, a sprinkle of turbinado sugar, and a dash of ground cinnamon. Serve right away.

262. Porridge With Rye Flakes And Abricot Compote

Serving: Serves 2-3 | Prep: | Cook: |Ready in:

Ingredients

- 1 cup rye flakes
- 1 cup rolled oats
- 2.5 cups water
- 1 pinch salt
- 3 ounces dried abricots
- 1 organic orange
- 1 tablespoon brown cane sugar

Direction

- Slice the dried apricots and add them to a pot. Grate the peel of the orange and add it to the pot as well as the juice of the orange. Lastly, add the sugar and let it simmer for 5-10 minutes.
- Add oats, rye flakes, water and salt to a pot and let it come to a boil. Once it is boiling it takes approximately 5 minutes.
- Serve the porridge with the apricot compote as topping. If you have a sweet tooth (like me), you can sprinkle a bit of sugar on top of the porridge as well.

263. Poule Au Pot

Serving: Serves 4 to 6 | Prep: | Cook: |Ready in:

Ingredients

- For the stuffing
- 1 cup oat groats
- 1 cup leeks, white part only, thinly sliced into half moons
- 2 tablespoons curly leaf parsley
- 1/3 cup pancetta, minced
- Kosher salt and pepper

- For the chicken
- 1   chicken, 3 to 3 1/2 pounds
- 2   yellow onions, peeled and quartered
- 4   leeks, white part only, trimmed
- 8   carrots
- 8   yukon gold potatoes
- 1   small head of green cabbage, cut into 6 wedges
- 2   celery hearts, root end trimmed but left intact
- 3   bay leaves
- 8   thyme sprigs
- 1 teaspoon   whole black peppercorns
- 2   whole cloves
- kosher salt
- Dipping sauce of your choice, my two favorites are Pommery mustard for the chicken and butter for the veggies

Direction

- Place the oats into a sauce pan. Add a heavy pinch of salt then cover with water by 2 inches. Place the pot over high heat and bring it to a boil. Boil two minutes then turn off the heat and cover the pan. Let the oats sit for two hours.
- The oats should be tender but chewy. Add the sliced leeks to the liquid and turn the heat to medium. Bring the oats to a boil and cook them another 10 minutes. Drain them, add the pancetta and parsley a good grinding of black pepper then let them cool.
- Give the oats a taste and adjust the seasoning as necessary.
- Rinse out, drain then stuff the cavity of the chicken with the oat stuffing. Depending on the size of you bird you may have a little extra stuffing but better they have too much than too little. Using a trussing needle, sew shut the cavity or you can pinch together the skin and run a toothpick through it much like a straight pin through a hem. Either way make sure you close the opening or the stuffing will wind up floating around in your broth.
- Truss the chicken legs and tuck the wing under the back. Place the chicken in a large pot and add the rest of the ingredients. Add cold water, make sure it is cold, to cover, and two teaspoons of salt. Place the pot over medium high heat. Bring to a boil then reduce the heat to a simmer.
- Simmer the chicken till done, about an hour and a half. It takes longer than if you just poach a whole chicken because you have stuffed this bird.
- When the bird is done, fish it carefully from the liquid to a cutting board, remove the skin and carve the bird. Use a spoon to dig out the stuffing and place it on a platter surrounded by the veggies and then attractively plate the chicken on top of the veg. Serve with plenty of Pommery mustard and any other dipping sauce you may want.

264.   Pumpkin Baked Oatmeal With Brandied Cranberries And White Chocolate

Serving: Serves 6-8 | Prep: | Cook: | Ready in:

Ingredients

- 1/2 cup dried cranberries
- 1/2 cup brandy
- 2 cups rolled oats
- 1/3 cup dark brown sugar
- 1 teaspoon cinnamon
- 1 teaspoon powdered ginger
- 1/2 teaspoon sea salt
- 1 teaspoon baking powser
- 1/2 cup pumpkin puree
- 1/3 cup apple or pear butter
- 1 tablespoon grated orange rind
- 1 tablespoon freshly squeezed lemon juice
- 1 teaspoon freshly grated ginger
- 1 cup milk
- 2 tablespoons unsalted butter
- 1 teaspoon vanilla extract
- 1   egg
- 1/2 cup white chocolate chips

- 1/2 cup toasted peacns, roughly chopped
- 1 cup heavy cream, milk, or eggnog

Direction

- Preheat the oven to 375°F. Grease a nine inch pie pan. Place the cranberries and brandy in a bowl and microwave on medium power for about a minute. Let stand for at least an hour. Drain before adding to the batter.
- Place in a food processor: the oats, brown sugar, cinnamon, powdered ginger, salt, and baking powder. Pulse until blended. Add butter and pulse a few times until blended.
- Add fresh ginger, pumpkin, vanilla, egg, milk, orange rind, lemon juice, and apple butter. Pulse until mixed in.
- Mix in very briefly the drained cranberries, white chocolate chips, and toasted pecans. Spread the batter into the greased pie pan.
- Bake for about 20 minutes, until the oatmeal has set and the top is golden. Serve warm, topped with a drizzle of cream, milk, or egg nog.

265. Pumpkin Almond Scones W/ Maple Yogurt Frosting

Serving: Serves 6 | Prep: | Cook: | Ready in:

Ingredients

- For the scones:
- 1 cup garbanzo bean flour
- 1 cup oat flour
- 1 tablespoon baking powder
- 1 teaspoon sea salt
- 1 1/2 teaspoons pumpkin pie spice
- 4 tablespoons cold butter
- 1 teaspoon vanilla extract
- 1/4 cup milk
- 1/3 cup coconut sugar
- 2/3 cup pumpkin puree
- For the maple frosting:
- 1/2 cup greek yogurt
- 2 tablespoons pure maple syrup

Direction

- Preheat oven to 425F and line a baking sheet with parchment paper.
- Whisk the pumpkin puree, coconut sugar, milk, and vanilla in a small bowl. Set aside.
- In a medium-large bowl, combine the flours, baking powder, sea salt, and pumpkin pie spice. Use a knife to roughly chop the butter into small cubes into the dry ingredients and mix.
- Slowly pour the wet ingredients into the dry and mix until just combined. If it sticks to your fingers at a light touch, add more oat flour by the tablespoon until the dough dries out just a bit.
- Sprinkle a small handful of oat flour over the parchment paper. Scoop the dough onto the paper, lightly roll it in the oat flour, and form into a circle about 1 1/2-2" tall (it shouldn't be flat). Cut into 6 triangles and distribute evenly over the baking sheet
- Bake for 15-17 minutes, or until golden brown on top and firm to the gentle touch. Remove from the oven and cool completely.
- In a small bowl, whisk together the Greek yogurt and maple syrup. Once the scones have cooled, scoop a dollop of frosting onto each scone and spread over the top. Finish with a sprinkle of cinnamon and serve immediately. Store leftovers in an airtight container in the fridge for 1-2 weeks.
- Enjoy!

266. Pumpkin Cornbread Muffins

Serving: Makes 9 | Prep: | Cook: | Ready in:

Ingredients

- 1/2 cup pumpkin puree
- 1/4 cup maple syrup

- 2 teaspoons cinnamon
- 1 cup unsweetened vanilla almond milk
- 1/2 teaspoon baking soda
- 1 cup cornmeal
- 1 cup almond flour
- 1/3 cup GF oat flour
- 1/4 cup Truvia brown baking sugar
- 1/4 teaspoon sea salt
- 1 tablespoon apple cider vinegar

Direction

- Preheat oven 350 degrees
- Prepare a muffin tin with cooking spray or liners (or baking dish if making the bread version)
- In a food processor, combine pumpkin, almond milk, apple cider vinegar, oats, sugar, honey & cinnamon and combine
- To the mixture, add by hand baking soda, cornmeal, almond meal & salt and combine well
- Let the batter sit 1 hour in the refrigerator to allow the batter to thicken, the cornmeal will absorb all the ingredients to make fluffier and thicker muffins (trust me!)
- Pour the batter into the cavities
- Bake 30 minutes until muffins appear golden & a toothpick can be inserted cleanly in the center
- Cool muffins before serving

267. Pumpkin Maple Oat Rolls

Serving: Makes a tin of rolls | Prep: | Cook: | Ready in:

Ingredients

- 3/4 cup milk
- 1/2 cup maple syrup
- 2 tablespoons (chopped) butter or olive oil
- 1/4 cup pumpkin puree
- 1 egg
- 3/4 cup rolled oats
- 2 teaspoons kosher salt
- 2 &1/2 – 3 cups all-purpose flour, plus extra to dust work top
- 1 teaspoon instant action yeast
- Maple flakes, to taste
- Extra 2-3 tablespoons of melted butter, mixed with 2 – 3 tablespoons of maple syrup, to glaze roll tops

Direction

- Scald milk and pour into a large bowl. To it, add the maple syrup, butter, pumpkin puree, stirring till the butter is melted. Then add the egg, rolled oats and salt. Allow to cool to lukewarm.
- Combine the flour and yeast and using a dough whisk or a wooden spoon, then gradually add the flour mix to the cooled 'liquid' - you may not need all 3 cups. The resulting dough should hold together, with no flour lumps/patches and should be soft/loose but not liquid! In typical lazy (and successful, might I add), no-knead fashion, cover with a lid/loosely with plastic wrap and refrigerate for a minimum of 2 hours or overnight. The resulting dough does not rise much.
- Turn out the chilled dough on a floured work surface and knead or fold and turn the dough slightly. Cut dough into 12 balls. Press each ball into a flat rectangle with your fingers, then roll up and tuck ends under.
- Brush all over with ½ of the melted butter-maple mix and sprinkle with the maple flakes. Let rise until doubled in size in a warm place, about two hours. I find my microwave is the best spot for 'rising dough' not to mention safe and away from hands and other random objects falling out of (the sky :-)) aka full cupboards!
- Once risen, preheat the oven to 170°C (350° F). Bake for 35-40 minutes or until rolls are nicely browned and sound hollow when you tap their tops. The internal temperature should be 190 degrees (I used my meat thermometer to check this!)

- Remove from the pan and brush generously with melted butter – maple mix. Let cool on a rack for 5-10 minutes. Serve warm…with salted butter, jam and anything else that tips your scales!

268. Pumpkin Pie Oatmeal

Serving: Serves 4 | Prep: | Cook: |Ready in:

Ingredients

- 1.5 cups Whole Milk
- 2 Eggs
- 1 tablespoon Cinnamon
- 1/4 teaspoon Nutmeg
- 7 ounces Pureed pumpkin
- 1/4 cup Dark brown sugar
- 1/4 cup Steel cut oats
- 1 teaspoon Vanilla extract
- 1/2 Lemon (zest and juice)
- Chopped almonds or walnuts (for garnish)
- Fruit, such as raspberries or diced apple (for garnish)

Direction

- Combine milk, eggs, spices, sugar and pumpkin to a heavy bottomed sauce pan over low heat. Whisking vigorously to prevent the eggs from scrambling.
- Add the oats when the custard thickens enough to coats the back of the spoon. Continue to stir occasionally as the oats cook according to the package instructions (about 5-7 minutes).
- Cut the heat. Incorporate the vanilla, butter, lemon zest and juice. Garnish with apple, almonds, and a dusting of cinnamon.

269. Pumpkin Pie Spice Squares

Serving: Makes 9-12 squares | Prep: | Cook: |Ready in:

Ingredients

- For the Crust
- 1 cup Ground Rolled Oats
- 1/4 cup Unsweetened Shredded Coconut
- 1/2 cup Pitted Dates
- 1-2 tablespoons Maple Syrup or Agave Nectar*
- 3 tablespoons Coconut Oil (liquified)
- 1 pinch Salt
- For the Filling
- 1.5 cups Fresh Pumpkin (Roasted or Boiled until tender.)
- 1/4 cup Palm Sugar
- 1/2 cup Coconut Oil
- 1 Fresh Vanilla Pod
- 1 teaspoon Ground Cinnamon
- 1/2 teaspoon Nutmeg (I used freshly grated seed)
- 1/2 tablespoon Grated Ginger Root (or 1/8 teaspoon Ground)
- 1 pinch Ground Clove

Direction

- For the Crust
- In a food processor pulse together the oat flour, shredded coconut, dates, maple syrup or agave, coconut oil and salt until a ball begins to form. *More or less maple syrup or agave may added or omitted according to personal taste.
- Transfer the mixture to a plastic wrap or parchment paper lined 8 inch square or 9x13 inch dish. Press and flatten the crust into one even layer and set aside.
- For the Filling
- Add the pumpkin, cinnamon, nutmeg, ginger, and clove to a food processor and pulse until the blades begin to move freely. Gradually add the coconut oil and vanilla mixture to the pumpkin and spices while they blend. It's

preferable that the pumpkin is at least at room temperature as adding liquefied coconut oil to cold (anything) pumpkin will make it seize and re-solidify.*
- Once the pumpkin filling is smooth and there are no longer any visible lumps, pour the filling over the already prepared crust. Without covering**, placing the dish in a refrigerator for at least 5-6 hours, or overnight, to chill and become firm. Use the plastic wrap or parchment paper as leverage to remove the layers from the dish and cut squares of the desired size.
- **The pumpkin filling will likely be warm from being processed for the extended number of minutes it takes for it to become smooth. As a result of this, covering it right away will cause condensation to collect and drip onto the surface. To avoid this, only cover after a few hours (3 approx.) of refrigeration.

270. Pumpkin Seed Oatmeal Raisin Cookie Bars

Serving: Serves 8 | Prep: | Cook: | Ready in:

Ingredients

- 3/4 cup all-purpose flour
- 1/2 cup nut butter
- 1/3 cup maple syrup
- 2 flax eggs
- 1 teaspoon vanilla extract
- 1 teaspoon baking soda
- 1 teaspoon pumpkin pie spice
- 1 teaspoon sea salt, plus more for sprinkling
- 1/2 cup pumpkin seeds
- 1/2 cup rolled oats
- 1/3 cup raisins

Direction

- Preheat the oven to 350F and coat a baking dish with oil. Any small-medium baking dish will work, just know that smaller pans will require longer baking times and medium pans will let the bars cook faster.
- In a medium-size bowl, stir together the wet ingredients - the nut butter, maple syrup, flax eggs,
- In a large bowl, combine the dry ingredients - flour, baking soda, pumpkin pie spice, sea salt, oats, and raisins. Pour the wet into the dry and stir until incorporated.
- Transfer the dough to the baking dish, gently pressing it in to ensure uniformity. Bake for 28-30 minutes if using a smaller dish, and less time if using a medium dish. Remove from oven when golden brown and crisp at the top and a toothpick comes out clean.
- Cool completely before slicing and serving. Store leftovers in an airtight container for up to one week.
- Enjoy!

271. Quick Simple Beef Stew

Serving: Serves 3-4 | Prep: | Cook: | Ready in:

Ingredients

- 0.5 pounds Lean Stewing Beef
- 10   Peeld Baby Carrots
- 2   Medium Red Potatoes (about 2/3 lb)
- 1   Medium Onion
- 3 tablespoons Quick Oats
- 1 teaspoon Salt
- 2 tablespoons Olive Oil
- 1 tablespoon Unsalted Butter

Direction

- Wash potatoes and cut into bite size. Peel and halve onion and slice thinly.
- In a large pot, heat olive oil and sauté onion over medium heat until tender. Add beef, carrots and potatoes and sauté for 1-2 minutes. Add 2 cups water and bring to boiling.

- Reduce heat to medium-low heat and simmer for 15 minutes or until potatoes and carrots are tender removing the scum periodically.
- Stir in oats and salt. Simmer for another 5 minutes or until slightly thickened.
- Lastly, add butter to the pot. When the butter is melted, turn off the heat and put the stew into each serving bowl.

272. Quinoa Porridge

Serving: Serves 2 | Prep: | Cook: |Ready in:

Ingredients

- 1/4 cup Quinoa
- 1/4 cup Oats
- 1 1/2 cups Almond milk
- 1 tablespoon Honey/Maple Syrup
- 1/4 cup Peaches or any seasonal fruits
- 1 cup Water

Direction

- Wash quinoa in water a couple of times and transfer to a saucepan with 1 cup of water.
- Bring it to boil and then simmer the heat for 5 minutes. Add in the rolled oats and almond milk and cook on simmer for another 10 minutes.
- Remove from heat and stir cardamom powder and in the desired sweetener.
- Serve in small mason jars topped with honey/maple syrup and sliced peaches.

273. Quinoa And Oat Breakfast Porridge

Serving: Serves 2 generously | Prep: | Cook: |Ready in:

Ingredients

- 2 cups unsweetened almond milk, divided, see notes above
- 1 cardamom pod, crushed with the flat side of a knife
- 1/2 a bay leaf, fresh is best
- 1/2 cup quinoa, red is nice for color
- 3/4 cup rolled oats, extra-thick if you can find them, see notes above
- 1 teaspoon coconut oil
- 2 tablespoons maple syrup
- 1/4 teaspoon kosher salt, plust more to taste
- toasted coconut, toasted almonds, fresh berries such as strawberries and blueberries, for garnish

Direction

- Place 1 cup of the almond milk, the lightly crushed cardamom pod, and the 1/2 bay leaf in a small pot. Bring to a simmer, reduce heat to low, and keep warm.
- In a medium pot, combine the quinoa with 1 cup of water. Add a pinch of salt. Bring to a boil, turn heat to low, cover, and cook until tender, about 20 minutes. Remove from heat, and let stand covered.
- In another medium pot, combine the oats, remaining 1 cup almond milk, ¼ cup water, coconut oil, maple syrup, and salt. Bring to a simmer, then turn heat to low and cook until oats are tender, about 10 minutes. Taste. Add more salt to taste if necessary.
- Add ½ cup of the cooked quinoa to the oats along with ½ cup of the infused almond milk, taking care to leave the bay leaf and cardamom pod (and any seeds) behind. Stir to combine. Taste. Add more salt if necessary. Add more quinoa to taste (or save extra quinoa in the fridge in an airtight container for porridge on a future morning).
- To serve, pour ¼ cup of the warm, cardamom-infused almond milk into each bowl. Spoon porridge over top. Top with toasted coconut, almonds, and berries if using.

274. Quinoa, Beet And Chickpea Burgers

Serving: Makes 6 large burgers, or 12-18 small sliders | Prep: | Cook: | Ready in:

Ingredients

- 1/2 cup dried chickpeas, soaked overnight in cool water (or 1 [14 ounce] can cooked chickpeas, drained and rinsed)
- 1 bay leaf (if using dried chickpeas)
- 1/2 cup raw quinoa
- 3 medium-sized red beets (about 10 ounces by weight)
- 1 tablespoon olive oil
- 1 medium yellow onion, finely diced
- 2 cloves garlic, minced
- 2 tablespoons cider vinegar
- 2-4 tablespoons finely chopped parsley
- zest from half a medium lemon
- juice from 1 medium lemon
- 1 large egg
- 1/2 cup quick (baby) oats
- sunflower oil or coconut oil for frying the burgers
- For serving the burgers (optional): 6 buns (such as Honey Oat Beer Buns), halved and toasted, mustard, mayonnaise, avocado, thinly sliced red onion, sprouts

Direction

- If using dried chickpeas, cook the beans: Drain the soaked chickpeas and place them in a medium saucepan with the bay leaf. Cover with 3 inches of water, bring to a boil, then reduce the heat and simmer, partially covered, until the beans are almost tender. At this point, add 1/2 teaspoon of salt to the pot. Continue cooking until the beans are very tender. This can take anywhere from 30 minutes to over an hour total, depending on the size and age of the beans. Add water to the pan as needed. When the beans are done, let them cool in their water until needed. If you like, you can slip the loose skins off the beans, though this isn't necessary.
- Cook the quinoa: Place the quinoa in a very fine mesh strainer, place the strainer in a bowl or measuring cup, and fill with water to cover the quinoa. Let soak 5-10 minutes, swishing occasionally, to rinse off the bitter coating. The water will turn a beige-yellow. Drain the quinoa well, discard the soaking water, and place the quinoa in a small saucepan with 1 cup of water and 1/4 teaspoon salt. Bring the mixture to a boil, immediately reduce the heat to very low, cover the pot, and let the quinoa steam until tender and all the water is absorbed, 15-20 minutes. Remove from the heat and let sit, covered, until ready to use.
- Cook the veg: Peel the beets with a potato peeler, then grate them on the large holes of a box grater. The beets will spray, so wear an apron and have your work area clear of things you don't want covered in tiny red specks. Heat the oil in a wide sauté pan (that has a lid that you will use later) over medium heat. When it shimmers, add the onion and cook, stirring occasionally, until tender, 5-10 minutes. Add the garlic, the grated beets, and a big pinch of salt. Give it a stir, then cover the pan and let the mixture cook, stirring occasionally, until the beet is tender, 5 minutes or so. Remove from the heat and deglaze by adding the vinegar and stirring up any good stuff that is stuck to the bottom of the pan.
- Make the burgers: In a large bowl, combine the cooked chickpeas, quinoa and beet mixture and mash with a potato masher to break up the beans slightly - the mixture should still be fairly chunky. Stir in the parsley, lemon zest and juice, egg, oats, and 1/4 teaspoon salt until combined.
- Cook the burgers: Divide the mixture into 6 equal portions (a large spring-loaded scoop works well) and shape into 1" thick rounds. Coat the bottom of a wide skillet with oil and heat over a medium flame until the oil shimmers. Carefully add the burger patties. Cook until the first side is golden, 2-3 minutes, then flip and cook on the second side until it is

golden and the burger is cooked through, 2-3 minutes, reducing the heat if the burger is browning too quickly. Serve the burgers on toasted buns slathered in any toppings you like.

275. Rainy Morning Oats

Serving: Serves 1 | Prep: | Cook: | Ready in:

Ingredients

- 1/2 cup water
- 3/4 cup whole milk
- 1/3 cup steel-cut oats
- 1 pinch salt
- 1 1/2 tablespoons dark brown sugar, divided
- 1/8 teaspoon vanilla extract
- 1 heaping tablespoons chopped dried cherries & chopped dried apples
- 1 tablespoon chopped pecans, toasted
- 1 tablespoon cream
- sprinkle of grated nutmeg

Direction

- Bring water, milk and oats to a boil; reduce heat and simmer stirring occasionally, until liquid mostly absorbed (but not totally dry).
- Remove from heat. Stir in 1 tablespoon of brown sugar and vanilla.
- Place dried fruits in the bottom of a small bowl. Heap cooked oats on top. Top with pecans, cream, remaining brown sugar, and grate nutmeg over all.

276. Raisin, Pecan, And Banana Oatmeal With Flax Seeds

Serving: Serves 1-2 | Prep: | Cook: | Ready in:

Ingredients

- 1/2 cup Old fashioned rolled oats (not instant)
- 1 cup Milk (will be used 1/2 cup at a time)
- 1/2 cup Water
- 1/4 cup Raisins
- 2 tablespoons Coarse ground flax seeds
- 2 tablespoons Pecan pieces
- 1 Banana
- Pinch Salt (optional)

Direction

- Put the oats, flax, raisins, and salt (if using) into a sauce pan and add the water and 1/2 cup of milk. Cook over medium-low until most of the liquid is dissolved.
- While the oats cook, cut the banana into small slices. I just slice it into my bowl.
- Pour the cooked oats over the banana slices, pour the remaining 1/2 cup of milk over the top, and sprinkle on the pecans. From here, I mix everything together and chow down with a mug of green tea.

277. Raspberry Multigrain Muffins

Serving: Makes 12 | Prep: | Cook: | Ready in:

Ingredients

- 3/4 cup (110g) sweet rice flour
- 1/4 cup (30g) amaranth flour
- 1/4 cup (30g) teff flour
- 1/4 cup (30g) almond meal
- 1/3 cup (40g) tapioca starch
- 1 1/2 teaspoons baking soda
- 1/2 teaspoon sea salt
- 1/4 cup (30g) gluten-free rolled oats
- 1/2 cup (100g) brown sugar
- 1 teaspoon whole chia seeds
- 1/2 cup canola oil
- 2 eggs

- 1/2 cup unsweetened soymilk, almond milk, or coconut milk
- 1 teaspoon apple cider vinegar
- 2 teaspoons fresh lemon juice
- 1 teaspoon lemon zest
- 3/4 cup fresh washed raspberries

Direction

- Preheat oven to 375F. Grease your muffin tin with coconut oil or shortening. Bring out your eggs so they're room temperature when you use them.
- Measure dry ingredients into a large bowl (use grams if possible!). Break up baking soda and brown sugar lumps, mixing flours well. In a separate bowl or glass measuring cup, measure out liquids and lemon zest. Beat in eggs very thoroughly.
- Mix wet ingredients into dry. Gently fold in fresh raspberries. Fill muffin cups nearly to the top, dust each with a few whole oats, and put them into the oven immediately. They're rise higher the faster you're able to do this.
- Bake about 20-25 minutes or until toothpick inserted into center of a muffin comes out clean. Let cool at least 10 minutes before moving them from the tin. Store in a sealed container for 3 days at room temperature or up to 1 week in the refrigerator.

278. Raspberry Oat And Yogurt Spelt Muffins

Serving: Makes 12 | Prep: | Cook: | Ready in:

Ingredients

- 1 3/4 cup whole spelt flour
- 1 cup rolled oats
- 1/4 cup hemp hearts
- 2 teaspoons baking powder
- 1/2 teaspoon baking soda
- 1/2 teaspoon salt
- 2 large eggs
- 1/2 cup greek yogurt
- 1/2 cup coconut oil, melted
- 1/2 cup honey
- 1 teaspoon pure vanilla extract
- 1 cup fresh or frozen raspberries

Direction

- Preheat oven to 375F and line or grease a standard muffin tin.
- In a medium sized bowl, whisk together the flour, oats, baking powder, baking soda, and salt. If you're using frozen raspberries, stirring them in to the flour mixture will help prevent colour bleeding.
- In a large bowl, lightly beat the eggs. Add the melted coconut oil, yogurt, honey, and vanilla.
- Add the dry ingredients to the egg mixture and mix until just combined.
- Fill each muffin cup all the way to the top, and bake 18-20 minutes, or until a toothpick comes out clean.

279. Raspberry And Honey Cranachan

Serving: Serves 4 | Prep: | Cook: | Ready in:

Ingredients

- 1/2 cup old-fashioned rolled oats
- 2 tablespoons whiskey (preferably scotch but whatever whiskey you have on hand)
- 1 cup heavy cream
- 2 cups fresh raspberries
- 2 tablespoons heather honey (or other favorite honey)

Direction

- Warm a small frying pan over medium-low heat. Add the rolled oats and stir until they are golden and toasted – keep a close eye on them, as they can burn easily. Transfer to a plate to cool.

- Stir the whiskey and cream together in a bowl and then whisk (by hand or with a hand blender) until the cream holds soft peaks. Lightly crush a few of the raspberries, so the juices run. Loosely fold the honey, oats, and raspberries into the cream, spoon into glasses, and serve right away.

280. Raspberry Rhubarb Crumble With Cracklin' Oat Bran Topping

Serving: Serves 6 to 8, maybe more | Prep: | Cook: | Ready in:

Ingredients

- 360 grams raspberries
- 420 grams rhubarb, chopped into bite-sized pieces
- 1/4 cup raw sugar, or more to taste
- 1 pinch salt
- 250 grams Cracklin' Oat Bran cereal
- 50 grams roughly chopped walnuts
- 50 grams roughly chopped pecans
- 4 tablespoons cold unsalted butter

Direction

- Preheat the oven to 350° F.
- In a medium bowl, mix together the raspberries, rhubarb, sugar, and salt. If your raspberries are not sweet, you might consider adding another 2 tablespoons or 1/4 cup of sugar. Set aside.
- Use a food processor to grind the Cracklin' Oat Bran into a powder that resembles oat bran. In a medium bowl, mix this with the walnuts and pecans. Using your fingers, work the butter into the dry ingredients until you have clumps.
- Dump the fruit into a 9- or 10-inch ovenproof skillet or baking dish. Top with the Cracklin' Oat Bran crumble. Bake for 30 to 40 minutes, until the fruit is bubbling and the top is golden-brown and crisp.
- Serve warm with vanilla ice cream.

281. Rhubarb Cherry Hibiscus Crumble

Serving: Makes 1, 8x8-inch square crumble | Prep: 0hours0mins | Cook: 0hours22mins | Ready in:

Ingredients

- For the fruit filling:
- 6 cups chopped rhubarb (~3/4? cubes), divided
- 20 Bing cherries, pitted and halved
- 1 cup packed brown sugar
- 2 tablespoons hibiscus tea leaves (I use The Republic of Tea Natural Hibiscus loose leaf herbal; you can also use 8 hibiscus flowers, as does Kim Boyce)
- For the topping:
- 1/2 cup whole wheat flour
- 1/2 cup all-purpose flour
- 1/2 cup rolled oats (not quick- or instant)
- 1/4 cup brown sugar, packed
- 1/2 cup sliced almonds
- 1/2 teaspoon cinnamon
- 1 pinch salt
- 6 tablespoons butter, set out on the counter when you start making this dessert- you want it to be cool but pliable

Direction

- For the fruit filling:
- Preheat the oven to 400, and get out an 8" square glass baking dish. In a medium, non-reactive, heavy-bottomed saucepan set over medium-low heat, put 4 cups of the chopped rhubarb, the cherries, 1 packed cup of brown sugar and the hibiscus. Stir to combine everything, cover, and cook until the rhubarb releases its liquid and starts to break down, about 10-12 minutes.

- Uncover the pot, add the remaining 2 c of chopped rhubarb, stir to combine, and remove from heat. Set aside.
- For the topping:
- In a medium mixing bowl, whisk together the whole wheat and all-purpose flours, the oats, brown sugar, almonds, cinnamon and salt. With your fingers or a pastry cutter, blend in the butter until you have a crumbly mixture in which the butter is as uniformly distributed as possible.
- Pour the fruit filling into your baking dish and then pour the crumble topping evenly over the top. Place the dish into the oven and bake for 22 minutes. (I turned the heat up to 425 after 20 minutes to give it an extra boost of heat at the end). Some of the crumble topping will sink into the fruit compote. Yum!
- Serve with vanilla ice cream or with a lightly sweetened whipped cream with a little almond extract blended in (I used about 1/4 tsp of almond extract in mine).

282. Rhubarb Ginger Downside Up Oatmeal Cake

Serving: Serves 8-10 slices | Prep: | Cook: | Ready in:

Ingredients

- For the rhubarb:
- 2 1/4 cups fresh rhubarb, 1/2 inch slices
- 1 tablespoon fresh ginger, grated
- 1 cup brown sugar
- 1/4 cup unsalted butter
- For the oatmeal cake
- 1/2 cup thick cut rolled oats
- 3/4 cup boiling water
- 1/4 cup unsalted butter, 1/4 inch cubes
- 1/2 teaspoon vanilla
- 1 large egg
- 1/2 cup brown sugar
- 1/2 cup sugar
- 1 cup unbleached all-purpose flour
- 1 teaspoon baking powder
- 1/4 teaspoon baking soda
- 1/4 teaspoon salt

Direction

- In a mixing bowl combine the oats with the boiling water. Add the 1/4 cup of butter. Set aside to cool.
- Preheat the oven to 350 degrees. Gently melt the butter in a 10 inch cast iron skillet. Remove it from the heat. Spread the brown sugar evenly across the bottom. In a large bowl mix the ginger and rhubarb. Spread the rhubarb evenly across the brown sugar. Set aside.
- In the empty rhubarb bowl combine the flour, baking powder, baking soda and salt.
- To the cooled oatmeal add the egg, both sugars, and vanilla. Mix to combine. Add the dry ingredients to the wet and mix until combined.
- Spread the cake batter evenly across the top of the rhubarb. Place into the oven and bake for 30-40 minutes.
- Remove from the oven when done and let cool for 5 minutes before inverting onto a cake plate. Let cool for 20 minutes before slicing.

283. Rhubarb, Cherry And Strawberry Crumble

Serving: Serves 5 | Prep: | Cook: | Ready in:

Ingredients

- Rhubarb Mix
- 3 Rhubarb Stalks, chopped
- 1 cup Dark red cherries
- 1 cup Strawberries
- 1/3 cup Light brown sugar, packed
- Crumble
- 1/3 cup Gluten-free Flour
- 1/3 cup Rolled Oats
- 2 tablespoons Almond Butter

- 3 tablespoons Coconut Oil
- 1/4 cup Almonds, chopped

Direction

- Pre-heat oven to 400 degrees.
- Place chopped rhubarb, cherries and strawberries in a saucepan over medium heat. Cover and heat for 2-4 minutes.
- Add brown sugar to heated fruit mix and stir until blended. Heat an additional 10-12 minutes or until the fruit juices are bubbling and rhubarb is soft.
- While the fruit continues to cook, prepare the crumble.
- In a mixing bowl, combine the almond butter, coconut oil, gluten-free flour, oats and almonds. Mixture should be 'crumbly'. If not, add a few more oats.
- When fruit mixture is ready, remove from heat and pour into a glass 8x8 dish. Top with crumble.
- Bake for 20-25 minutes. Serve warm or room temperature.

284. Rich And Creamy Swiss Style Muesli

Serving: Serves 2 | Prep: | Cook: | Ready in:

Ingredients

- 3-4 ounces rolled oats
- 3-4 ounces orange juice
- 3-4 raspberry yogurt
- 2 tablespoons cranberries
- 6 pieces strawberries, hulled

Direction

- Place oats, orange juice, yogurt and cranberries in a plastic container. Mix well and keep refrigerated overnight.
- Take the container out of the fridge, beat the mixture lightly with a spoon and add hulled strawberries. Spoon the mixture into each glass and top it off with strawberries.

285. Roasted Squash Salad With Pomegranate And Spiced Oat Clusters

Serving: Serves 4 to 6 | Prep: | Cook: | Ready in:

Ingredients

- 3/4 teaspoon ground cinnamon
- 1/2 teaspoon paprika
- 3/4 teaspoon plus 1 pinch sea salt, divided
- 1 small buttercup squash, peeled, cored, and seeded
- 2 teaspoons heat-tolerant vegetable oil, such as grapeseed
- 1/2 cup freshly squeezed orange juice
- 1/4 cup sweetened dried cranberries
- 1 cup pomegranate arils
- 3 tablespoons extra virgin olive oil
- 1 handful KIND Snacks Cinnamon Oat Clusters or granola of choice

Direction

- Preheat oven to 425° F. Slide two rimmed baking sheets in to preheat as well.
- In a small bowl, combine the cinnamon, paprika, and 3/4 teaspoon sea salt.
- Slice squash into even 3/4-inch thick wedges, and then cut each wedge into thirds. Set in a large bowl and toss with vegetable oil. Tossing with hands, sprinkle in spice mixture until each piece of squash is coated. Arrange squash on hot baking sheets, allowing 1 to 2 inches of space between each piece. Roast for 20 minutes, carefully flip squash, and roast for 10 to 15 minutes longer, or until edges are crisp and centers are tender.
- Meanwhile, combine orange juice and dried cranberries in a small bowl; set aside for 20 minutes, then remove cranberries from orange juice. In a small bowl, measure 2 tablespoons

of the cranberry soaking liquid. Use a fork to whisk in a pinch of sea salt, followed by the olive oil.
- Just before serving, toss warm squash, cranberries, and pomegranate arils with a few drizzles of dressing and top with oat clusters. Arrange on plates, and serve immediately.

286. Rockin RAW Nut Granola The Best RAW Granola....Ever

Serving: Makes 7 cups | Prep: | Cook: | Ready in:

Ingredients

- 1 1/2 cups walnuts (soaked for 4 hours & drained)
- 1 1/2 cups cashews (soaked for 4 hours & drained)
- 1 1/2 almonds (soaked for 4 hours & drained)
- 1 1/2 raw sunflower (soaked for 2 hours & drained)
- 3/4 cup oat flour (grind oats in blender until fine powder)
- 2 tablespoons tbsp ground flax seed (grind in a coffee grinder)
- 3/4 cup dried unsweetened coconut
- 1/2 cup cranberries or raisins
- 2 medium granny smith apples, cored and chopped
- 10 large medjool dates, pitted (soaked in hot water for 30 min)
- 1/4 cup coconut oil
- 1 tablespoon freshly squeezed lemon juice
- 2 tablespoons tahini
- 1/2 cup agave OR 100% REAL maple syrup (not pancake syrup)
- 2 teaspoons vanilla extract
- 1 teaspoon cinnamon
- 1/2 teaspoon sea salt

Direction

- Pulse soaked nuts in food processor until chopped. Place nuts in a large mixing bowl. Add ground oats & flaxseeds to the bowl and combine with the processed nuts and seeds. Stir in coconut and cranberries (or raisins).
- Without cleaning the food processor, add chopped apples, soaked dates, lemon juice, coconut oil, tahini, agave (or REAL maple syrup), vanilla, cinnamon and salt and process until smooth.
- Pour mixture into the bowl and stir into the nut mixture until thoroughly combined. Spread out onto 2 or 3 Teflex sheets and dehydrate for 8 to 12 hours at 115 degrees F. Flip over onto mesh tray, remove Teflex sheets and dehydrate for another 8 to 12 hours or until dry and crisp. Remove from dehydrator and let cool.
- When cool, break up into small pieces and store until needed in an air tight container. Refrigerated, it will last for a few weeks.

287. Rosemary Cayenne Granola Bars

Serving: Makes 12 granola bars | Prep: | Cook: | Ready in:

Ingredients

- 2 cups old fashioned rolled oats
- 1/2 cup cashews
- 1/2 cup peanuts
- 1/2 cup pecans
- 1/2 cup almonds
- 1/2 cup honey
- 1/4 cup brown sugar, packed
- 3 tablespoons unsalted butter
- 1 teaspoon vanilla extract
- 1/2 teaspoon salt
- 2 tablespoons fresh rosemary, chopped
- 1/4 teaspoon cayenne

Direction

- This recipe calls for raw and unsalted nuts, but you can adjust as needed to use what you have on hand. Preheat the oven to 300 degrees Fahrenheit.
- Spread onto a half-sheet pan and toast in the oven for 15 minutes, stirring occasionally. If you're working with any already roasted nuts, omit them from this step
- While the oats and nuts are toasting, combine the brown sugar, butter, vanilla extract, salt, rosemary and cayenne in a small saucepan over medium heat. If the nuts you're using in the previous step are already salted, use less salt than this recipe calls for in this step or skip the salt entirely.
- Stir over the heat until the butter is melted and the brown sugar is completely dissolved. Remove from heat and set aside.
- When the oats and nuts are a finished toasting in the oven, combine everything in a mixing bowl and stir until well combined.
- Pour into the greased baking dish and bake at 300 degrees for 20 minutes. The bars will still have a bit of chewiness to them, so if you prefer a crunchier bar, extend the baking time an additional 5 minutes. The bars went the extra 5 minutes. Remove from oven and let cool until completely hardened, about an hour.
- Remove from the oven and let cool until completely hardened, about an hour.
- Use the sides of the parchment paper to lift the granola bars out of the baking dish and onto a cutting board. Cut into bars and store them in an airtight container for up to a week, placing parchment paper between layers to keep them from sticking to each other.

288. Rosemary, Fig, Walnut, And Honey Granola

Serving: Makes about 4 cups | Prep: | Cook: | Ready in:

Ingredients

- 3 cups oats
- 1 teaspoon sea salt
- 1 dash black pepper
- 1 tablespoon fresh rosemary, finely chopped
- 1 cup walnuts, chopped (not pre-toasted)
- 1 teaspoon cinnamon
- 2 tablespoons olive oil
- 1/4 cup honey
- 1/2 cup dried figs

Direction

- Preheat the oven to 350°F. Line a rimmed baking sheet with tinfoil or parchment paper. Set aside.
- In a large bowl, combine the oats, salt, rosemary, walnuts, cinnamon, and pepper. Fold and stir the ingredients until thoroughly combined.
- In a separate, smaller bowl, combine the olive oil and honey. Vigorously whisk with a fork to combine the two. Drizzle this evenly over the dry oat mixture, and then continue to fold the ingredients until all of the oats are covered. It may seem difficult at first, but just keep mixing and it will eventually get there (the mixture should be no more than moist).
- Spread the granola mixture out over the prepared baking sheet. You want everything to be laid out in a nice flat layer. Place this in the oven for about 10 minutes.
- Carefully remove the pan, stir and flip the granola, and bake for another 10-15 minutes, or until the oats are crisp and golden.
- While the granola is baking, chop your figs into fine pieces, about 1/2 inch thick. This is harder than it looks, so use a sharp knife.
- Let the granola cool on the sheet before stirring in the figs. Store in a sealable jar or container, at room temperature, for up to two weeks.

289. Russet Rollscuits With Herbs And Cheese

Serving: Serves 20 - 24 | Prep: | Cook: |Ready in:

Ingredients

- 1 large russet potato (about ½ pound / 226 grams, before peeling), peeled
- Pinch of salt for cooking the potato
- 55 grams (½ cup / 120 ml) quick oats
- 12 grams / 15 ml / 1 tablespoon brown sugar
- 330 grams (660 ml / heaping 2 ¾ cups) bread flour (it's best not to use all-purpose)
- 7 grams (2 teaspoons + heaping 1/2 teaspoon) instant yeast (also called, "rapid-rise")
- 253 grams (253 mil / 1 cup + 1 tablespoon) water, lukewarm (use as much potato cooking water as you can)
- 5 grams kosher salt (1 ½ teaspoon Diamond Crystal brand)
- 42 grams (heaping 1/3 cup / 1 ½ ounces) grated fresh Parmigianno-Reggiano, Pecorino Romano or similar cheese
- 1 tablespoon / 15 ml dried oregano or marjoram
- Extra flour for kneading, if necessary
- Extra olive oil for your proofing bowl, and for brushing on the rollscuits before baking
- Flaky sea salt for sprinkling on, just before baking

Direction

- Cut the peeled russet into three or four large chunks. Cover with cold water and a pinch of salt and bring to a boil; reduce heat and simmer until the potato is tender. Remove from the cooking water, put in a bowl, and mash well. Let cool.
- Measure potato cooking water with enough filtered water to make 253 grams / 253 ml / 1 cup + 1 tablespoon.
- Put it in the bowl of your stand mixer along with the oats, wheat germ, bread flour, instant yeast, olive oil and brown sugar. Using a spoon, stir together to incorporate the wet and dry ingredients. Put the bowl on your mixer, and using the dough hook, mix at low speed for about five minutes, scraping the sides down after the second and fourth minutes.
- Remove the dough hook and cover the bowl with a damp tea towel. Let it sit for about 25 minutes. We're letting the gluten form, undisturbed by the other, non-flour ingredients.
- Add the mashed potatoes, cheese and herbs and knead with the dough hook for about ten minutes, scraping down occasionally. After 7 or 8 minutes, if the dough seems very wet and sticky, and does not pull away from the side of the bowl, add one or two more tablespoons of flour, one at a time, letting the dough hook incorporate the first before adding the second (or more, if necessary).
- Drizzle a teaspoon or two of olive oil into the bottom of a large mixing bowl. Put the dough into the bowl and flip it over so the top is coated with oil. Cover the bowl with a damp tea towel or plastic wrap. Let rise for at least 1 ½ hours.
- Form the dough into 22 – 24 small free-standing rolls. I do this by shaping the dough into a circle, cutting it into fourths with a bench scraper, and then cutting 6 skinny wedges from each quarter. Then I roll each wedge up and pull the sides down to the bottom, stretching to create surface tension, giving a gentle pinch on the bottom.
- Set the rollscuits on a parchment-lined baking sheet with at least one open side. Cover with plastic wrap or a damp tea towel and let rise for at least 45 minutes.
- Meanwhile, heat a baking stone on a rack in the lower third of your oven at 400 degrees.
- When the rolls have nearly doubled in size, brush them ever so gently with a bit of olive oil and sprinkle with flaky salt.
- Slide the rolls, still on the parchment, onto the hot stone, through the open side of the baking sheet. Bake for 23 minutes. Remove to a cooling rack; let sit for at least ten minutes. I hope you like these. Yours truly, Antonia James

- Variation: These can also be made with 3 ounces of well drained feta, crumbled, with ¼ cup each chopped dill and sliced chives. You'll need an additional ¼ - 1/2 cup of flour, depending on the moisture level of the cheese; add that flour once the cheese and potato have been incorporated into the dough, after at least 5 minutes of kneading. These rolls will be a bit more dense than the dry cheese and oregano variety described above (which you'll find smells and tastes for all the world like a particularly good pizza crust).

290.   SUGAR FREE Barley Oats Quinoa Cashew Orange Cake With Blackberry And Peach Puree

Serving: Serves 12 | Prep: | Cook: | Ready in:

Ingredients

- The Cake Batter
- 1 1/4 cups barley
- 1/2 cup oats
- 1/2 cup quinoa
- 1 1/4 cups water
- 1 cup raisins soaked in water
- 1 1/2 cups cashews
- 1 1/4 cups deglet dates sliced & soaked in water
- 2 tablespoons coconut oil
- 1/2 cup golden flax meal
- 1 tablespoon nutritional yeast
- 1 tablespoon tahini
- 1 tablespoon soy lecithin
- 1/8 cup club soda
- 7 drops orange essential oil

Direction

- The Cake Batter
- Module 1 - Boiling the Barley, Oats and Quinoa: Pour 1/2 c barley, 1/2 c oats and 1/4 c quinoa in a pot of boiling water with salt. Cook the grains until soft but not too mushy. Drain and set aside.
- Module 2 - Soaking the Dried Fruits: Soak the raisins and dates in water.
- Blend all the ingredients except 3/4 c soaked dates and 1/2 c soaked raisins (which will be used in making the blackberry and peach puree) in a powerful blender (I used a Blend etc., but you can use a food processor too).
- Module 3 - Baking the Cake: Oil and sprinkle almond flour, or any flour, at the side and bottom of a non-stick baking pan. Line the bottom with a parchment paper (for double protection).Pour all the blended/processed mixture/batter in the baking pan. Bake in a 300 degree oven for 3 hrs. or until toothpick comes out clean. I used a 9 inch spring form baking pan. Note: When the top becomes golden brown, cover with a foil to stop it from burning. Cool. Serve with the Blackberry and Peach Puree
- Module 4 - Making the Blackberry Puree: Ingredients: 3/4 cup thawed frozen blackberries 1/2 cup raisins soaked 1/2 cup water. Procedure: Blend. Strain the seeds of the blackberries by putting the blended liquid in a produce bag or a nut-milk bag (we got ours from The Container Store) and squeezing the juice out. Throw the seeds. Drizzle the blackberry syrup over your cake slice, then, drizzle with the peach puree.
- Module 5 - Making the Peach Puree: Ingredients: 3/4 cup thawed frozen peach slices3/4 cup soaked pitted deglet dates sliced1/2 cup water1 tablespoon tahini
- Module 6 - Plating: Pour some Blackberry Puree on a plate. Place the cake on top of the puree. Garnish with Peach Puree and orange segments (optional).Enjoy.

291. Salted Caramel Chocolate Protein Bites

Serving: Serves 15 balls | Prep: | Cook: | Ready in:

Ingredients

- 3 tablespoons tbsp almond butter (stir before measuring if it's separated)
- 1 Scoop vegan chocolate protein powder (I use Plant Fusion)
- 1 teaspoon Sea Salt
- 1 tablespoon Chia Seeds
- 1/2 cup Rolled Oats

Direction

- Pulse dates in food processor until they start to get creamy, but small pieces remain.
- Add almond butter, protein powder, sea salt, chia seeds, and oats. Pulse until everything is well combined.
- Quickly roll into 1-inch balls and place each one on a parchment-lined baking sheet. Transfer to the refrigerator and allow them to set up for at least 30 minutes.
- I like to store mine in the fridge, but they will last for 1 week in an airtight container.

292. Sara's "Granola Bars"

Serving: Makes about 30 2-inch bars | Prep: | Cook: | Ready in:

Ingredients

- 1 1/2 cups old fashioned rolled oats
- 1 cup raw sunflower seeds
- 1 cup raw sliced almonds
- 1 cup raw pumpkin seeds
- 3 cups brown rice crispies (you can substitute regular rice crispies or puffed rice)
- 1 cup dried apricots, sliced thinly
- 1 cup dried cranberries
- 1 cup almond butter
- 1 cup honey
- 1 tablespoon sea salt
- 2 teaspoons cinnamon

Direction

- Heat the oven to 350 degrees. Toast the oats, sunflower seeds, almonds, pumpkin seeds. (Sara recommends toasting them all separately because of different burn rates -- I found that the pumpkin seeds took the least amount of time, at 7 minutes, and the sunflower seeds the most, at about 15 minutes.)
- When all the items are sufficiently toasted, toss them with the brown rice crispies, sliced apricot and cranberries in a large bowl.
- In a small saucepan, heat the almond butter and honey just to get melty, not cooked. (This is your glue and if it boils or even comes close, it gets hard and yucky.) Stir in the salt and cinnamon, then pour over the oat and nut mixture and stir. You want to get everything incorporated and 'glued' together without crushing the tender crispies.
- Turn into a 9x13 baking dish lined with parchment and press the mixture evenly and firmly -- again, try not crush the crispies too much. Cover with plastic wrap and refrigerate for several hours. Cut into 2-inch squares before serving.

293. Savory Breakfast Oat Bowl With Grana Padano

Serving: Serves 1 | Prep: | Cook: | Ready in:

Ingredients

- 1 1/2 cups water
- 1/2 cup milk of choice
- 1/2 cup steel cut oats
- 1/2 teaspoon salt (divided)
- 1 tablespoon butter or coconut oil
- 1 teaspoon olive oil
- 1 teaspoon balsamic vinegar

- 1 sprig rosemary, finely chopped
- 1/4 cup loosely packed arugula
- 1/4 cup sautéed carrots
- 1 soft boiled egg (6 min boil)
- 1 handful grated Grana Padano cheese (use a vegetable peeler for thin shavings)

Direction

- In small to medium saucepan, combine the water and milk and bring to a simmer over medium-high heat.
- Stir in oats and reduce heat to medium low, simmering gently for about 20 minutes, stirring occasionally, until the mixture is very thick.
- Meanwhile, gently toss arugula, olive oil, balsamic and rosemary; sauté carrots until golden brown; boil egg for 6 mins and add to ice bath. Set arugula, carrots and egg aside.
- When oats are thick, stir in salt and butter/coconut oil. Continue to simmer the mixture, stirring occasionally until almost all of the liquid is absorbed and oatmeal is creamy and smooth.
- Remove from heat and let rest for 5 minutes.
- Stir in arugula and carrots.
- Remove egg from shell and cut in half. Add to bowl.
- Top with salt, pepper and Grana Padano.
- Enjoy!

294. Savory Oatmeal With Ham, Poached Eggs, And Hollandaise Sauce

Serving: Serves 2 | Prep: | Cook: | Ready in:

Ingredients

- For the hollandaise sauce:
- 200 grams (about 14 tablespoons) butter
- 3 egg yolks
- 1 tablespoon lemon juice
- 1/2 tablespoon salt
- 1 pinch cayenne pepper
- For the porridge:
- 1 cup oats
- 2 cups water
- 1 pinch salt
- 1 pinch pepper
- 1 tablespoon green pesto
- 1 tablespoon Parmesan or cheddar cheese
- 1/2 avocado
- 4 slices of ham
- 2 eggs
- 1 pinch cayenne pepper

Direction

- Start by making the hollandaise sauce. Melt butter (don't heat it too much), and in the meantime, mix all of the other ingredients in a bowl until the mixture becomes lighter in color. Very slowly add the butter to this mixture and blend until everything is well combined.
- In a cooking pot, place oats and water, season with salt and pepper, and cook for about 10 minutes over a medium heat. When the porridge is thick, it's done. Mix in a tablespoon of pesto.
- Make two poached eggs. Making a poached egg is not the simplest thing in the world, but it's not as difficult as most people think. It helps to add 1 tablespoon of vinegar and 1/2 tablespoon of salt to the boiling water and then, just before adding an egg, stir the water to create a whirlpool motion.
- Divide the porridge between two bowls. Sprinkle some grated cheese over top, and place avocado, ham, and a poached egg on each bowl. Finally, pour over the hollandaise sauce and sprinkle each bowl with cayenne pepper.

295. Savory Oats With Roasted Red Pepper Sauce, Baby Broccoli And Poached Eggs

Serving: Serves 2-4 | Prep: | Cook: | Ready in:

Ingredients

- For the oats
- 2 tablespoons grass fed butter
- 3 tablespoons finely chopped shallot
- 1 cup old fashioned rolled oats
- 2 cups vegetable stock, warmed
- grated cheese*
- kosher salt to taste
- For the red pepper sauce
- 1 very large roasted red pepper
- 1 cup raw, unsalted whole cashews
- 2-4 tablespoons filtered water
- dash white pepper
- kosher salt and hot sauce to taste

Direction

- Soak cashews in water at least four hours.
- Drain cashews and continue to rinse until the water runs clear (this step is really important).
- Drain red pepper and pat dry. Throw it in the blender with the cashews, white pepper and 2T water.
- Blend until smooth and add more water if needed.
- Season with salt and hot sauce (I used maybe 1/2 teaspoon sriracha) to taste. Your red pepper sauce is done! You'll have some leftover, but it's great as a dip for raw vegetables or tossed with shells and cheese.
- To make oats, melt butter in a small pot over medium heat. Add shallot with a big pinch of salt and cook until translucent and slightly soft, about three minutes.
- Add oats to pan and make sure they are evenly coated with butter. Stir them around until they are toasted, about five minutes (you'll know they're done when they have the faint smell of popcorn).
- Pour in vegetable stock and boil until oats are cooked through.
- Grate in cheese to taste, then add more salt if needed. Serve immediately; this does not keep well. For this I really like a hard, nutty cheese like parmesan or pecorino, but a sharp white cheddar would be good, too. I used some Thomasville Tomme from Sweet Grass Dairy since I had it on hand. The amount of cheese you use will depend on the type, so taste as you go.
- Steam baby broccoli.

296. Savory Ris Oat To With Poached Egg

Serving: Serves 1 | Prep: | Cook: | Ready in:

Ingredients

- 1/2 teaspoon coconut oil
- 3 to 4 medium/large shiitake mushroom caps, sliced
- 1 teaspoon rice vinegar
- 1/2 cup almond or coconut milk (carton not can)
- 1/2 cup "quick-cooking" steel-cut oats
- 1 large egg
- 1 splash white vinegar
- 1 pinch salt
- 1 tablespoon tamari
- 1 tablespoon thinly sliced scallions
- 1/2 teaspoon sesame seeds, to garnish

Direction

- In a small saucepan, melt coconut oil on medium heat. Add shiitake mushrooms and toss, cooking for 30 seconds.
- Add rice vinegar to mushrooms and toss again. Let cook another 2 minutes or so, until all oil and vinegar has been absorbed and parts are starting to brown. Remove from heat and set aside.

- As mushrooms are cooking, heat the almond milk with added 1/2 cup of water to boiling in a medium pot.
- Once boiling, lower heat to a simmer and add oats. Stir, then cover. Stir occasionally and keep an eye on it to keep it from boiling over (the milk likes to foam up from the heat), cooking until desired thickness. About 10 to 12 minutes.
- Towards the last few minutes of cooking, poach the egg: In a small pot, bring water to a boil with a splash of white vinegar and a pinch of salt. Crack egg open into a small dish. Once water is boiling, reduce to a simmer and use a spoon to get the water going in a swirling motion. With a gentle flick of the wrist pour egg directly into the middle of the pot. Let cook for 2 to 3 minutes, until the white has firmed up but the yolk still feels runny when poked with your finger.
- When oats are done, place into a bowl. Top with shiitake mushrooms. Pour over tamari and scatter scallions all over. Add the poached egg on top. Sprinkle with sesame seeds to garnish. Enjoy!

297. Savory Oat, Leek, And Pecorino Scones

Serving: Makes 16 | Prep: | Cook: |Ready in:

Ingredients

- 1 1/2 cups butter
- 3 cups flour
- 1 cup rolled oats
- 6 teaspoons baking powder
- 1/2 teaspoon salt
- 2 teaspoons za'atar or finely chopped fresh thyme
- 1 cup milk
- 2 eggs
- 1 cup coarsely grated pecorino
- 1 long or 2 small leeks
- Zest from 1 lemon

Direction

- Preheat oven to 375°F. Line a baking sheet with parchment and butter generously.
- In a small saucepan, melt the butter over low heat. Set aside.
- In a large bowl, mix together the flour, oats, baking powder, salt, and za'atar (fresh thyme).
- In a medium bowl, whisk the eggs and add the milk and melted butter. Combine this with the oat/flour mixture until all the flour is absorbed.
- To clean the leek remove the coarse outer leaves, rinse thoroughly under running water, opening up the inner leaves slightly to make sure no sand remains. Slice the leek very thinly.
- Add the leek, ground pecorino, and lemon zest to the dough. Stir to combine well.
- With a large soup spoon, scoop out balls of dough and place them on the baking sheet.
- Bake for 22 minutes. The outside should be starting to turn golden and feel slightly resistant to the touch but not firm (it will become harder as it cools).
- Serve quickly, while still warm, with delicious butter and orange marmalade… (These scones are really very delicious when warm, so they should be eaten immediately, or toasted or reheated in the oven later.)

298. School Morning Muesli

Serving: Serves 2, well | Prep: | Cook: |Ready in:

Ingredients

- 1 cup rolled oats
- 1 cup milk
- 1/4 cup dried cranberries, roughly chopped
- 1 apple, grated or roughly chopped
- 1 peach or nectarine, roughly chopped
- 1/4 almonds, roughly chopped

- Honey (optional)

Direction

- The night before, mix together the oats and the dried cranberries and then stir in the milk. Cover and refrigerate overnight.
- In the morning, remove the soaked oats from the fridge and toss with the apple and the peach or nectarine. Serve in individual bowls with the chopped almonds on top plus a drizzle of honey, if desired.

299. Silly Good Oatmeal Cookies With Golden Raisins (flourless And Vegan)

Serving: Makes 15 large cookies | Prep: | Cook: | Ready in:

Ingredients

- 1 1/2 cups rolled oats
- 1/2 teaspoon baking soda
- 1/4 teaspoon kosher salt
- 3 tablespoons granulated sugar
- 3 tablespoons pure maple syrup
- 2 tablespoons canola oil
- 1/4 cup golden raisins
- 1 teaspoon pure vanilla extract
- 1-2 tablespoons almond milk

Direction

- Pre-heat oven to 375F and lightly grease a cookie sheet.
- Using a blender or food processor (I used an immersion bender), blend oats, sugar, baking soda and salt together until mostly floury with still some larger bits of oatmeal visible. Pour into a large mixing bowl and set aside.
- In a smaller bowl, mix together oil, maple syrup and vanilla.
- Add the wet ingredients into the oat mixture and combine well. Add in raisins and mix.
- Using a cookie scoop or heaping tablespoon, scoop out onto cookie sheet and flatten slightly into a cookie shape. Make sure they are 2 inches apart, as they will spread a bit.
- Bake for 7-10 minutes, until edges are nicely browned and centers are soft. Let cook on the pan for at least 5 minutes before transferring to a cooling rack.

300. Simple Gifts Granola

Serving: Makes about 6 cups | Prep: | Cook: | Ready in:

Ingredients

- 3 cups rolled oats (I like Bob's Red Mill Extra Thick Rolled Oats.)
- 1 cup roughly chopped walnuts (or a mixture of walnuts and pecans)
- 1/2 cup pumpkin seeds
- 1 tablespoon kosher salt (I use Diamond Crystal. If you use another brand or table salt, use 1/2 tablespoon.
- 1/2 teaspoon cinnamon
- 1/2 teaspoon allspice
- 1/4 teaspoon clove
- 1/2 cup dark brown sugar
- ~2 tablespoons maple syrup
- ~2 tablespoons honey
- ~1 tablespoon molasses
- 1/4 cup olive oil
- 1 cup dried sour cherries

Direction

- Heat oven to 275. In a large bowl, mix together the oats, walnuts, pumpkin seeds, salt and spices.
- Place the sugar, syrup, honey, molasses and olive oil into a small saucepan and warm over low heat until the sugar has just dissolved. Fold liquids into the mixture of oats, stirring well so that the dry ingredients are thoroughly coated.

- Line 2 large rimmed baking sheets with parchment paper or aluminum foil, and spread granola over it. Bake until dry and golden, 45-50 minutes, stirring granola about every 15 or 20 minutes. Remove granola from oven, and let it cool. Mix in the dried sour cherries, and store in an airtight container.

301. Slow Cooker Granola With Spicy Molasses Glazed Nuts

Serving: Makes 2 1/2 quarts | Prep: | Cook: | Ready in:

Ingredients

- Spicy Molasses Candied Nuts
- 2 cups mixed nuts
- 1 cup maple syrup
- 1/2 cup blackstrap molasses
- 1/2 teaspoon cayenne
- 1 teaspoon coarse sea salt
- Slow Cooker Granola
- 2 cups spicy molasses nuts
- 4 cups gluten-free oats
- 1/2 cup diced dates
- 1/2 cup roasted sunflower seeds
- 1/2 cup diced dried apricots
- 1/2 cup whole flax seeds
- 1/2 cup of each, mixed: walnut oil, molasses & maple syrup

Direction

- In a medium non-stick fry pan, heat nuts and maple syrup/molasses mixture to a simmer and add in 2 cups of mixed nuts (I used pecans and peanuts). Stir constantly for about 10 minutes until a thicker syrup begins to coat each nut. When all liquid has been cooked off and a syrupy coating is on the nuts, remove from heat to let cool. Break nut candies into smaller pieces and cool completely.
- For the granola, mix together all the dry ingredients except for the candied nuts in a large mixing bowl. Combine oil, molasses and maple syrup and then pour over your mixed dry ingredients. Stir gently to combine and coat completely. The oats and fruit should be saturated with the wet. Add in additional oil if needed.
- Oil the sides of a large slow cooker (I used a 7 quart) Line the bottom of the cooker with parchment paper and heat on high. Pour the granola into the slow cooker and spread along the bottom. The granola will be about 2-3 inches thick. Place lid on cooker and vent slightly to reduce moisture (I used a chop stick under the lid to create a 1/4-inch gap). Heat on high for 3 hours stirring occasionally. The granola will crispen after cooling. Carefully pour your cooked granola out onto a large sheet pan and spread out to one layer thick. Cool and store in a sealed container. Serve with nut milks or eat plain. Makes a great ice cream topping as well.

302. Smoked Apple Streusel

Serving: Makes 4 | Prep: 0hours30mins | Cook: 1hours0mins | Ready in:

Ingredients

- Apples
- 4 medium sized apples
- 1/2 cup applewood or hickory smoking chips
- 3/4 cup water, warm
- Streusel and Sauce
- 2 tablespoons rolled oats
- 3 tablespoons unsalted butter
- 1/3 cup all purpose flour
- 1/3 cup brown sugar or coconut sugar
- 1/4 teaspoon ground cinnamon
- Pinch ground nutmeg
- Pinch sea salt
- 1/4 cup sugar
- 1 teaspoon lemon juice

Direction

- Set up a charcoal grill for indirect cooking. Move charcoal to one side of the grate and a disposable pan filled with water to the other side. Start charcoal to build a bed of hot coals.
- With a melon baller, scoop out the stem, seeds and core of the apples leaving the bottom intact for the streusel. Place scooped apple pieces in 3/4 cup warm water and set aside for sauce.
- Wrap smoking chips in tin foil and place on top of the charcoal. Place hollowed apples on the grill over the disposable pan side. Cover and smoke for 20 minutes.
- While the apples smoke, make the streusel. Combine oats, 2 tablespoons butter, flour, brown sugar, cinnamon, nutmeg and salt. Mash in butter and mix altogether. Don't worry if it looks dry, the apples will add moistness.
- While the apples smoke, make the streusel. Combine oats, butter, flour, brown sugar, cinnamon, nutmeg and salt. Mash in butter and mix altogether. Don't worry if it looks dry, the apples will add moistness.
- Make the caramel apple sauce. Strain apple pieces from water. Place sugar, lemon juice and half of reserved apple water in saucepan. Cook over medium high heat stirring occasionally to dissolve sugar. Continue cooking to boil off water until it is a light golden color then remove from heat. Let stand for 5 minutes. Carefully add the remaining apple water and 1 tablespoon butter. Stirring to incorporate. Cover with a lid.
- Remove tinfoil from apples and cook for an additional 5-10 minutes until they are golden brown and soft to the touch.
- Once done, remove apples from the oven and transfer to a serving dish. Spoon caramel apple sauce over apples. Serve warm.

303. Soda Bread With Walnuts And Rolled Oats

Serving: Serves 4-6 | Prep: | Cook: | Ready in:

Ingredients

- 1 cup rolled oats
- 1 cup whole wheat flour
- 1 cup unbleached white flour
- 1 cup semolina, or another cup of white or whole wheat flour, or a mix (NB if semolina is used, you may not need all the liquid)
- 1 teaspoon salt
- 1 teaspoon baking soda
- 2 teaspoons baking powder
- 2 cups buttermilk or yogurt thinned with milk or whole milk soured with lemon juice
- 1 handful walnuts broken up a bit with your fingers

Direction

- Preheat oven to 375.
- Mix up all the dry ingredients in a large bowl. You can play around with the grains a bit, but some whole wheat flour is important; I've used all whole wheat, which works, but makes it a bit heavier. Do use real rolled oats in all their chewy integrity, not quick cooking ones. Toss in the nuts when the flour, salt and leavening ingredients are well mixed up. I never actually measure the nuts, just keep breaking them into the bowl till it looks right.
- Add the acidulated dairy product slowly. Start with 1 and 1/2 cups, and stop when you have a workable dough. Especially if semolina is used - or other unusual flours, or if the buttermilk is unusually liquid - you may not need all of it. Stir, then mix with your hands to thoroughly incorporate the liquid. You can dump out on a floured board, but you don't have to. If you knead in the bowl, you can flour your hands and/or sprinkle the dough with a little flour if it looks too gloppy to touch at first. Be careful not to over mix, and knead as little as possible.

- Sprinkle a layer of rolled oats on the bottom of a dry cast iron pan or pie pan or baking sheet. Gather dough into a ball and drop it into the pan, forming it into a slightly flattened round shape. You need to cut into it to help it expand; the standard cut is a cross on top, but two slashes work as well.
- Put in oven and bake 45-50 minutes. Cool on rack, slice when no longer hot. Stays good for a few days.

304. Soft Oat Cookies

Serving: Makes 20 cookies | Prep: | Cook: | Ready in:

Ingredients

- 1 teaspoon vanilla extract
- 100 grams butter
- 85 grams honey (if possible not runny)
- 200 grams oats
- 150 grams whole wheat flour
- 1 pinch salt
- 150 grams sugar
- 2 eggs
- 100 grams milk chocolate
- sea salt

Direction

- Preheat your oven to 200°C. Line a baking sheet with baking paper.
- Melt the butter on a low heat in sauce pan. Whisk in the honey and the vanilla extract. Set aside to cool. Then add the eggs and stir until smooth.
- Put half of the oats in a food processor and whiz them up to oat flour. Mix with remaining oats, whole wheat flour, sugar and salt.
- Use a wooden spoon to mix the dry ingredients into the butter-honey-mixture. The dough should hold together while still being a bit wet.
- Use a teaspoon to heap the dough onto the baking paper. Bake for 10 minutes until the bottoms of the cookies are lightly browned and the tops are still soft to touch. Let them cool down completely before decorating them.
- Gently melt the chocolate over a bain-marie. Top each cookie with a generous teaspoon of chocolate and sprinkle with a bit of sea salt.

305. Spiced Cranberry Orange Maple Breakfast Porridge

Serving: Serves 1-2 | Prep: | Cook: | Ready in:

Ingredients

- 2 cups almond milk
- 1/2 cup whole cranberries
- 1 orange (juice and peel)
- 1/4 teaspoon cinnamon
- Pinch ground clove (a little less than 1/8 teaspoon)
- Pinch ground ginger (a little less than 1/8 teaspoon)
- 1/8 teaspoon freshly grated nutmeg
- 1 cup whole grain old-fashioned rolled oats (gluten free for a gluten-free recipe)
- 2 tablespoons maple syrup
- 1 tablespoon chia seeds (optional)
- Pinch of salt

Direction

- In a sauce pan, place the almond milk, cranberries, and peel of 1/2 an orange and the juice of a whole orange, and bring to a boil.
- Add the oats, chia seeds, maple syrup, and salt and reduce the heat to low. Cook the oats, stirring occasionally, for about 10-15 minutes until most of the liquid is absorbed and the oats are cooked through (time will depend on the consistency you like and the cooking instructions). Add more milk or water as needed.
- Remove the orange peel and pour the oats into a bowl and top with anything you like. I like mine with sliced almonds. Enjoy!

306. Spicy Shorties

Serving: Serves about 2 dozen | Prep: | Cook: | Ready in:

Ingredients

- 3/4 cup rolled oats
- 1/2 pound salted butter (2 sticks)
- 1 cup dark brown sugar, packed (like Muscovado)
- 1/4 teaspoon salt
- 1 teaspoon freshly ground cardamom
- 1/2 teaspoon freshly ground black pepper
- 1 1/2 cups whole wheat pastry flour
- 1 teaspoon fresh ginger, finely grated
- 1 cup candied ginger, chopped fine

Direction

- Preheat the oven to 350 degrees.
- Process the oats briefly in a food processor, just to break them up slightly.
- Beat the butter and sugar until light and fluffy, then add the salt, spices and oats. Work in all the flour well, and mix in the fresh and candied ginger.
- Press the dough into a 9x12 pan and score the surface in squares as you would with shortbread. (You can make any shape you like but these are rich, so smaller pieces are best.) Bake until surface is lightly browned, 30-35 minutes. Baking them longer will result in a drier, crisper cookie (which is also nice).
- Remove and cut through along the score lines, then set aside to cool. (These freeze well.)

307. Steel Cut Oats Mash Up

Serving: Serves 4 | Prep: | Cook: | Ready in:

Ingredients

- 1 cup steel cut oats
- 1 cup milk/soy milk
- 2 cups water
- 1 handful hemp seeds
- 1 handful wheat germ
- 1 handful flax seeds
- 1-2 tablespoons jam/agave
- 1-2 tablespoons almond butter/cashew butter or both
- 1 handful unsweetened coconut
- 1 handful dried fruit/fresh fruit of your choice!
- 1 handful nuts

Direction

- Add milk and water to steel cut oats in pot. Let cook until most oats absorb the liquid (about 7-10 min). Add the rest of the ingredients and mix well. Be as generous as you want with the add-ins. Remember all the addition are options. This is one loaded batch of steel cut oats! Enjoy

308. Steel Cut Oats With Baked Apple

Serving: Serves 2 | Prep: | Cook: | Ready in:

Ingredients

- 1 Leftover Baked Apple (Link to recipe in intro)
- 2 cups Whole Milk
- 1 cup Water
- 1 pinch Salt
- 1/2 cup Steel Cut Oats
- 2 tablespoons Chia Seeds (Optional)

Direction

- Bring milk, water, and salt to a boil.
- Stir in steel cut oats and bring the mixture to a simmer. Continue simmering over low-

medium heat for 20-30 minutes or until you reach your desired consistency.
- Take your baked apple and cut it into bits. I did this quite easily and without a mess by leaving it in the glass jar I had used to contain it in the fridge, and simply slicing it up from the top using kitchen shears.
- Once the oats are finished, stir in the bits of baked apple, and (optional) stir in chia seeds. You do NOT need the chia seeds, however, I try to throw these into the mix when I can because they are high in Omega 6s, Omega 3s, and Fiber. They also make your hair and skin glow--bonus! This recipe can be made ahead and simply reheated over medium for 5-7 minutes the day after. Enjoy!

309. Strawberry Goat Cheese Oat Pie With Whipped Goat Cheese

Serving: Serves 8 | Prep: | Cook: |Ready in:

Ingredients

- Strawberry Goat Cheese Oat Pie
- 2 cups rolled oats, certified gluten-free
- 3 tablespoons olive oil
- 2 tablespoons honey
- 2 tablespoons dark brown sugar
- 1/4 cup yogurt
- 1/4 cup heavy cream
- 3 ounces goat cheese
- 3 eggs
- 1/2 teaspoon vanilla extract
- 1 1/4 teaspoons baking powder
- 1/4 teaspoon baking soda
- 1/4 teaspoon kosher salt
- 1 handful fresh strawberries
- Whipped Goat Cheese
- 4 ounces heavy cream
- 2 ounces goat cheese
- 1 dash honey

Direction

- Strawberry Goat Cheese Oat Pie
- Preheat oven to 375° F. While oven is preheating, toast your oats (for a nuttier flavor). Spread oats out on large, parchment-lined pan. Let toast for 15 minutes, stirring every 5 minutes.
- In the bowl of your food processor or a medium bowl, combine olive oil, honey, dark brown sugar, yogurt, heavy cream, goat cheese, eggs and vanilla. Process or whisk thoroughly, until creamy.
- In a large bowl, whisk together oats, baking powder, baking soda and salt.
- Stir the wet ingredients into the dry ingredients and mix well.
- Pour into a greased 9" pie pan. [The pan should be at least 2" deep or there will be overflow.]
- Place sliced strawberries in three concentric circles on the oat mixture.
- Bake for 20 minutes or until a toothpick tester comes out clean.
- Let fully cool [at least 4 hours] before slicing. Top with whipped goat cheese and fresh strawberries.
- Whipped Goat Cheese
- Combine heavy cream and goat cheese in a medium bowl and whip with an electric mixer [or large whisk] until airy and doubled in size.
- Add the dash of honey [a small drizzle to cut the goaty tang] and mix thoroughly. Chill until serving.

310. Strawberry Oatmeal Breakfast Shake

Serving: Serves 1 | Prep: | Cook: |Ready in:

Ingredients

- 1 cup strawberries
- 1/2 cup rolled oats
- 1 tablespoon ground flax

- 1 tablespoon honey
- 1/2 teaspoon lemon juice
- 1/4 teaspoon lemon zest
- 1/4 teaspoon ground cinnamon
- 1 teaspoon unsweetened coconut flakes

Direction

- Add everything to your blender and blend until smooth
- Alternately, add the oats to the blender first and grind them fine. Then add the rest of the ingredients and blend until smooth

311. Strawberry Oatmeal Cookie Cobbler

Serving: Serves 15-20 | Prep: | Cook: | Ready in:

Ingredients

- Oatmeal Cookie Crust
- 1 cup unsalted butter, cubed (plus more for the pan)
- 1 cup brown sugar
- 1 cup granulated sugar
- 2 eggs
- 1 teaspoon vanilla extract
- 2 cups all-purpose flour
- 1 1/2 teaspoons cinnamon
- 1/2 teaspoon baking powder
- 1/2 teaspoon kosher salt
- 3 cups old fashioned oats (not quick cooking)
- Strawberry, Pear and Apple Filling
- 2 cups strawberries, hulled and halved
- 2 pears, cored and chopped
- 1 green apple, cored and chopped
- 1 cup brown sugar
- 1 tablespoon tablespoon cornstarch
- 1 teaspoon vanilla extract

Direction

- Combine the filling ingredients in a large bowl and set aside.
- Preheat your oven to 350 degrees F. Beat together your butter and sugars for at least 5 minutes, until light and fluffy. Add in the eggs, one at a time, until fully combined, scraping down the bowl as needed. Beat in the vanilla.
- Whisk together your flour, cinnamon, baking powder and salt. Add to the bowl with the sugar and butter and beat until just moistened. Add in the oats and mix to combine, scraping down the bowl as needed.
- Butter a 9x13-inch pan well. Press a little less than half of the dough into the bottom of the pan, then pour the fruit mixture over the top. Drop dollops of the remaining dough on top of the fruit (it doesn't have to be perfect), then sprinkle with decorative sugar (if you like - this is optional). Bake for 60 minutes or so, until golden and bubbling. Allow to cool a bit before serving warm, or cool completely, cover with foil and refrigerate for up to 2 days.

312. Strawberry Rhubarb Crisp

Serving: Serves 6-8 | Prep: | Cook: | Ready in:

Ingredients

- Crisp Topping
- 1 cup all-purpose flour
- 3/4 cup rolled oats
- 1/2 teaspoon kosher salt
- 3/4 cup dark brown sugar, packed
- 7 tablespoons unsalted butter, chilled and cut into pea-sized pieces
- Strawberry Rhubarb Filling
- 19 ounces rhubarb, peeled and cut into 1-inch pieces
- 18 ounces fresh strawberries, stemmed and quartered
- 1 zest of one naval orange
- 1/2 cup granulated sugar
- 1 tablespoon tapicoa starch

Direction

- Crisp Topping
- Move a rack to the middle of the oven and preheat oven to 375 degrees Fahrenheit.
- Place the flour, rolled oats, salt and brown sugar in the bowl of a food processor and pulse to combine.
- Add the butter and pulse until the mixture is coarse and crumbly looking.
- Set aside or place in the freeze in an airtight container (the topping can go directly from the freezer to the oven once you are ready to bake your crisp; there is no need to defrost it).
- Strawberry Rhubarb Filling
- In a large mixing bowl, carefully toss the rhubarb, sliced strawberries, granulated sugar, and orange zest in a large mixing bowl and let stand for 5 to 10 minutes. Transfer the filling to an 8x8 glass baking dish.
- Sprinkle the topping evenly over the fruit and bake for 30-40 minutes, or until the topping is just beginning to turn golden brown and the fruit is bubbling.
- Let the crisp cool for 20-25 minutes before serving. Serve warm with vanilla ice cream.

313. Strawberry Rhubarb Crumble Parfait

Serving: Serves 8 | Prep: | Cook: | Ready in:

Ingredients

- Crumble
- 2/3 cup old-fashioned oats
- 1/2 cup all-purpose flour
- 1/4 teaspoon salt
- 1/3 cup packed light brown sugar
- 1/4 cup butter, melted
- Ice Cream
- 1 1/4 cups packed light brown sugar, divided
- 1/4 cup fruity red wine
- 1 1/2 cups finely diced rhubarb
- 2 cups diced fresh strawberries
- 3 cups half & half
- 2 large eggs
- 1 teaspoon vanilla

Direction

- Preheat oven to 350° F.
- In a medium bowl, combine oats, flour, salt and cup brown sugar. Add melted butter and stir until mixture is crumbly. Pour onto a large baking sheet and spread out with your hands. Bake at 350° F for 10 minutes. Stir, and return to the oven for another 5 minutes, or until golden brown. Cool and put into an airtight container.
- In a medium saucepan, add ½ cup brown sugar, wine, rhubarb and strawberries. Bring to a boil and cook until rhubarb is tender and mixture is syrupy, about 8-10 minutes. Remove from heat and set aside to cool. Cover and refrigerate until chilled.
- Prepare an ice bath in a large bowl.
- Heat the half & half in a large saucepan over medium heat until tiny bubbles start to form around the edge.
- In the meantime, beat the eggs and ¾ cup brown sugar in a large bowl with an electric mixer for 3 minutes. Gradually add small amounts of the half & half until about a third of it has been added. Then pour in the rest and mix thoroughly.
- Put the mixture back into the saucepan and cook over medium heat, stirring constantly with a wooden spoon, until it coats the back of the spoon (about 175°).
- Remove from heat and pour the mixture into a bowl with a pouring spout. Add vanilla and place the bowl in the ice bath to chill. Cover and refrigerate until very cold (overnight if possible).
- When the ice cream base has chilled, churn in an ice cream maker, according to manufacturer's instructions. Spoon ½ of the ice cream into a freezer-safe container, followed by ½ the rhubarb/strawberry sauce. Repeat with another layer of ice cream and sauce. Place sealed container in the freezer to bloom for at least 3 hours.

- Just before serving, remove from freezer and allow to rest 5-10 minutes. Scoop ice cream into a parfait glass, layering in crumbles after every scoop. Grab a long spoon and prepare to go to rhubarb heaven!

314. Strawberry And Almond Crumble (gluten Free)

Serving: Serves 4 - 5 | Prep: | Cook: | Ready in:

Ingredients

- For the fruit prep:
- 400 grams strawberries, hulled and halved
- 2 tablespoons granulated sugar
- 1/2 teaspoon ground cinnamon
- 1 teaspoon corn flour
- 1 teaspoon lime juice
- Vanilla ice cream/cream, to serve
- For the crumble topping:
- 250 grams ground almonds
- 80 grams un-salted butter (at room temperature), cubed
- 2 tablespoons oats
- 3 tablespoons demerara sugar
- 1/4 teaspoon salt
- 2 tablespoons flaked almonds (optional)

Direction

- Preheat oven to 180 C / 360 F.
- Toss together halved strawberries, granulated sugar, cinnamon, lime juice and corn flour in a bowl and tip into an oven-proof dish.
- In another bowl, combine ground almonds, flaked almonds, demerara sugar, oats, salt, and butter. Using your fingertips, rub the butter into the mixture until it starts to resemble coarse breadcrumbs (I like to have a combination of small clumps and fine bits for texture).
- Sprinkle the crumble topping evenly over the strawberries and bake for 30 - 40 minutes, or until slightly golden on top and the fruit juices are bubbling to the surface. Let the crumble cool for at least 10 minutes before serving.

315. Summer Berry & Fig Muffins

Serving: Makes 1 dozen | Prep: | Cook: | Ready in:

Ingredients

- 1 1/4 cups almond milk
- 2 teaspoons apple cider vinegar
- 1 cup whole wheat flour
- 1/2 cup oat flour
- 1 cup rolled oats
- 1 teaspoon baking powder
- 3/4 cup turbinado sugar
- 1 cup mixed summer berries
- 1/2 cup figs
- 1/2 cup coconut oil
- 1 flax egg
- 2 lemons, juiced

Direction

- Preheat the oven to 350° F. Line a dozen muffin pan with muffin tins or apply a thin coat of oil to prevent muffins from sticking to the side.
- In a medium-sized mixing bowl, whisk together almond milk and apple cider vinegar. Let rest for 5 minutes.
- While the milk is thickening, mix flour, oats, baking powder and sugar together in a food processor. Transfer to a large mixing bowl and set aside.
- Whisk oil, flax egg, and lemon juice together with almond milk and apple cider vinegar.
- Make a well in your flour mixture and pour in wet ingredients. Thoroughly incorporate the wet and dry ingredients before gently mixing in your mixed berries and figs.
- Fill each muffin tin 2/3 of the way full, topping with slices of figs or berries, and bake for 25-30 minutes, or until golden.

316. Sundried Tomato And Olive Bread

Serving: Makes 6-10 slices | Prep: | Cook: |Ready in:

Ingredients

- 2 cups almond pulp (wet)
- 1/3 cup Irish Moss Paste
- 2 tablespoons flax meal
- 1/4 cup oat flour sifted
- 1 tablespoon lemon juice
- 1/2 cloves of garlic
- 2 teaspoons garlic powder
- 3 dates or date syrup
- 1 teaspoon sea salt
- 1 tablespoon heaped of tomato powder
- 1/4 cup finely chopped sundried tomatoes (soaked)
- 1/4 cup black or green olives
- 1 tablespoon oregano

Direction

- Blend the almond pulp, oat flour, tomato powder, garlic and salt. Then add the Irish Moss paste, and then the rest of the ingredients. Shape into a bread load and slice thinly. Dehydrate for 5 to 8 hours at 40 degrees. You can also dehydrate for longer if you wish a biscotti type texture.

317. Susan's Health Bomb Muffins

Serving: Makes 18 - 24 muffins | Prep: | Cook: |Ready in:

Ingredients

- 1 1/2 cups whole wheat flour
- 3/4 cup flaxseed meal
- 3/4 cup oat bran
- 1/4 cup brown sugar
- 2 teaspoons baking soda
- 2 teaspoons baking powder
- 1/2 teaspoon salt
- 2 teaspoons cinnamon
- 1 1/2 cups finely grated carrots
- 1 cup unsweetened applesauce
- 3/4 cup golden raisins
- 1 cup chopped pecans (or walnuts)
- 1 cup milk
- 2 beaten eggs
- 1 teaspoon real vanilla extract

Direction

- Preheat oven to 350 degrees. Mix the flour, flaxseed meal, oat bran, brown sugar, baking soda, baking powder, salt, and cinnamon in a large bowl. Stir in the carrots, applesauce, raisins, and nuts.
- Combine the milk, beaten eggs, and vanilla in another smaller bowl. Pour the liquid ingredients into the dry ingredients. Stir until all ingredients are moistened. Do not over mix.
- Fill the muffin tins a little more than 3/4 full. Let the batter rest a few minutes before putting in oven. Bake at 350 degrees for 25 minutes. I ended up with 18 muffins. I may have overfilled a few. Enjoy!

318. Sweet Potato Banana Pancake & Strawberry Glaze

Serving: Serves 3-4 | Prep: 0hours0mins | Cook: 0hours0mins |Ready in:

Ingredients

- Strawberry Glaze
- 2 cups Strawberries (sliced)
- 1 tablespoon Coconut Ool
- 1/2 tablespoon Maple Syrup
- 1/8 teaspoon Salt

- Sweet Potato Banana Pancake
- 1/2 Baked Sweet Potato
- 1 Ripe Banana (mashed)
- 3 Large Eggs
- 1/2 cup Gluten Free Oat Flour
- 1/2 teaspoon Baking Soda
- 1/8 teaspoon Cinnamon Powder
- 1 tablespoon Maple Syrup
- 1 tablespoon Coconut Oil (for cooking)
- 2-3 tablespoons Coconut Milk (if needed)

Direction

- Place all the ingredients in an oven safe dish & bake at 375 for about 10-12 minutes. It can bake while you prep & cook the pancakes. Remove from oven & let cool for a few minutes.
- Mash bananas & sweet potato in a mixing bowl with the back of a fork. Add eggs, maple syrup, & coconut milk to the mixture & whisk to incorporate. Combine oat flour, cinnamon & baking powder to the bowl & whisk again to incorporate. Melt 1/2 tbsp coconut oil. On a large nonstick pan or pancake griddle, drop 1/4 cup batter & cook until golden brown on both sides. Serve with a drizzle of the strawberry glaze & plain yogurt as a topping.

319. Sweet And Savory Whole Oats And Sweet Brown Rice Porridge

Serving: Serves 4 to 6 | Prep: | Cook: | Ready in:

Ingredients

- 2/3 cup whole oat groats
- 2 bay leaves
- 1 cinnamon stick, split in 2
- 1 two-inch piece of vanilla bean
- Small pinch of salt
- ½ cup sweet brown rice
- ¼ - ½ cup homemade almond or cashew milk, or for a non-vegan porridge, half-and-half, or whole cream to taste (See note below.)
- Yellow raisins (optional)
- Jaggery or brown sugar, to taste
- Toasted cashews, or (for a non-vegan dish) Cashew Infused Chhena, or both (recipe for the latter is on food52)

Direction

- Simmer the oat groats uncovered in 4 cups of water with the bay leaves, cinnamon stick, vanilla bean and salt for about an hour, or until nearly all the water is absorbed, i.e., until there is a very thin layer of water covering the groats.
- Add the rice and another cup of water. Bring to a boil, then turn down the heat to very low and cover. Cook for 45 minutes, then turn off the heat and let the porridge sit for about fifteen minutes.
- Remove the bay leaves, cinnamon stick and vanilla bean. For a stronger vanilla flavor, scrape out the vanilla seeds. (I find that they overwhelm the other flavors in this, so I don't do that.)
- Stir in the nut milk or half-and-half and the raisins and heat through.
- Serve with jaggery or brown sugar, to taste, and cashew-infused chhena, if using. Garnish with toasted cashews or other nuts, or pine nuts.
- Enjoy!! ;o)
- NB: This is also delicious with my Sweet Almond Chhena.
- For vegans, you can leave out the dairy and stir in some cashew or almond butter, or use a rich homemade nut milk.

320. Thai Inspired Turkey Burgers

Serving: Makes 10 burgers | Prep: | Cook: | Ready in:

Ingredients

- 1/3 cup rolled oats, ground
- 1 tablespoon peanut butter
- 2 egg whites
- 1 1/3 pounds ground turkey
- 1 pound ground turkey breast
- 1 medium zucchini, shredded
- 1 cup grated carrots
- 1/2 teaspoon grated fresh ginger
- 1 lime, zest and juice
- 4 tablespoons cilantro
- 1 tablespoon fish sauce
- 1 1/2 teaspoons Srirarcha
- 2 teaspoons soy sauce
- 2 teaspoons toasted sesame oil
- 1/2 teaspoon salt

Direction

- Place oats in a food processor and pulse a few times, you don't want to make it into flour, you want a course crumb. Then mix oats, peanut butter and egg whites in small bowl, set aside
- Cut zucchini lengthwise and scoop out seeds/center; discard seeds and grate zucchini, this should result in about 1 1/2 cups
- Grate carrots, or if bought already grated, just run your knife through them for a course chop
- Zest lime, you can zest right into the carrots or zucchini, cut lime in half
- In small bowl, juice 1/2 the lime (you should get about 1Tbs of juice), whisk in fish sauce, Sriracha, soy sauce, ginger, sesame oil and salt; set aside
- Place both lbs of turkey in a large mixing bowl, add zucchini, carrots and the contents of the two small bowls that you've set aside (oatmeal/peanut butter mixture & lime/Sriracha mixture), and also add the fresh cilantro
- Using your hands, mix everything together well
- Form into patties (I get 10). I then place on a sheet of waxed paper, evenly spaced and place a second piece of waxed paper over the burgers. Cut in between each burger and then place burgers into a large freezer bag. Freeze.
- To cook: If frozen, thaw first. Spray burger with olive oil or cooking spray (they can stick) and grill over medium heat for about 4 minutes a side...they can be fragile so move and flip carefully. If they stick too much to your BBQ, they cook easily stovetop in a skillet.
- Footnotes: For the THAI-PEANUT MAYO: Use your favorite mayonnaise (regular, lite, fat-free or mayonnaise substitute such as Greek yogurt) and mix with House of Tsang- Bangkok Padang Peanut Sauce. The ratio is up to you, I use about 2 parts mayo to 1 part peanut sauce. I sometimes add chopped cilantro and/or Sriracha to kick it up. This mayo is great on the burgers, but also on pretzels, chips, tomatoes, sandwiches, or anything you can get your hands on....I think it could even be a dip served at a party.
- Footnote 2: An alternative great topping is an Asian Slaw: Sauté some broccoli-slaw with a splash each of rice wine vinegar, soy sauce and then stir in 2 or so tablespoons of the House of Tsang- Bangkok Padang Peanut Sauce. Serve right on top of burger.

321. The Best Breakfast Pancakes To Touch My Lips

Serving: Makes 8-10 pancakes | Prep: 0hours0mins | Cook: 0hours0mins | Ready in:

Ingredients

- 1 tablespoon ground flax seeds
- 1 cup full-fat, unsweetened coconut milk
- 1/3 cup oat flakes (quinoa flakes are a great gluten-free option)
- 1/3 cup millet flour
- 1/3 cup buckwheat flour
- pinch sea salt
- 1 egg

- 1.5 tablespoons maple syrup
- 1 tablespoon coconut oil warmed to liquid, (plus more for the pan)
- 1 medium zucchini, finely shredded
- 1 cup fresh/frozen blueberries

Direction

- In a bowl, mix coconut milk and flax seeds well. Set aside
- In a large bowl, combine flours, oats, salt, and chocolate.
- In a medium bowl, beat the egg with maple syrup until creamy and doubled in volume. Pour the milk and chia mixture into the large bowl with flours. Mix well.
- On medium heat, warm a skillet with a small amount of coconut oil. Ladle 1/4 cup of the batter into the pan to form 4 inch pancakes.
- Scatter blueberries on top of each pancake and gently press into the batter with a spatula. Cook until bubbles form (about 1 minute). Flip the pancakes and cook for another minute, or until golden.
- Serve with maple syrup, berries, yogurt, or coconut whip cream

322. The Easiest, Creamiest (One Ingredient!) Homemade Oat Milk

Serving: Makes about 4 1/2 cups oat milk | Prep: 0hours20mins | Cook: 0hours0mins | Ready in:

Ingredients

- For Plain Oat Milk (Unsweetened)
- 1 1/2 cups old fashioned rolled oats
- 4 cups water (room temperature), plus more if needed to thin
- For Chocolate and Vanilla Varieties (Optional)
- 3 tablespoons plus 1 teaspoon maple syrup, divided into 2 tablespoons and 1 tablespoon plus one teaspoon
- 1 teaspoon vanilla extract
- 1 small pinch of salt plus 1 large pinch of salt (plus more to taste)
- 1 tablespoon plus 2 teaspoons Dutch-processed cocoa powder

Direction

- In the bowl of a food processor fitted with its blade, soak oats in water for 15 minutes.
- Then, blend for about 45 seconds, until it looks homogenous and opaque. (There will still be very small shards of oat floating in the liquid.) Pour through a fine mesh sieve into a container (ideally one that has a pour spout), using a spatula to push as much liquid through as you can. You should get about 4 1/2 cups of liquid, the consistency of cream – this is your unsweetened oat milk. If you would like to thin it, just stir in additional water to your desired consistency.
- From here, the possibilities are endless – you could make a sweetened variety by adding maple syrup, agave, honey, or any soluble sweetener you like (to taste), plus a pinch of salt. You could add some cinnamon. Or, you could divide the batch in two, and make vanilla and chocolate flavors to drink with an amusingly patterned straw, as follows:
- Into one half-batch, whisk 1 tablespoon plus 1 teaspoon of maple syrup, 1 teaspoon of vanilla extract, and 1 small pinch of salt. (This is the vanilla flavor.)
- In a separate container, make chocolate syrup: Whisk together 2 tablespoons of maple syrup, 1 tablespoon plus 2 teaspoons of cocoa powder, and a large pinch of salt, until the cocoa powder has dissolved. Add the remaining half-batch of oat milk to the chocolate syrup and whisk to combine. (This is the chocolate flavor.)
- Note: Oat milk should be stored covered in the refrigerator. It keeps up to a few days. The milk will separate as it sits; just stir from the bottom to recombine.

323. The Healthiest Pumpkin Pie Ever

Serving: Serves 8 | Prep: | Cook: | Ready in:

Ingredients

- For the crust:
- 2 handfuls mixed nuts (almonds, walnuts, hazelnuts)
- 2 handfuls dates
- 3 tablespoons oats (substitute with rice flour for gluten-free version)
- 1 cm thick piece of fresh ginger
- 1 pinch salt
- 1 splash olive oil
- For the filling:
- 1/2 medium pie pumpkin
- 1 tablespoon brown sugar
- 1 teaspoon ground cloves
- 3 teaspoons cinnamon
- 1 teaspoon cardamom
- 1 teaspoon nutmeg
- 1 teaspoon ground ginger
- 1/2 teaspoon ground hot pepper
- 1 egg
- 1 tablespoon rice flour

Direction

- Preheat the oven to 200 C. Cut a medium pie pumpkin in half, you will need just a half of it. Take one half and cut it in 4 pieces. Place the pumpkin pieces in the oven and roast for 30-40 minutes until the pulp softens.
- While the pumpkin is in the oven let's make the pie crust. We will need a blender or a food processor. Take 2 handfuls of mixed nuts. We used almonds, walnuts and hazelnuts, you can choose any nuts you love. Take 2 handfuls of dates and 3 tablespoons oats. Place all the ingredients in the food processor, add your ginger, a pinch of salt and drizzle with a little bit of olive oil. Blend the ingredients until they turn into a crumbly crust. You can test it by rolling a small amount of it in your hands: if the crust sticks together then it's perfectly ready. Line a tart mould with parchment paper, press the crumbs into the mould and place in the fridge while preparing the pie filling.
- For the filling put the pumpkin out of the oven and turn the heat down to 180 C, we will need it for baking the pie. Scrape the pumpkin pulp off the peel, let it cool for a while, add to the food processor together with an egg, sugar, rice flour and spices. Puree the ingredients and pour them into the cooled pie crust.
- Put the pie in the oven and cook it for 25-30 minutes until the filling thickens. Let cool and serve with a spoon of crème fraiche on top, it greatly balances the sweetness of the pie.
- Bon Appétit!

324. The Pantry Cookie

Serving: Makes about 20 cookies | Prep: | Cook: | Ready in:

Ingredients

- 8 tablespoons (1 stick) butter
- 2/3 cup white or whole wheat flour
- 2/3 cup rolled oats
- 1/2 teaspoon kosher salt
- 1/2 teaspoon baking soda
- 1 egg
- 1/3 cup brown sugar
- 1/4 cup granulated sugar
- 1/2 teaspoon vanilla extract
- 1/2 cup toasted pecans, chopped (or other toasted nuts or seeds)
- 1/2 cup dried cranberries (or other dried fruit, chopped if large)
- 1/2 cup chocolate chips (or other chips, or chopped chocolate)

Direction

- Heat the oven to 350° F. Lightly butter a baking sheet or line it with parchment.

- Melt the butter on the stove or in the microwave. Set it aside briefly to cool. In a bowl, mix together the flour, oats, salt, and baking soda. Set it aside too.
- Using a standing mixer with a whisk attachment, or a large mixing bowl and a whisk, thoroughly beat the egg with the sugars and the vanilla extract, ideally until it thickens slightly and begins to form a ribbon. Add the melted butter and stir. Then add the flour mixture and stir until it is just combined. Gently mix in the pecans, dried cranberries, and chocolate. (If you want to stop at this point, you can refrigerate the dough for a week or freeze for longer.)
- On the prepared baking sheet, place small mounds of dough, about two tablespoons worth (just a bit larger than a ping-pong ball). Flatten very slightly. Bake for about 12 minutes, or until the cookies are golden, rotating the baking sheet midway. Let the cookies sit for a minute and then remove them from the baking sheet and let cool. If they survive the day, pack away in an airtight container.

325. The Toast With The Most Toasted Oat Sourdough

Serving: Makes 10 loaves | Prep: | Cook: | Ready in:

Ingredients

- Preferment
- 600 grams Bread flour
- 600 grams Harvest Grains Blend (King Arthur Flour)
- 1,200 grams Water
- 84 grams Sourdough starter
- Final Dough
- 1,400 grams Bread flour
- 400 grams Light buckwheat flour (toasted and cooled)
- 1,000 grams Semolina flour
- 2,060 grams Water
- 12 grams Yeast (instant active)
- 84 grams Salt
- 480 grams Oats (toasted and cooled)
- 2,460 grams Preferment

Direction

- Preferment
- Mix all ingredients together in a large bowl until smooth. The mixture will be very wet; this is normal.
- Cover the mixture tightly with plastic wrap.
- Let the mixture ferment overnight. If you notice that the mixture is too active (growing very large or producing too much gas), you can move the mixture to the refrigerator to finish fermenting. Make sure to remove it from the refrigerator and bring it up to room temperature before using to make the bread dough.
- Final Dough
- Gather and measure all of your ingredients.
- The Desired Dough Temperature for this recipe is 75 F. It is best to use the DDT formula ((DDT x 4) minus flour temp, room temp, preferment temp, and friction factor = proper water temp.) with the factors of the kitchen currently being used to find your desired water temperature. Our machine's friction factor was 30, and if the mixing bowl was cold or the preferment was not up to room temperature, we also factored this in and added 4 to 6 degrees to the final desired water temperature.
- Toast the light buckwheat flour and oats at 425 F, until a medium golden brown. Remove from the oven and let cool before using.
- Add all of the ingredients to the bowl of a spiral mixer (starting with liquid ingredients and ending with dry ingredients).
- Mix on 1st speed for 4 - 5 minutes.
- Mix on 2nd speed for 2 minutes 30 seconds.
- Using a dough scraper, remove the dough from the mixer and place it into a covered bin that has been sprayed lightly with pan spray and ferment the dough for 1 1/2 hours. In this

fermentation time, fold the dough a total of two times, one fold 30 minutes after finishing the dough, the second fold 30 minutes after the first fold. Make sure to flour your bench/table heavily, along with your hands, when folding the dough, as it will be wet and shaggy.
- Divide the dough into 779 g. pieces and very loosely pre-shape for boules (though if you prefer a different shape for your loaves, this will not affect the bread).
- Rest the dough, loosely covered with plastic, for 20 minutes.
- Shape your dough pieces into boules, place them onto a lightly floured baker's couche (as many as needed to fit all of your loaves) on a flat surface and cover loosely with plastic or place onto a covered baking rack. Proof loaves in a warm section of your kitchen for 1 to 1 1/2 hours.
- Score and/or stencil your loaves as desired.
- Load the loaves into a deck oven and bake with steam at 460 F for 40 to 45 minutes, venting the oven after 20 minutes, until the crust has developed a deep brown color.
- Remove the loaves from the oven, let cool, and enjoy!

326. The Treasure Loaded Peanut Butter Cookie

Serving: Makes 12 | Prep: | Cook: | Ready in:

Ingredients

- ½ teaspoons baking soda
- 1 teaspoon ground cinnamon
- 1 teaspoon salt
- 1 cup gluten free rolled oats
- 1 cup organic peanut butter, chunky or smooth; whatever your fancy
- ½ cups white sugar
- ½ cups packed dark brown sugar
- 2 whole eggs (I am at altitude. You may find you only need to use 1.)
- 1 teaspoon real vanilla extract
- ½ cups chocolate chips
- ½ cups dried cherries
- ½ cups roasted and salted peanuts

Direction

- Day One:
- In bowl, combine baking soda, salt, cinnamon, and oats. Set aside.
- In another bowl, combine peanut butter and sugars and whip with electric beaters until creamy.
- Add one egg at a time and beat in thoroughly. Then add vanilla.
- Stir in oatmeal mix, chocolate chips, cherries, and peanuts until combined.
- Cover and refrigerate for at least 12 hours to allow flavors to develop.
- Day 2:
- Set oven to 350 degrees F.
- Set up sheet pan with parchment or silpat mat.
- Wet hands with cool water.
- Using a spoon or an ice cream scoop, form dough in to a ball. Use wet hands to shape dough into disk shape and place disk on to parchment.
- Bake for 8 to 15 minutes depending on your oven's efficiency. You are looking for GBD (golden brown deliciousness).
- I only make enough cookies for my fika, one or two, and save rest of dough in fridge for another day. Use dough up within five days.

327. Throwback Oatmeal Muffins

Serving: Makes 6-12 muffins | Prep: | Cook: | Ready in:

Ingredients

- 1 cup nondairy milk such as almond milk
- 1 teaspoon apple cider vinegar
- 1 tablespoon ground flax seed
- 3 tablespoons water

- 1/3 cup unsweetened applesauce
- 1 cup rolled oats (not quick or instant)
- 1 cup whole wheat pastry flour
- 1 teaspoon baking powder
- 1/2 teaspoon baking soda
- 1/2 cup chopped walnuts
- 1/2 cup raisins

Direction

- Preheat the oven to 400°F. Grease or line a standard 12-cup muffin tin with paper liners, or use a 6-cup tin for big breakfast muffins!
- In a measuring cup, combine the nondairy milk and vinegar. Set aside to "curdle." (This will act like buttermilk in the batter.)
- In a medium mixing bowl, whisk the flaxseed and water together until thickened. Add the nondairy milk mixture, the maple syrup and the applesauce and stir to combine.
- Add the oats, flour, baking powder and baking soda and mix until just combined. The batter will be lumpy.
- Fold in the nuts and raisins (or, if you prefer, omit the raisins and add 1/2 cup vegan chocolate chips). Divide batter among muffin cups until each is about 2/3 full. Bake for 20 minutes, or until a toothpick inserted in the center comes out clean.

328. Toasted Oat & Pecan Oatmeal

Serving: Serves 2 | Prep: | Cook: | Ready in:

Ingredients

- 1/2 cup old-fashioned oats
- 1/4 cup chopped pecans
- 1 1/2 cups unsweetened vanilla almond milk
- 1 tablespoon agave nectar
- 1 teaspoon cinnamon
- 1 teaspoon vanilla extract
- dash   sea salt
- dash   nutmeg
- 1 cup fresh berries (optional)

Direction

- In a medium-sized pot on low-medium heat, toast oats and pecans for about five minutes, shaking the pot a couple of times to spread the mixture.
- After they oats and pecans are nice and toasty, stir in remaining ingredients and increase heat to medium.
- Cook uncovered until mixture reaches a boil, stirring occasionally. After the milk is boiling, let cook for two minutes, then remove from heat.
- Let cool for a couple of minutes and serve with toppings of your choice, or enjoy plain.

329. Toasted Oatmeal With Fruit & Spice

Serving: Makes 4 - 6 portions | Prep: | Cook: | Ready in:

Ingredients

- 2 cups quick-cook/instant oats
- 1 whole apple (pears, stone fruit), chopped
- 2 – 3 tablespoons whole nuts (almonds, pecans, walnuts, etc), roughly chopped
- 2 tablespoons dried fruit (cranberries, blueberries, raisins, currants, etc)
- 1/2 teaspoon spice, or to taste (cinnamon powder, ground cardamom, turmeric, etc)
- Pinch of salt
- 1 cup milk (I use Soy most times)
- 1 cup water, room-temperature
- Sweetener to taste: Sugar, Agave syrup, Maple syrup, etc

Direction

- Place a large skillet on medium heat.
- Put the following ingredients in. In no particular order. Oats, apples, nuts, dried fruit, spices, and a pinch of salt. I love the

combination of cinnamon and apple, with a pinch of freshly ground cardamom.
- Using a spoon, stir the mixture to combine. Continue stirring and tossing, for 8 - 10 minutes, till the oats take on a bronzed color. (Note that at this point, you can choose to continue and cook up the entire batch {or you can remove what you don't need right away and store it in the fridge (for a couple of days) or deep freezer (for a few weeks)}.
- Turn the heat down to low and add half the milk and half the water. Stir, to combine and continue to cook on low heat. It takes about 10 minutes for it to get to the consistency I like which is creamy but with some texture to the oats. Yours might take longer. Or shorter. It's up to you.
- Continue cooking, adding more liquid till you're happy. (Permission given to adjust recipe. This should make for a tick!)
- Remove from heat and serve with your sweetener of choice

330. Toasty Brown Butter Steel Cut Oats

Serving: Serves 3 to 4 | Prep: | Cook: | Ready in:

Ingredients

- 1 cup steel-cut oats (regular or quick-cooking)
- 2 tablespoons unsalted butter
- 1 tablespoon dark brown sugar, plus more for serving, if desired
- Tiny pinch of salt
- 1/4 teaspoon ground cinnamon
- 1/8 teaspoon ground allspice (optional, or use freshly grated nutmeg, or the tiniest pinch of cloves -- whatever you like)
- A small piece of best-quality cinnamon stick (you'll need a fine microplane-style grater for this)
- Add-ins: Dried fruit (raisins, dried sour cherries, and dried cranberries are my go-to add-ins), spiced applesauce, toasted chopped nuts, or whatever strikes your fancy
- Sweeteners to taste: Maple syrup, sorghum, or honey
- Almond milk (ideally homemade) or cream, to taste

Direction

- For regular steel-cut oats, boil 4 cups of filtered water. If using quick-cooking oats, boil whatever other amount is recommended on your package.
- Put a heavy 2- or 3-quart saucepan on the stove over a medium flame while you measure the oats. When the pan is good and hot, add the oats and shake the pan a bit. Let them toast, shaking every 30 seconds or so (Be patient! They need time to darken a bit.), for about 3 minutes.
- Turn the heat off and remove the oats from the pan. (I put them in one of the bowls in which I'll be serving the porridge.)
- Add the butter to the hot pan, stirring briskly. It will melt immediately and start to evaporate. Turn the heat back on to medium. Keep stirring!
- When the foaming subsides and the solids have started to darken, add the one tablespoon of brown sugar. Stir it for about a minute to get a mild toffee flavor.
- Add the oats and a tiny pinch of salt and stir thoroughly, letting the ingredients brown, stirring all the while, for one minute. Turn the heat off and continue to stir for another minute.
- Very carefully and slowly, pour the hot water into the pan. It will send off a lot of steam, so be careful. Stir the oatmeal thoroughly and let it come to a full boil. Keep an eye on it so it doesn't boil over.
- At this point, I usually add about half of the dried fruit we plan to use.
- Once the oats start to boil briskly, turn them down to a slower boil. If you let them cook too fast, the water will evaporate before enough of it has been absorbed.

- Cook for about 15 minutes, or as long as necessary to absorb the water to your desired consistency. (Quick-cooking oats should require only about 6 to 8 minutes) Sprinkle the ground spices on and stir them in.
- Top with whatever add-ins you like. Use a microplane-style grater to grate a touch of cinnamon over each bowl.
- Serve with whatever sweeteners you like, and almond milk or cream, as desired.
- Enjoy! ;o)

331. Trail Mix Oatmeal

Serving: Makes 20 | Prep: | Cook: |Ready in:

Ingredients

- 2 cups flour
- 2 cups rolled oats
- 1 teaspoon kosher salt
- 1 teaspoon baking soda
- 1/2 teaspoon ground cinnamon
- 2 sticks unsalted butter
- 1 cup brown sugar, packed
- 1/2 cup sugar
- 2 large eggs
- 2 teaspoons vanilla
- 1/2 cup white chocolate chips
- 1 1/4 cups trail mix

Direction

- Preheat oven to 350. In a medium bowl stir together the flour, oats, salt, baking soda and cinnamon.
- In a mixer cream the butter and sugar. Beat in the eggs, one at a time, then add the vanilla. Add the flour mixture and mix on low speed until combined. Stir in the chocolate chips and trail mix until incorporated.
- I use a small ice cream scoop to form uniform balls of dough. You can also just use a regular spoon and portion accordingly on a baking sheet lined with a silpat or have it lightly greased. Bake for about 12 to 14 minutes, don't over bake. You want them very light brown. Cool on wire rack.

332. Tuna Tartare With Cottage Cheese And Crumble

Serving: Makes 3-4 | Prep: | Cook: |Ready in:

Ingredients

- 1/4 cup flour
- 1/4 cup oats
- 1/4 cup hazelnut powder
- 3 tablespoons Butter (semi-salted is fine)
- 150g fresh red tuna
- 2 tablespoons olive oil
- 1 cup cottage cheese
- 1 handful chives, snipped
- 1 small shallot, thinly cut

Direction

- Cut the tuna into 1/4 inch dices. In a bowl, combine the olive oil, lemon juice, salt and pepper to make the marinade. Place the tuna in the marinade and set in the fridge for a 30 min-1 hour.
- Combine flour, ground hazelnut, oats, dices of cold butter, wasabi and a little bit of pepper. Combine well, preferably by hand. You can dilute the wasabi paste a little bit of water if it is too thick
- Spread the crumble on greaseproof paper and put in the often for 12-15 minutes. Make sure the crumble does not burn. Set aside and let cool
- In the meantime, whisk together, snipped chives, cottage cheese and shallot. Season to taste. I do not usually add a lot of salt because I find the tuna naturally salty.
- To assemble the verrine, place the diced tuna at the bottom of the glass, add some cottage cheese then top with savoury crumble. Enjoy

333. Ultimate Superfoods Breakfast Bars

Serving: Makes 8-12 bars | Prep: | Cook: | Ready in:

Ingredients

- 1/2 cup oat flour (1/2 cup ground oats)
- 2 cups old fashion rolled oats
- 1/2 cup hemp seeds
- 1/2 cup brown sugar
- 1 tablespoon cinnamon
- 1/4 teaspoon salt
- 1.5 teaspoons baking powder
- 1/3 cup chia seeds
- 1 cup unsweetened vanilla almond milk (or other non dairy milk)
- 1 whole mashed large banana
- 1/2 cup almond butter
- 1 teaspoon vanilla extract
- 2 cups cooked quinoa

Direction

- Preheat oven to 350F
- Start by cooking the quinoa according to package directions, 1 cup uncooked should make about 2-3 cups cooked. While your quinoa is cooking on the stove you can assemble the rest of the ingredients.
- Combine dry ingredients including oat flour, oats, hemp seeds, brown sugar, cinnamon, salt, and baking soda in a large bowl and mix well.
- In another medium size bowl combine chia seeds, milk, mashed banana, almond butter and vanilla and whisk until smooth and well combined. Chia seeds will start to gel thickening the ingredients.
- When the quinoa is done add it to the dry ingredients, then add the wet ingredients and mix till well combined.
- Spread evenly in a 9 x 13 greased baking dish and compact with a spatula. Just press the back of the spatula across the bake so everything is well combined together.
- Bake 40-45 minutes until browned around the edges. A toothpick should come out clean and it should feel firm. Let cool 30 minutes before cutting into bars.

334. Underrated Oats Peanut Ginger Eggplant And Sweet Potato With Coconut Oats

Serving: Serves 2 | Prep: | Cook: | Ready in:

Ingredients

- 1 cup quick oats
- 1 medium eggplant
- 1 medium sweet potato
- 1 medium onion, sliced
- 2 large garlic cloves
- 1 large knob ginger, equivalent size to garlic cloves
- 2 tablespoons peanut butter (just peanuts!)
- 1 tablespoon low sodium soy sauce
- 1 cup full fat coconut milk
- sesame oil and olive oil for cooking
- salt, pepper, chili flake to taste

Direction

- Chop the eggplant into 1 – 2 inch-ish cubes and sprinkle with coarse salt. Let stand for 20 minutes.
- Chop the sweet potato into 1 – 2 inch-ish cubes and boil in water on medium heat for 15 – 20 minutes or until tender. Set aside.
- Once the eggplant is ready, rinse off the salt and use a paper towel to dry them off and soak up any excess water. Place the eggplant and onion in a baking pan, and add a generous helping of olive oil, and a tiny dash of salt and pepper. Use your hands to mix the olive oil around, making sure the eggplant pieces are coated. Cook at 350F/180C for 20 –

- 30 minutes or until the eggplant is soft and cooked through.
- When the sweet potato and eggplant are cooked you can prepare to serve. In a bowl, add the oats and 1/2 c coconut milk. Let stand for a few minutes and then add 1/2 c boiling water. Stir a few times to incorporate and then let sit.
- In a pan on medium-high heat, add a dash of sesame oil and into it grate the ginger and garlic. Add a pinch of chili flake. Sautee until just starting to brown. Lower the heat to medium/medium-low and add the soy sauce, peanut butter, and a tbsp. or so of lukewarm water. Stir to incorporate.
- To that, add 1/2 c coconut milk and combine. Add the sweet potato and eggplant, and combine. Add a little spoonful of water as needed to help the sauce coat the vegetables.
- Serve with the coconut oats and a light cilantro and mint salad (dressed here with a light dash of sesame oil and lemon juice).

335. Vanilla Berry Baked Oatmeal

Serving: Makes 4 generous or 6 small servings | Prep: 0hours20mins | Cook: 0hours30mins | Ready in:

Ingredients

- 1 tablespoon ground flax meal
- 3 tablespoons warm water
- 2 1/2 cups rolled oats
- 1 teaspoon baking powder
- 1/4 teaspoon salt
- 1 teaspoon cinnamon
- 1/2 teaspoon vanilla powder or the seeds of 1 vanilla bean, scraped (or substitute 1 teaspoon vanilla extract)
- 1/3 cup maple syrup, plus more for serving
- 2 1/4 cups almond or soy milk, plus more for serving
- 1 tablespoon canola oil or melted coconut oil
- 1 1/2 cups fresh mixed berries, plus a few extra for topping
- 1/4 cup sliced almonds or chopped pecans
- 2 tablespoons organic brown sugar
- Jam and/or nut butter, for serving (optional)

Direction

- Preheat the oven to 350° F and lightly oil an 8- or 9-inch square baking dish. Mix the flax meal and the water together in a small bowl. Allow them to thicken for a few minutes.
- In a large mixing bowl, mix together the rolled oats, baking powder, salt, cinnamon, and vanilla powder or vanilla bean (if you're substituting vanilla extract instead, add it to the wet ingredients).
- Whisk together the prepared flax mixture, the maple syrup, almond milk, and oil. Add the wet ingredients to the oat mixture and stir to combine. Fold in the berries.
- Turn the mixture out into your baking dish. Top with a few additional berries. Transfer the oatmeal to the oven and bake for 15 minutes. Sprinkle the almonds or pecans and brown sugar over the top and bake for an additional 10 minutes, or until most of the liquid is absorbed and the oats are spongy, but solid. Allow them to cool.
- You can serve the baked oatmeal either warm or cold. Cut the oatmeal into squares and drizzle with additional non-dairy milk and some fresh jam or maple syrup, if desired. A schmear of almond or cashew butter is also delicious!

336. Vanilla Porridge

Serving: Serves 1 | Prep: | Cook: | Ready in:

Ingredients

- 1 piece vanilla pod
- 7 pieces cranberries
- 1/2 piece nectarine

- 10 grams dried apricots
- 160 milliliters almond milk
- 45 grams oats
- 1 teaspoon maple syrup
- 10 grams walnuts
- 1/2 piece small banana

Direction

- Split the vanilla bean and scrape out the inside, then place in a saucepan with the oats and almond milk. Heat over a medium heat for 5 minutes, stirring regularly.
- Meanwhile, slice the nectarine, banana and crush the walnuts.
- When the porridge is ready, top with the fruit, nuts and maple syrup.

337. Vanilla Spice Granola

Serving: Makes approx. 3 quarts | Prep: | Cook: | Ready in:

Ingredients

- 4 cups rolled oats
- 1/2 cup dark brown sugar
- 1/2 cup canola oil
- 1/3 cup honey
- 1 tablespoon granulated sugar
- 2 tablespoons vanilla extract
- 1 cup raw almonds
- 3/4 cup raw pecans (halved)
- 1/2 cup raw pistachios
- 1/2 cup raw, chopped walnuts
- 1/2 cup unsweetened coconut chips
- 1/4 cup pepitas
- 1/4 teaspoon kosher salt
- 1/4 teaspoon ground cinnamon
- 1/4 teaspoon ground allspice
- 1/4 teaspoon ground cardamom
- 1/3 cup raisins
- 1/3 cup dried cranberries
- 1/3 cup dried blueberries
- 1/3 cup date pieces

Direction

- Pre-heat oven to 300°
- Place canola oil, honey and granulated sugar in a small sauce pan and heat over a medium flame until the sugar has melted. Remove from heat, add the vanilla extract and set aside to cool.
- In a large bowl, combine the oats, brown sugar, nuts and seeds, coconut, salt, and spices, and mix well. Add the cooled canola oil and honey mixture, and stir to coat the dry ingredients. Pour the mix onto a large (I use a 20x12), rimmed, non-stick baking sheet (or a regular sheet with a Silpat 11-5/8-by-16-1/2-Inch Nonstick Silicone Baking Mat) and spread to an even thickness.
- Place the baking sheet into the oven on the center rack and cook for around 40 - 45 minutes until nicely browned, removing the sheet at 15-minute intervals to stir the granola.
- Once cooked, remove the sheet tray and place it on a rack to cool. When the granola has completely cooled, break it up into a large bowl, mix in the dried fruits and place in a large air tight container for storage.
- Have fun with this recipe by adding different fruits, nuts and spices to your liking.

338. Vanilla Bean Oatmeal Ice Cream With Oat Cookie Crumbs

Serving: Serves 4 | Prep: | Cook: | Ready in:

Ingredients

- 1/2 cup rolled oats
- 3 cups whole milk
- 1 cup heavy cream
- 2/3 cup sugar
- 1 pinch salt
- 4 teaspoons cornstarch
- 1 tablespoon agave syrup
- 1 vanilla bean
- 50 grams cream cheese

- 75 grams crushed oat cookies

Direction

- Toast the oats in a 375F oven for 5-10min until fragrant and golden brown (stirring them once in a while as to not burn them).
- Dissolve the cornstarch in 1/2 cup milk, leave to rest.
- In a small saucepan combine the leftover whole milk, the heavy cream, sugar, agave syrup, pinch of salt, place on medium heat, bring to a boil, throw in the toasted oats and cook for 15-20min until the oats are cooked. Strain the mixture through a fine sieve lined with a cheesecloth, getting rid of the oats. Return the strained mixture back into the saucepan, add the seeds of 1 vanilla bean, bring to an almost boil, add the cornstarch milk and cook on medium stirring constantly until thickened. Take off heat, mix in the cream cheese, mix until fully smooth and combined. Cool to room temperature, then transfer to the fridge overnight.
- Freeze in your ice cream maker according to the manufacturer's instructions. Add the crushed oat cookies at the last minute of churning. Store in an airtight container in the freezer or spoon right away.

339. Vegan Almond And Toasted Oat Jam Bars

Serving: Makes 8 | Prep: | Cook: |Ready in:

Ingredients

- For the base
- 1/2 cup whole wheat flour
- 1 cup almond meal
- 1 tablespoon brown sugar
- 1/3 cup coconut oil, solid
- 2 tablespoons almond milk (or other vegan milk)
- Pinch salt
- 1/2 cup jam
- For the oat topping
- 3/4 cup quick oats
- 1 1/2 teaspoons cinnamon
- 1 tablespoon brown sugar
- 1 1/2 tablespoons coconut oil, solid or melted

Direction

- Preheat the oven to 350F. Line an 8×8-inch pan with parchment paper and set aside.
- First make the base. In a food processor (or using a bowl and fork), pulse the whole wheat flour, almond meal, brown sugar, and salt until combined. Add the coconut oil and pulse until evenly distributed. Add the almond milk, one tablespoon at a time, and pulse until the mixture forms large clumps.
- Press the dough evenly into the pan, using your fingertips to pat down until smooth. Spread the jam evenly across the top of the dough.
- Now make the topping. In a small bowl, mix together the oats, cinnamon, sugar, and coconut oil. The mixture will not form clumps. Spread the oat mixture across the top of the jam until covered.
- Bake for 40 minutes until golden brown. Let cool until slicing.

340. Vegan Apple Crisp

Serving: Serves 6 | Prep: | Cook: |Ready in:

Ingredients

- Topping
- 1 cup old fashioned rolled oats
- 3/4 cup pecans
- 3/4 cup all-purpose flour
- 3/4 cup packed light brown sugar
- 1 tablespoon ground cinnamon
- 1/2 teaspoon kosher salt
- 6 tablespoons canola oil
- Filling

- 6 large apples, peeled, cored, and sliced
- 1/2 cup packed light brown sugar
- 1 tablespoon cornstarch
- 2 teaspoons ground cinnamon
- 2 lemons, juiced

Direction

- Preheat oven to 375 degrees F. In a medium bowl, stir together oats, pecans, flour, sugar, cinnamon, and salt until well combined. Add oil and stir until clumps of various sizes form. Set aside.
- In a large bowl, combine apples, sugar, cinnamon, cornstarch, and lemon juice. Stir until all of the apples are well coated.
- Pour the apple mixture into an 8-inch square pan. Sprinkle the topping evenly over the apple mixture. Place pan on a large foil lined baking sheet to catch any juices that may bubble over during baking. Bake 30-35 minutes until the top is golden brown and the juices are bubbling.
- Crisp is best served warm out of the oven, but may be stored in the refrigerator in an airtight container for up to 3 days. It may be eaten cold or reheated in the microwave for about 1 minute.

341. Vegan Banana Chocolate Muffins

Serving: Makes 12 muffins | Prep: | Cook: | Ready in:

Ingredients

- 3/4 cup rolled oats
- 1 1/3 cups all-purpose flour
- 1/4 cup granulated sugar
- 2 1/2 teaspoons baking powder
- 1/4 teaspoon salt
- 1/2 cup unsweetened vanilla almond milk, or other non-dairy milk
- 1/4 cup canola oil
- 1/2 teaspoon vanilla extract
- 2 bananas, mashed
- 2 tablespoons unsweetened applesauce
- 1 small bar (roughly 1.5 oz) of vegan dark chocolate

Direction

- Preheat oven to 350 degrees.
- In a large bowl, mix together the oats, flour, sugar, baking powder, and salt. In a separate bowl, combine the almond milk, canola oil, vanilla, bananas, and applesauce. Once mixed well, stir the wet mixture into the dry ingredients. Stir in the chocolate.
- Spoon into a greased muffin tin and bake for 20 minutes.

342. Vegan Beetloaf

Serving: Serves 6-8 | Prep: | Cook: | Ready in:

Ingredients

- 3/4 cup raw unsalted sunflower seeds
- 1/2 cup rolled oats
- 1/2 pound mushrooms
- 1 cup cooked adzuki beans
- 1-1/2 cups (packed) grated beets
- 1 small onion, coarsely chopped (about 1/2 c.)
- 2 teaspoons tomato paste
- 2 teaspoons smoked paprika
- 1 teaspoon salt

Direction

- Pre-heat oven to 375 degrees. Lightly oil a 9x5" loaf pan (silicon is best for extracting the loaf later).
- Place sunflower seeds, oats and mushrooms in a food processor and run until a crumbly uniform texture is achieved. Add in beans and pulse a few times to integrate them.
- Place sunflower seed mixture in a large mixing bowl and add beet and onion. Stir well with a

heavy wooden spoon. Once vegetables are well-distributed, stir in tomato paste, smoked paprika and salt.
- Transfer beet loaf mixture to the greased loaf pan, using a spatula to smooth the top evenly. Bake for 55-65 minutes, until top is firm and just slightly crisp. Remove beet loaf from oven and let it cool 8-10 minutes before slicing and serving.
- Beet loaf can be made ahead and refrigerated. When ready to serve, reheat at 350 degrees for 15-18 minutes.

343. Vegan Chocolate Chunk Cookies With Flaky Sea Salt

Serving: Makes 26-28 cookies | Prep: | Cook: | Ready in:

Ingredients

- 1 cup plus 3 tablespoons (150) grams all purpose unbleached flour
- 3/4 cup plus 1 tablespoon (80 grams) oat flour
- 1/2 teaspoon salt (I use fine sea salt)
- 1/4 teaspoon baking powder
- 3/4 cup (150 grams) packed (not too firmly) organic light brown sugar
- 1/4 cup plus 1 tablespoon (80 grams) almond butter (the kind you have to stir)
- 2 tablespoons (30 grams) water
- 1 1/2 teaspoons pure vanilla extract
- 1/2 cup (112 grams) virgin coconut oil, melted and warm
- 3/4 cup (130 grams) chocolate chips, or coarsely chopped chocolate
- 3/4 cup (75 grams) coarsely chopped walnuts
- Flaky sea salt

Direction

- Position racks in the upper and lower thirds of the oven. Preheat a non-convection oven to 350F (or adjust accordingly for convection). Line two baking sheets with parchment.
- In a medium bowl, whisk the all-purpose and oat flours, salt, and baking powder until thoroughly blended. Set aside.
- In another bowl, combine the brown sugar, almond butter, water, and vanilla. Add the warm coconut oil and whisk until thoroughly blended.
- Pour in all of the flour mixture and stir with a spatula or wooden spoon just until all of the flour is incorporated.
- Add the chocolate chips and walnuts and stir only until they are distributed.
- Place slightly rounded tablespoons (28 grams) of dough 2 inches apart on the lined baking sheets. Press each mound of dough until it's about 1/2 inch thick and 2 inches in diameter. I do this roughly with my fingers so that cookies don't look too flat or smooth. Sprinkle each cookie with a tiny pinch of the flakey salt.
- Bake 10-12 minutes, or until the cookies are very slightly golden brown at the edges (they will still be very soft to the touch, but will firm up after they cool).

344. Vegan Cookie Dough Pops

Serving: Makes 8 | Prep: | Cook: | Ready in:

Ingredients

- 3/4 cup certified gluten-free oats
- 1/2 cup almonds
- 4 large medjool dates, pitted and chopped
- 1 14-ounce can coconut milk
- 1 teaspoon vanilla extract
- 1 tablespoon agave syrup
- 1/4 teaspoon salt
- 2 1/2 ounces dark chocolate, shaved into curls with a vegetable peeler (check the label for dairy)

Direction

- Get your Popsicle mold ready and set aside.

- Pour oats into a bowl and cover with water. Do the same with the almonds. Refrigerate both bowls at least 4 hours or overnight to allow oats and nuts to soften. When you're ready to blend, drain oats in a sieve and pour into your blender. (They'll be quite mushy.)
- Drain almonds. (Skip this next step if using blanched almonds.) Set a kettle on to boil and put almonds back in their bowl. When water is boiling, pour over almonds and allow to stand 5 minutes until just warm. Skin almonds by breaking skin gently with your fingernail and squeezing out the nut.
- Add almonds, dates, coconut milk, vanilla, stevia, and salt to blender. Blend ingredients for 2 minutes until creamy, scraping down sides occasionally with a spatula. Pour in chocolate shavings and mix with a spatula to distribute evenly.
- Pour mixture into prepared molds. Push in sticks and freeze according to manufacturer's directions. Invert mold and run under or dip in warm water to loosen popsicles. Store in freezer for up to a week.

345. Vegan Dark Chocolate And Gogi Berry Oatmeal Cookies

Serving: Makes 12 cookies | Prep: | Cook: | Ready in:

Ingredients

- 3/4 cup flour
- 1/2 teaspoon baking soda
- 1/2 teaspoon salt
- 3/4 teaspoon ground ginger
- 1/2 cup brown sugar
- 1/4 cup white sugar
- 1/2 cup vegetable oil
- 1 teaspoon vanilla extract
- 1/4 cup applesauce
- 1 1/2 cups quick oats
- heaping 1/2 cups dried goji berries
- 1/2 cup dark chocolate chunks or chips

Direction

- Preheat oven to 350 degrees. Sift flour, baking soda, salt, and ginger into a small bowl. Set aside.
- In a large bowl, combine sugars, oil, vanilla and applesauce. Gradually add flour mixture and stir well. Mix in oats, berries and chocolate. Spoon onto greased baking sheet and bake for 12-15 minutes, until cookie edges have browned and crisped. (They will still be soft in the middle). Transfer to a baking sheet to cool, and serve warm. Store any leftover cookies in the fridge.

346. Vegan Dark Chocolate Gingerbread Thumbprint Cookies

Serving: Makes 14 large cookies | Prep: 0hours30mins | Cook: 0hours50mins | Ready in:

Ingredients

- Candied Ginger
- 1 cup coconut sugar, plus 3 tablespoons
- 2 cups water
- 1 3-inch piece of ginger, peeled and sliced into coins about 1/8-inch thick
- Cookies & Chocolate Ganache
- 1 1/2 cups oat flour (store-bought works best) (180 grams)
- 1/2 cup (68 grams) super-fine almond flour
- 1/2 cup (72 grams) coconut sugar
- 1 teaspoon (4 grams) baking powder
- 2 teaspoons (6 grams) ground cinnamon
- 1 tablespoon (7 grams) ground ginger
- 1/4 teaspoon (1 gram) ground nutmeg
- 1/4 teaspoon (1 gram) ground cloves
- 3/4 teaspoon (3 grams) kosher salt
- 7 tablespoons (77 grams) refined coconut oil, melted

- 6 tablespoons (132 grams) blackstrap molasses
- 4.2 ounces Hu Simple Dark Chocolate (2 bars), roughly chopped into shards
- 3 tablespoons unsweetened coconut cream

Direction

- Make the candied ginger: Combine 1 cup coconut sugar with 2 cups water in a small saucepan, and heat over a medium low flame, stirring every minute or so, until the sugar dissolves (a few minutes total). Add the ginger coins and let it come to a rolling simmer for about 30 to 35 minutes, stirring every few minutes, until the liquid starts to bubble and cook down into a thick syrup. Drain the ginger pieces (you can reserve the syrup to use in cocktails later!), and toss them in 3 tablespoons of coconut sugar, then set aside in the refrigerator to cool and dry. This can be done several days in advance—just be sure to cover the candied ginger coins in the fridge. (You'll only need 14 of them for the cookies; save the extras for snacking.)
- Heat the oven to 350°F. Line two baking sheets with parchment paper.
- In a large bowl, combine the oat flour, almond flour, coconut sugar, baking powder, cinnamon, ginger, nutmeg, cloves, and salt. Whisk to thoroughly mix. Add the coconut oil and molasses and mix together with your hands or a wooden spoon until a moist ball of dough forms.
- Divide the dough into 14 roughly equal pieces. Roll each into a ball. Arrange evenly on the prepared cookie sheets, and use your thumb to make a deep indentation in the center of each, almost down to the cookie sheet but not quite. (If the sides around the thumbprint start to split, just pinch them back together to create a retaining wall.) Chill the cookie sheets in the freezer for 15 minutes, then place into the oven. Bake for 14 minutes, peeking after 10 minutes to check on your indentations—if they're starting to fill in, briefly pull out the trays and press the indentations in with a teaspoon before returning to oven. Once you remove them from the oven, press down the centers one final time as they cool on their tray.
- While the cookies are cooling, make the chocolate ganache. In a small saucepan, heat the coconut cream until melted and just barely simmering around the edges. Remove pan from heat and add the chocolate shards. Stir to combine until the chocolate has melted. Use a spoon to fill the centers of the cookies, and top each well of chocolate with one piece of candied ginger. Let sit at room temperature (or pop into the fridge for about 20 minutes, to expedite) until the chocolate centers have set.
- To store, chill in a covered container for 2 to 3 days.

347. Vegan Strawberry Cream Pie

Serving: Serves 12 | Prep: | Cook: | Ready in:

Ingredients

- Biscuit Base
- 1 cup raw oat flour
- 1 cup raw dehydrated almond pulp flour
- 1/2 cup cashew flour
- 1/2 cup maple syrup
- 1/4 cup melted coconut butter
- 1 pinch salt
- 2 tablespoons strawberry powder (dehydrated)
- 1 tablespoon vanilla essence
- Strawberry Cream Topping
- 1 cup young coconut flesh (from a green or thai coconut) or tin of celebs coconut cream
- 1 cup coconut butter melted
- 1/4 cup raw honey
- 1 punnet of thoroughly washed organic fresh strawberries
- 1 cup Vegeset prepared as instructed.
- 1 pinch salt
- 1 cup raw coconut flour

Direction

- First line a 9 inch flan tin with non PVC plastic wrap. Then in a food processor blend all the biscuit base ingredients. To make the flours you need a dehydrator. I use oat groats soaked overnight and then dehydrated till dry and then milled, same process with the almond pulp flour. You can make almond pulp flour with what is left over from making almond milk. Once the mix has been nicely blended, transfer the crumbly mix into the tin and flatten with either your hands or a spoon. Put in freezer to set while you start on the topping. If you are gluten free, omit the oat flour and use more almond flour instead.
- In a Vitamix blend all the ingredients except for the coconut flour until really smooth and creamy, once blended add the coconut flour and use the prodder to mix well, the texture should resemble a light fluffy mix. Take the tin out of freezer and add the topping. You can use celebs coconut cream which though tinned is very good quality, I used about half a tin. Transfer to the freezer for 10 minutes and then in the meantime slice more Strawberries to decorate as you wish, you can also use raspberries or mixed berries. To glaze with a vegetarian Jelly make up the Vegeset as instructed, it is carrageen based and sets as a jelly. Take the cake out of the fridge and decorate with the fruits then add the jelly once it has cooled enough for your small finger to feel slightly warm but not boiling. The trick is to work fairly quickly at the final stage before the jelly sets too much so don't go on the phone at this point.

348. Vegan Sweet Potato Casserole

Serving: Serves 10-12 | Prep: 0hours30mins | Cook: 0hours20mins | Ready in:

Ingredients

- Sweet Potato Mash
- 4-5 large sweet potatoes
- 3 tablespoons pure maple syrup
- 1 teaspoon vanilla
- 1 teaspoon cinnamon
- 1/8 teaspoon nutmeg
- 1/2 teaspoon salt, or to taste
- Pecan Crumble Topping
- 1 cup rolled oats
- 1 1/3 cups chopped pecans
- 3 tablespoons maple syrup
- 1 teaspoon cinnamon
- 1/2 teaspoon salt

Direction

- Peel and roughly chop sweet potatoes into large chunks. Place into a large pot and cover with water. Bring water to a boil, reduce heat to medium-high, and gently boil for 10 to 20 minutes, until the potatoes are fork tender.
- Preheat oven to 375°F. Lightly spray 9x11 casserole dish or use one that is non-stick.
- Prepare the crunchy nut topping: Pour oats into a food processor and pulse until coarsely chopped. In a mixing bowl, add the chopped pecans, oats, cinnamon, salt and stir to combine. Pour in the maple syrup. Mix until combined, using your hands if needed. Set aside.
- Drain the cooked sweet potatoes and place in a large mixing bowl and mash until smooth.
- Stir in the maple syrup, vanilla, cinnamon, nutmeg, and salt. Adjust to taste if needed. Dump into casserole dish and evenly smooth out.
- Sprinkle the crunch nut topping all over the sweet potato mixture, evenly.
- Bake, uncovered, at 375°F for 20 minutes, until the dish is hot throughout. Plate and serve immediately.

349. Vegan Coconut Chocolate Chip Oat Cookies!

Serving: Serves 12 large cookies | Prep: | Cook: |Ready in:

Ingredients

- 100 grams coconut sugar (3/4 cup)
- 150 grams medium-sized oats (1 + 1/2 cup)
- 120 grams oat flour (1 + 1/4 cup)
- 80 grams smaller vegan dark chocolate chips (1/2 cup)
- 30 grams unsweetened coconut flakes (1/3 cup)
- 125 milliliters solid coconut oil (1/2 cup solid)
- 300 milliliters coconut-rice beverage (1 cup + bit less than 1/4 cup)
- 1/2 teaspoon baking soda
- Pinch of sea salt

Direction

- Place your solid coconut oil in a fitted cooking pot & let it completely melt on lower heat. Stir often. Turn heat off & set aside. In a medium bowl, pour coconut oil & add coconut sugar. Mix well with a spoon. Now, add oats, oat flour, pinch of sea salt & baking soda. Mix well through. Now, add coconut-rice milk, chocolate chips & coconut flakes. Mix well. Taste! You must taste the coconut & chocolate chips. The dough tastes a bit sweet but not too sweet either, just right! ;) Place cling film over the top & place to rest in the fridge for 30 minutes. This way, the dough will stiff up in the fridge.
- After the resting time, take your bowl out of the fridge & remove cling film. Preheat your oven to 180°C (350oF) for 10 minutes. I always use a fan-oven. With your hands, take bigger pieces of your dough, a bit less than the inner palm of your hand & roll balls. Flatten them with your hands & place on a Silpat & do the same with remaining dough. Space them apart & my Silpat could hold 9 bigger cookies. Place in the lower end of your oven & bake for about 18 minutes. The cookies must be cooked through & browned on the tops. Take them out of the oven & leave them for about 5 minutes on the Silpat. This will give a lovely shine on the bottom of the cookies. Then, move them to wire racks to get crisp & to cool down completely! ;) Enjoy, just like that, as a nice breakfast, snack or as a lovely dessert with a good café latte or an enjoyable tea! :) When cold, pack them nicely to give as a lovely food gift! ;)

350. Vegan, Gluten Free And Refined Sugar Free Granola Bars With A Chocolate Dip

Serving: Makes 8 bars | Prep: | Cook: |Ready in:

Ingredients

- 1 tablespoon psyllium husk
- 1 1/2 tablespoons chia seeds
- 4 tablespoons water
- 1 1/2 cups (GF) oats
- 1/4 cup hazelnuts
- 1/2 cup almonds
- 1/4 cup raisins
- 1/8 cup coconut oil
- 1/2 cup maple syrup
- 1 teaspoon vanilla paste
- 1 cup unsweetened apple puree
- 1/8 teaspoon salt
- 100 grams dark chocolate, melted (+ tempered if necessary)

Direction

- In a little bowl, combine chia seeds and water. Stir and set aside until a gel forms.
- In a big bowl, combine oats, salt, hazelnuts, almonds, pecans, flaxseeds, and raisins.
- In another bowl, combine psyllium husk, coconut oil, maple syrup, vanilla, and apple puree. Stir until combined. Add the chia gel and stir again.

- Pour wet into dry and using either a wooden spoon or your hands, thoroughly mix/knead until everything is coated and combined.
- Grease a baking tin (9 x 9, for short bars) or loaf pan (9 x 5, for higher bars) with coconut oil and line with parchment paper.
- Press the granola mixture into the pan, spreading it out evenly. Let it rest for about 10-15 minutes.
- Preheat oven to 180 C.
- Bake granola bars for about 50-60 minutes, until golden brown and completely cooked through.
- Let cool completely.
- Trim the bar if necessary and cut 1, 5 inches/4 cm bars. Dip one side into the melted chocolate. Place in the fridge to set completely.
- Wrap/Pack/Serve/Eat!

351. Vegetable Crumble With Chorizo

Serving: Serves 4-6 | Prep: | Cook: | Ready in:

Ingredients

- 800g butternut squash
- 2 parsnip
- 1 onion
- 1 leek
- 2 garlic cloves
- 100g chorizo
- olive oil
- 1 cup oats
- 1/3 cup Butter
- 2/3 cup grated mozzarella or parmesan
- 3/4 flour
- 1/3 cup pine nuts

Direction

- Peel and dice the butternut and parsnip. Also peel the onion and mix together with the garlic. Cut the leek into thin slices. Dice the chorizo into bit size pieces
- Heat the oil in a wok. Fry the onion on medium heat for 5 minutes; Add the leek, chorizo and cook for five more minutes. Now add the parsnip and butternut. Season with some pepper. Add a little bit of water and cook for 20-30 minutes.
- For the crumble, put the flour, Parmesan, oat and pine nuts in a bowl. Add the diced butter. Knead with the tip of your fingers and until dough is crumbly.
- Preheat oven on 400FPut all the vegetables in an oven dish and cover with crumble. Bake in the oven for 20 minutes until top is golden.

352. Very Almond Raspberry Oatmeal Bars (Gluten Free)

Serving: Makes 24 | Prep: | Cook: | Ready in:

Ingredients

- 1/2 cup coconut oil
- 1 cup brown sugar
- 1/2 cup almond paste
- 2 drops bitter almond oil
- 1/4 teaspoon salt
- 2 eggs
- 8 ounces jar simply fruit raspberry spread
- 1/4 teaspoon cinnamon
- 2 1/2 cups gluten free rolled oats
- 3 tablespoons white sugar or Penzey's vanilla sugar
- 1 cup blanched almonds (optional)

Direction

- Lightly grease a 9x13 pan with coconut oil. Preheat oven to 350.
- On low to medium speed, beat coconut oil and almond paste until smooth. Add brown sugar, almond oil, eggs, salt, and cinnamon. Add rolled oats. Spread the dough in an even layer in the pan. Top with raspberry spread. Sprinkle with almonds and white sugar.

- Bake at 350 for 25 min. Let cool. Cut into squares. Makes 24 bars.

353. Walnut, Oat & Apricot Squares

Serving: Makes 20 squares | Prep: | Cook: | Ready in:

Ingredients

- 1 cup Oat Flakes
- 1 cup Walnut Halves, heaping
- 8 Organic Dried Apricots
- 2 tablespoons Organic Brown Rice Syrup or other sweetener of choice
- 1 tablespoon Cold Pressed Sunflower Oil (unflavoured/odourless) or other neutral baking oil of choice
- 1/2 teaspoon Pure Organic Bourbon Vanilla Powder

Direction

- Grind the walnuts into a medium fine meal, a little bit at a time, being careful not to over process and overheat the mixture, otherwise it will turn into walnut butter. Set aside.
- Add oats to a food processor and pulse into a flour.
- Add walnut meal and dried apricots to the oat flour in the food processor and pulse to combine and break down the apricots.
- Add vanilla, rice syrup, oil and a pinch of salt, if using and pulse to combine. By now the mixture should be clumping together a bit.
- Press mixture firmly into an 11x 9 baking dish and bake in a preheated oven at 180 C (356 F) for about 20 minutes. Baking times vary by oven, so you will want to adjust the baking time accordingly. You could also make these in a smaller pan (8x8 for example) to get slightly thicker squares, but again, be sure to adjust the baking time accordingly. You will know they're ready when the edges start to brown.

- Remove from the oven and let cool enough to handle without burning your fingers, then slice into squares and serve. Store them in an air tight container.

354. White Bean & Chicken Sweet Potato Casserole

Serving: Serves 12-16 people | Prep: | Cook: | Ready in:

Ingredients

- Mashed Sweet Potato Topping
- 6 medium sweet potatoes
- 1/2 cup milk, or as needed
- White bean & Chicken Filling
- 3/4 cup steel cut oats/quick oats/instant oatmeal
- 1 cup water
- 1 teaspoon salt
- 1 tablespoon olive oil
- 1 celery stalk, diced
- 1 onion, diced
- 2 cups fresh mushrooms, diced
- 1 pound boneless chicken meat, diced (or ground chicken meat)
- 2 cans of white beans
- 3/4 cup stock (vegetable or chicken)
- 1 tablespoon soy sauce
- 3 teaspoons smoked paprika
- 1/4 cup parsley, chopped
- 1 cup mozzarella cheese, shredded
- 2 cups mozzarella cheese, shredded (optional)

Direction

- Wrap sweet potatoes in aluminum foil and bake at 180 degrees Celsius for 45 minutes to an hour, until very soft to the touch.
- Remove skins from the sweet potatoes and mash them till smooth. Add milk if the potatoes are too dry or not creamy enough and whisk till smooth.
- Cook oats with water and salt. If using steel cut oats, simmer for 25 to 30 minutes. If using

quick cook or instant oatmeal, follow directions on the package.
- Heat 1 tbsp. of olive oil over medium heat in a saucepan. Add celery, carrot, onion and mushrooms. Saute till onions are soft and translucent.
- Add chicken, white beans, stock, soy sauce, paprika, and parsley and cooked oats. Stir till well combined and simmer for 5 minutes.
- Turn off the heat and stir in 1 cup of mozzarella. Spread onto a 9x13 inch baking dish.
- Spread mashed sweet potato over the mixture in the baking dish.
- (Optional) Sprinkle 2 cups of mozzarella over the sweet potato.
- Bake at 180 degrees Celsius for 30 to 35 minutes. Serve hot and enjoy!

355. Whole Bean Vanilla Almond Granola

Serving: Makes five cups of granola | Prep: | Cook: | Ready in:

Ingredients

- 3 cups rolled oats
- 1/4 cup butter
- 1/2 cup sugar
- 1 vanilla bean, roughly chopped
- 1 pinch salt
- 1 tablespoon vanilla extract
- 1 cup whole almonds, roughly chopped
- 1 cup pitted dates, roughly chopped

Direction

- Preheat oven to 375 F.
- Melt butter in a medium saucepan over medium heat. Continue to heat until butter turns brown and fragrant. Remove from heat.
- Combine sugar, vanilla bean pieces, and salt in a small food processor or clean coffee or spice grinder and pulse until no large vanilla bean pieces remain.
- Add sugar mixture and vanilla to brown butter and stir to combine. Add water, 1 tablespoon at a time until sugar is dissolved.
- Add oats and almonds to brown butter vanilla syrup and stir to coat.
- Spread oat mixture on a parchment lined baking sheet and bake for 20-30 minutes until deep golden brown, stirring halfway.
- Allow granola to cool, add chopped dates, and store in an airtight container.

356. Whole Grain Banana Bread

Serving: Makes 1 9"x 5" loaf | Prep: 0hours15mins | Cook: 1hours15mins | Ready in:

Ingredients

- 4-5 Over ripe bananas, thoroughly mashed
- 1/2 cup mild tasting oil, such as vegetable, walnut oil, avocado oil etc.
- 1/2 cup Brown sugar
- 1/2 cup maple syrup
- 2 Large eggs
- 1 teaspoon Vanilla extract
- 1 cup All-purpose flour
- 1 cup Whole wheat flour
- 1/2 cup Rolled Oats
- 1 teaspoon Baking soda
- 1/2 teaspoon Baking powder
- 1/2 teaspoon Ground cinnamon
- 3/4 cup Chopped walnuts
- 1 tablespoon Golden flax seeds
- 1 tablespoon granulated sugar, for topping

Direction

- Oven rack placed in the center, pre-heat the oven to 350°F. Lightly grease a 9"x 5" loaf pan and set to the side
- In a large bowl, stir together the mashed banana, oil, sugar, eggs, and vanilla. Set aside

- In a separate bowl, whisk the flours, oats, baking soda, baking powder, salt, cinnamon till evenly combined.
- Mix the dry ingredients into the banana mixture, making sure to scrape the bottom and sides of the bowl. Once the batter it fully incorporated, fold in the flax seeds and walnuts
- Pour the batter into prepared baking dish and evenly sprinkle remaining sugar over the top before baking. Option to sprinkle some extra oats and seeds on the top, along with the sugar
- Bake for about 75 minutes or until golden and feels firm to a light touch. To be confident it's cooked through, using a thin knife, insert it into the center and if it comes out clean, or with just a few moist crumbs (but no wet batter) your bread is done. If the bread seems to be browning too quickly, tent it with aluminum foil for the final 15 to 20 minutes of baking. Side Note: If baking in a glass pan, increase the baking time by 15 to 20 minutes and drop the temp to 325°F
- Once finished, remove the bread from the oven and let it cool it in the pan for 15 minutes. Using a knife, loosen the edges and turn it out onto a rack to cool completely. Do not cut or package until fully cooled! It may be tempting to tear off a chunk, but I promise the wait it well worth it! Enjoy!

357. Whole Grain Sourdough Rye Bread

Serving: Makes 2 loaves | Prep: 48hours0mins | Cook: 1hours30mins | Ready in:

Ingredients

- Preferment and Mash
- 1 cup active sourdough starter (200g)
- 2 cups whole grain rye flour (256g)
- 3/4 cup lukewarm water (171g)
- 1 cup cracked rye berries, or whole rye berries pulsed in spice grinder (150g)
- 2/3 cup rolled oats (60g)
- 1/3 cup corn meal (50g)
- 1/8 cup amaranth, millet, or quinoa (50g)
- 1 1/2 cups water (342g)
- oil, for coating bowls and misting dough
- Final Dough
- all of preferment
- all of mash
- 6 cups whole grain rye flour (764g)
- 3 teaspoons salt (22g)
- 1 cup unsalted, raw sunflower seeds or pepitas (100g)
- 1/4 cup molasses (60g), optional
- 3 tablespoons cocoa powder (15g), optional
- 3 cups lukewarm water (695g)
- oil, for coating bowls and misting dough
- Special equipment: sourdough starter, 9x4x4 loaf pans

Direction

- DAY 1: Make the preferment. Mix the sourdough starter, rye flour, and lukewarm water together in a bowl until all the ingredients are combined. The dough should be a little sticky and slightly shaggy.
- Place dough in a lightly oiled bowl, cover with plastic wrap, and let sit at room temperature for about 2 hours, or until the dough has noticeably swelled. Place covered bowl in refrigerator overnight.
- Make the mash. Preheat oven to 200 F. Mix together the cracked rye berries, rolled oats, corn meal, and amaranth in an oven safe bowl.
- Bring 1 1/2c water to 165 F, and stir it into the mixed grains with a wooden spoon.
- Lower the oven temperature to the warm setting, cover the bowl with foil, and place in the oven for one hour.
- After one hour, remove the bowl from the oven and let sit, covered, at room temperature overnight.
- DAY 2: Take the preferment out of the refrigerator one hour before you make the final dough. Use a pastry scraper or a knife to

- chop the preferment into 10 pieces. Cover the pieces with plastic wrap and let sit one hour to take off the chill. Alternatively, you can take the bowl out two hours before you make the final dough and let the preferment sit in the bowl in one piece for two hours.
- Make the final dough. Stir together the flour, salt, and cocoa powder together in a large mixing bowl. Add the preferment, mash, sunflower seeds, molasses, and lukewarm water. Stir with your hands or with sturdy wooden spoon until the ingredients are well combined, all the flour is hydrated, and no streaks of molasses are visible. The dough will be very sticky and shaggy.
- Oil another large mixing bowl. Or turn the dough onto floured counter and oil the original bowl. Gather the final dough up into a ball, transfer it to the oiled bowl, and turn it around a few times to coat in oil.
- Cover the bowl with plastic wrap, and let dough ferment at room temperature for 4-6 hours. The dough should almost double in size, however, rye dough does not rise in the smooth, buoyant way wheat flour rises. Rye dough will swell, and it may not seem as obvious a change in the first couple of hours.
- When the dough is almost ready, prepare two 9x4x4 loaf pans. Cut parchment paper to fit into the bottom of the pans, and oil the sides. Alternatively you can omit the parchment paper and just oil the pans, but you may need to run a knife around the sides to loosen the loaves after baking.
- Sprinkle the counter generously with rye flour. Turn dough out into the counter. You should see that the underside of the dough has lots of little holes from bubbles that formed during the rise, and the dough should smell pleasantly tangy and fruity.
- Using a pastry scraper or knife, split the dough into two equal portions. Use your hands to quickly shape each portion of dough to fit into the prepared loaf pans. Working quickly helps with sticky dough, but you can wet or oil your hands to decrease sticking.
- Spray the tops of the loaves with oil, or use your fingertips or a brush to lightly oil the tops of the loaves. Gently pat the dough so it fills the corners and smooth the top. The dough should fill the pans about 2/3 of the way.
- Cover pans in plastic wrap or foil, and place in the refrigerator overnight. You can also let the pans rest for another two hours at room temperature to rise a little after you shape the loaves, and bake on Day 2. However, having tried both ways, I find the last cold fermentation adds a lot of flavor.
- DAY 3: Take pans out of the fridge, and let sit at room temperature for about 2 hours to take off the chill. The dough will have risen a little more, and the pans will be about 3/4 full. The bread will not rise any more during baking.
- Preheat oven to 350F.
- Place loaf pans in the oven, uncovered, and bake until the inside reaches 200 F. This takes about 1 1/2 hours, but check the temperature after one hour. The bread will be a rich brown on top, and start to pull away from the sides of the pans.
- Once baked, turn the loaf pans upside down on a cooling rack. The bread should fall out easily, and sound hollow when tapped. Peel off the parchment paper if it stuck to the bottom of the loaves, turn right side up, and let cool completely before slicing. Ideally, the bread should sit at room temperature overnight before slicing. The bread can be stored at room temperature for a few days, and 1-2 weeks in the refrigerator, loosely wrapped. This bread freezes well.

358. Whole Wheat Oatmeal Banana Bread

Serving: Makes 1 loaf | Prep: 0hours10mins | Cook: 1hours10mins | Ready in:

Ingredients

- 1 cup mashed banana (about 4 small very ripe bananas, it's ok if you have more than a cup)
- 1/3 cup honey
- 1/2 cup applesauce (one individual cup)
- 1 egg
- 3/4 cup half and half (you can use any milk you like, but I love the richness of half and half here)
- 1 1/5 cups whole wheat flour
- 1 cup old-fashioned oats
- 3/4 teaspoon baking soda
- 1/4 teaspoon salt
- 1 teaspoon ground cinnamon
- 2/3 cup dark chocolate chips

Direction

- Preheat the oven to 350F and spray a loaf pan with cooking spray.
- In a large bowl combine the banana, applesauce, honey, egg, milk, and vanilla until creamy. Make a well in the center of the wet ingredients and add the remaining ingredients, reserving a few oats for sprinkling over the top if you'd like. Combine the dry ingredients gently, then fold into the wet mixture until just mixed. Pour into a loaf pan and sprinkle with extra oats.
- Bake for 60-70 minutes until a toothpick inserted in the center of the loaf comes out clean. Let cool for 5 minutes in the pan, then remove from the pan to a rack to cool completely before covering or slicing and serving.

359. Zucchini Chocolate Espresso Brownies

Serving: Serves 12 | Prep: | Cook: | Ready in:

Ingredients

- 1 1/2 cups shredded zucchini, ~2 small zucchini
- 1/2 cup almond or hazelnut butter
- 1/4 cup maple syrup
- 1/2 cup unsweetened applesauce
- 1 teaspoon vanilla extract
- 1/2 cup unsweetened dutch cocoa powder
- 1 1/2 teaspoons espresso powder
- 3/4 cup gluten free rolled oats
- 1 teaspoon baking soda
- 1/4 teaspoon salt
- 2 tablespoons almond butter for swirl

Direction

- Preheat oven to 350 degrees F and prepare an 8x11 baking pan with nonstick cooking spray.
- Place oats in food processor or blender and process until ground.
- In a large bowl, mix together almond butter, applesauce, honey and vanilla until smooth.
- Next add zucchini, cocoa powder, ground oats, baking soda, espresso powder and salt and mix ingredients together until well combined.
- Pour batter into the prepared baking pan. With a toothpick swirl in the 2 tbsp. of almond butter into the batter.
- Bake 25-30 minutes until a toothpick can be inserted into middle of the brownies and comes out clean. Remove from the oven and allow to cool in the pan 30 minutes prior to slicing into 12 brownies and devouring!

360. Zucchini Sausage Walnut Bread

Serving: Makes 2 loaves | Prep: | Cook: | Ready in:

Ingredients

- 1 pound flavorful breakfast sausage
- 1 cup whole wheat flour
- 1 cup all-purpose flour
- 1 teaspoon baking soda
- 1/2 teaspoon baking powder
- 1 teaspoon salt
- 1/2 cup quick-cooking oats

- 3 eggs, beaten
- 1/2 cup neutral oil
- 1/2 cup plain yogurt
- 1/3 cup brown sugar
- 4 tablespoons granulated white sugar
- 2 cups shredded, drained, packed zucchini
- 1 cup walnuts, toasted then ground

Direction

- Preheat the oven to 350°. In a pan, brown the sausage well, drain on a paper towel, and crumble into small pieces.
- In a large bowl, combine the flours, baking soda, baking powder, salt, and oats.
- In a separate bowl, mix together the eggs, oil, yogurt, and sugars. Stir in the zucchini, then add the mixture to the dry ingredients. Stir until just combined. Fold in the nuts and sausage and pour into 2 greased loaf pans. Bake for about 50 to 60 minutes or until a toothpick comes out clean.
- Enjoy as is, or brown slices of the bread in butter.

361. B[EAT] Burgers

Serving: Makes 8 patties | Prep: | Cook: | Ready in:

Ingredients

- 2 pounds beets, thoroughly washed
- 1 medium red onion, peeled
- 1.25 cups rolled oats
- 4 cloves garlic, minced
- 1 tablespoon fresh rosemary, minced
- 2 cans (15 ounces each) cannellini beans, thoroughly drained and rinsed
- .5 cups raw walnuts
- 4 tablespoons olive oil, divided

Direction

- In a food processor fitted with a grater attachment (or using a handheld box-grater), finely grate beets and red onion. Transfer to a fine-mesh strainer or cheese cloth and press out as much excess liquid as possible. Transfer to a large bowl. Add rolled oats, garlic, and rosemary and (using hands), thoroughly combine. Set aside.
- In a high speed blender or food process fitted with an S blade, process cannellini beans and walnuts until very smooth. Scoop into large bowl with beet mixture, then using your hands, thoroughly combine. Form mixture into 8 even balls, then flatten until about 1 inch thick patties. Allow patties to sit for about 30 minutes, allowing the oats to absorb some of the moisture.
- Preheat oven to 350 degrees F, rack in the middle. Line a baking sheet with foil and lightly grease with olive oil. Bake patties for 15 minutes, flipping gently after 5 minutes. Remove from oven.
- Preheat 1 tablespoon olive oil over medium-high heat in a non-stick skillet. Add 2 patties to pan and cook for 2 minutes. Gently flip and cook for an additional 2 minutes. Remove from heat, then repeat (adding 1 tbs. oil per 2 burgers) for the remaining 6 patties. Enjoy!

362. Best Healthier Chocolate Chip Cookies

Serving: Makes 36 | Prep: | Cook: | Ready in:

Ingredients

- 1 cup Oat four
- 1/2 cup Garbanzo bean flour
- 1/2 cup White wheat flour
- 1 teaspoon Baking soda
- 1 teaspoon Salt
- 8 tablespoons Butter slightly hard
- 1/4 cup Coconut oil cold
- 3 tablespoons Plain Greek yogurt
- 2 Eggs
- 2 teaspoons Vanilla

- 3/4 cup Mini chocolate chips

Direction

- To make oat flour put oats in high speed mixer grind till fine.
- Sift flours, sugar, baking soda and salt. Set aside
- In large bowl or with stand mixer. Mix Greek yogurt, butter and coconut just till blended. Add vanilla.
- To the yogurt mixture slowly add the dry ingredients and eggs one after the other. Just till blended.
- Fold in chocolate chips.
- Place in fridge to set for at least 20 minutes.
- Bake in preheated oven at 350 for 10 minutes or till edges are brown.

363. Coconut Cashew Oatmeal Cookies| Gf + Vegan

Serving: Makes 12 cookies | Prep: | Cook: |Ready in:

Ingredients

- 1/2 cup flour (all purpose or whole wheat or for gluten free: 1/4 cup coconut flour, 1/4 cup oat flour)
- 1/2 teaspoon baking soda
- 1/4 teaspoon salt
- 1/4 teaspoon ground cinnamon
- 1/2 cup cashew butter (or other nut butter)
- 1/4 cup dark brown sugar
- 1/4 cup almond milk
- 1/2 teaspoon vanilla extract
- 1/2 cup old fashioned rolled oats, toasted
- 1/2 cup flaked coconut, toasted (use half this amount if you have shredded coconut)
- 1/2 cup chopped pecans (I used 1/4 cup and put them only in the blueberry version)
- optional: 1/4 cup white chocolate chips (if not vegan)

Direction

- Heat oven to 350 degrees.
- On two separate rimmed baking sheets, toast the coconut and oats. The coconut will take under 5 min and should be watched carefully, the oats will be about 5-8 min - toast both until just starting to get golden. Set aside.
- Line a large baking sheet with a baking mat or parchment paper for the cookies.
- In a small bowl, whisk together flour(s), baking soda, salt, and cinnamon. Set aside.
- With an electric mixer, combine the nut butter and brown sugar. Mix until smooth and light, about 2-3 minutes. Mix in the almond milk and vanilla extract, scraping down the sides.
- Turn the mixer to low and add the dry ingredients. Mix until just combined. Stir in the oats, dried fruit, coconut and optional nuts and/or white chocolate chips.
- Roll cookie dough into tablespoon balls and place on prepared baking sheet, about 2 inches apart. Gently flatten the dough balls with the palm of your hand.
- Bake cookies for 10 minutes or until they are set and golden brown around the edges. Let the cookies cool on the baking sheet for 2 minutes. Transfer to a wire cooling rack and cool completely.

364. Orange Oat Cookies

Serving: Makes 16 cookies | Prep: | Cook: |Ready in:

Ingredients

- 1/2 cup all purpose flour
- 1 1/2 cups cups cook cooking oats
- 1/2 cup cup sugar
- 1 large egg
- 1 teaspoon baking powde
- 1 teaspoon tbsp orange zes
- 1 tablespoon sugar .
- 6 tablespoons orange juice.

Direction

- In a sauce pan bring orange juice and 1 table spoon of sugar and orange zest to boil on a low heat for 8 mins.
- Sift the flour with baking powder and salt then mix with the oats.
- Mix the melted butter with sugar well, add an egg and keep mixing.
- Now add 2 tbsps. of orange mixture without orange peel.
- Now add the dry ingredients into the egg mixture.
- Make small balls and set on the baking sheet then press a little on each one.
- Pre-heat the oven on 170 degrees.
- Bake the cookies for 15 -20 mins.

365. "Fudgy" No Bake Chocolate Oatmeal Cookies

Serving: Makes 18 cookies | Prep: 0hours0mins | Cook: 0hours0mins | Ready in:

Ingredients

- 2/3 cup raw agave nectar
- 1/4 cup vegetable oil
- 5 tablespoons unsweetened cocoa powder
- 1 teaspoon ground cinnamon
- 1/2 cup raw almond butter
- 1 cup rolled oats {not instant}
- 1 teaspoon vanilla extract

Direction

- In a saucepan over medium heat combine the agave nectar, oil, cocoa and cinnamon. Boil for three minutes, stirring constantly. Remove from heat and stir in the almond butter, rolled oats and vanilla until well blended. Drop by heaping spoonfuls onto waxed paper and chill to set, about 30 minutes.

Index

A

Almond 3,4,5,6,7,11,12,13,35,53,58,63,65,70,72,73,83,87,90,96,98,103,110,114,115,127,133,138,152,156,161,162,179,181,188,193,200,202

Anise 3,12

Apple 3,4,5,6,7,13,14,15,16,17,21,22,28,35,38,47,65,77,81,123,134,172,175,177,193

Apricot 3,5,7,18,35,114,201

Arborio rice 103

Asparagus 5,119

Avocado 3,4,6,9,63,132

B

Bacon 6,129

Baking 10,24,35,73,105,125,127,166,175,181,192,201,202,206

Banana 3,4,5,6,7,8,10,23,24,25,35,41,42,55,59,65,73,74,75,83,117,136,158,180,181,194,202,204

Barley 6,35,166

Beans 5,99,116

Beef 6,155

Beer 157

Berry 3,4,5,7,27,63,70,80,125,179,191,196

Bicarbonate of soda 10

Biscuits 4,52

Blackberry 3,6,31,32,166

Blueberry 3,5,6,25,33,34,35,102,106,139

Bran 3,4,6,9,65,66,151,160

Bread 3,4,5,6,7,8,9,10,23,40,53,65,68,74,86,101,114,120,121,124,127,134,173,180,185,202,203,204,205

Broccoli 6,7,135,169

Brown sugar 67,202

Buckwheat 4,5,84,111

Buns 3,31,157

Burger 3,6,7,8,29,30,31,157,181,206

Butter 3,4,5,6,7,10,11,20,21,38,40,41,45,46,52,57,60,63,67,70,71,78,79,95,100,105,107,117,118,119,125,143,144,145,155,161,177,186,188,189,200,206

C

Cake 3,4,5,6,14,15,17,24,26,37,44,45,46,55,71,78,88,111,113,139,148,161,166

Caramel 3,6,7,42,43,129,167

Cardamom 3,4,6,33,46,72,84,125,142

Carrot 3,6,37,44,45,46,132,155

Cashew 3,4,6,8,46,60,90,166,181,207

Cava 3,47

Cheese 4,5,6,7,46,48,88,89,133,165,176,189

Cherry 4,5,6,48,54,125,138,160,161

Chicken 7,201

Chickpea 6,157

Chips 4,24,49,73,105

Chocolate 3,4,5,6,7,8,23,24,26,28,41,49,53,54,55,56,57,58,59,66,67,69,73,84,89,105,113,117,124,127,144,151,167,183,194,195,196,197,199,205,206,208

Chorizo 7,200

Cider 17

Cinnamon 3,4,6,13,21,22,35,36,48,60,65,67,70,73,127,134,137,138,154,162,181

Clarified butter 72

Coconut 3,4,5,7,8,14,23,35,46,54,61,62,63,64,74,106,138,154,162,180,181,190,199,206,207

Coffee 3,5,17,116

Condensed milk 57

Coulis 6,133

Crab 4,65

Crackers 5,91

Cranberry 4,5,7,61,66,67,68,96,110,174

Cream 3,4,5,6,7,14,17,32,33,34,38,39,46,48,62,76,78,88,89,90,128,130,132,143,162,178,183,192,197

Crumble 3,4,5,6,7,17,19,21,32,33,34,58,81,93,101,116,140,146,160,161,178,179,189,198,200

Curd 5,104

D

Date 3,4,11,25,70,71,72,154

Dried apricots 115

Dried fruit 188

E

Egg 5,7,24,35,57,105,125,141,154,168,169,181,190,206

F

Fig 3,4,6,7,33,64,164,179

Fish 34

Flapjacks 3,37

Flour 4,24,33,53,57,82,84,85,105,125,161,181,185

Fruit 3,4,5,6,7,14,32,57,78,87,95,133,134,146,154,166,187

Fudge 5,113

G

Game 4,78

Ghee 72

Gin 3,4,6,7,14,31,35,61,66,80,81,142,154,161,190,196

Gnocchi 5,119

Grain 5,7,54,89,185,202,203

Grapes 4,55

H

Ham 7,168

Hazelnut 4,61,65

Heart 5,94,138

Herbs 6,165

Honey 4,5,6,24,35,67,81,83,90,97,98,99,105,127,156,157,159,164,171

J

Jaggery 72,181

Jam 3,5,7,33,111,122,165,191,193

Jelly 6,143,198

Jus 20,34,163,179,190,207

L

Leek 7,170

Lemon 4,5,6,27,61,102,103,104,133,154

Lettuce 30

Lime 5,102,105

M

Mace 88

Mango 4,5,62,105,106

Maple syrup 25,137,188

Marmalade 5,115

Meat 4,51

Milk 4,7,10,24,27,35,57,65,72,73,137,138,154,158,175,181,183

Millet 3,28

Molasses 7,172

Muesli 3,4,5,6,7,36,48,114,116,138,142,162,170

Muffins 3,4,5,6,7,9,10,15,33,37,41,55,56,61,73,115,152,158,159,17

9,180,186,194

N

Nectarine 3,5,35,110

Nut 4,5,6,7,68,75,80,82,111,154,163,172

O

Oatcakes 4,71

Oatmeal 3,4,5,6,7,8,13,15,20,21,22,23,27,35,38,39,40,43,45,49,50,51,55,61,62,65,66,67,68,69,74,80,82,89,94,95,100,107,108,109,112,117,125,126,127,128,129,130,131,132,133,134,137,138,139,142,145,151,154,155,158,161,168,171,176,177,186,187,189,191,192,196,200,204,207,208

Oats 3,4,5,6,7,10,24,26,32,35,37,43,53,57,59,60,63,65,68,70,72,73,93,101,105,118,125,136,138,143,149,154,155,156,158,161,166,167,169,171,173,175,181,185,187,188,190,202

Oil 5,6,24,28,35,53,117,118,127,135,137,154,155,162,166,172,181,201,204

Olive 3,5,6,7,9,25,40,117,127,135,155,180

Onion 3,43,155

Orange 3,4,6,7,8,32,33,48,70,125,166,174,207

P

Pancakes 3,4,5,6,7,24,25,65,92,105,123,129,132,137,182

Parfait 6,7,149,178

Parmesan 168,200

Peach 3,4,5,6,15,31,32,33,34,71,109,132,139,140,141,142,143,156,166

Pear 3,5,6,30,101,146,147,148,177

Pecan 3,4,5,6,7,25,35,55,57,68,108,158,187,198

Pecorino 7,165,170

Peel 15,33,37,82,91,106,155,157,198,200,204

Pepper 3,7,30,169

Pie 3,4,5,6,7,27,38,57,79,81,100,108,141,146,154,176,184,197

Pistachio 3,4,18,70

Pizza 5,96,97

Plum 6,142,149

Pomegranate 6,149,162

Potato 3,5,7,31,88,155,180,181,190,198,201

Pulse 13,20,22,31,91,141,149,152,163,167

Pumpkin 3,5,6,7,23,36,38,93,118,119,151,152,153,154,155,184

Q

Quinoa 3,4,5,6,30,31,37,63,107,109,138,156,157,166

R

Raisins 5,7,114,115,158,171

Raspberry 3,4,6,7,21,56,82,158,159,160,200

Rhubarb 4,5,6,7,80,86,87,138,160,161,177,178

Rice 3,7,28,36,73,90,181,201

Ricotta 3,43,135

Risotto 5,103

Rosemary 6,147,163,164

S

Salad 3,6,38,162

Salt 3,5,7,25,30,35,43,52,65,70,103,105,116,125,127,135,138,154,155,158,167,175,180,185,195,206

Sausage 8,205

Savory 7,167,168,169,170,181

Seasoning 80

Seeds 3,5,6,36,37,70,101,149,158,167,175

Semolina 185

Shortbread 4,5,6,74,89,133

Soda 5,6,7,24,101,105,125,134,173,181

Spelt 6,159

Squash 3,6,41,162

Stew 3,6,47,133,155

Strawberry 5,6,7,87,161,176,177,178,179,180,197

211

Sugar 3,6,7,10,17,27,38,39,52,53,54,57,105,125,127,134,154,187,199

Syrup 36,73,105,138,154,156,180,181,201

T

Tahini 3,44

Tapioca 122

Tea 5,101,112,160

Tomato 7,180

Turkey 7,181

V

Vanilla extract 70,127,154,202

Vegan 4,5,7,8,77,94,171,193,194,195,196,197,198,199,207

Vegetable oil 129

Vegetable shortening 92

W

Waffles 4,83,85

Walnut 3,4,5,6,7,8,10,24,25,27,35,48,57,59,71,109,125,128,164,173,201,205

Wholemeal flour 115

Y

Yeast 185

Yuzu 80

Z

Zest 70,125,132,170,182

Conclusion

Thank you again for downloading this book!

I hope you enjoyed reading about my book!

If you enjoyed this book, please take the time to share your thoughts and post a review on Amazon. It'd be greatly appreciated!

Write me an honest review about the book – I truly value your opinion and thoughts and I will incorporate them into my next book, which is already underway.

Thank you!

If you have any questions, **feel free to contact at:** *author@shellfishrecipes.com*

Debra Boone

shellfishrecipes.com

Printed in Great Britain
by Amazon